Oxford Handbook of
Medical Statistics

Janet L. Peacock

Professor of Medical Statistics
King's College London
UK

Philip J. Peacock

Academic Clinical Fellow in Paediatrics
University of Bristol
UK

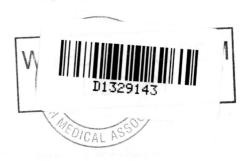

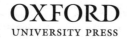

OXFORD
UNIVERSITY PRESS

OXFORD
UNIVERSITY PRESS

Great Clarendon Street, Oxford OX2 6DP

Oxford University Press is a department of the University of Oxford.
It furthers the University's objective of excellence in research, scholarship,
and education by publishing worldwide in

Oxford New York

Auckland Cape Town Dar es Salaam Hong Kong Karachi
Kuala Lumpur Madrid Melbourne Mexico City Nairobi
New Delhi Shanghai Taipei Toronto

With offices in

Argentina Austria Brazil Chile Czech Republic France Greece
Guatemala Hungary Italy Japan Poland Portugal Singapore
South Korea Switzerland Thailand Turkey Ukraine Vietnam

Oxford is a registered trade mark of Oxford University Press
in the UK and in certain other countries

Published in the United States
by Oxford University Press Inc., New York

British Library Cataloguing in Publication Data
Data available

Library of Congress Cataloging in Publication Data
Data available

Typeset by Glyph International, Bangalore, India
Printed in China
on acid-free paper by C&C Offset Printing Co., Ltd
Asia Pacific Offset Ltd.

ISBN 978–0–19–955128–6

10 9 8 7 6

Foreword

All health care professionals want to provide safe and effective care to their patients. This means that everyone has to keep up with the speed of innovation and be in a position to apply the findings of new research. Historically individuals have tended to delegate the assessment of the quality of research to journal editors, the peer review system and guideline developers. However for many reasons this may not be sufficient. All professionals have to make a judgement call on whether the research findings or guideline recommendations that they are assessing are relevant to the patient in front of them. They will have to decide whether the drug trial designed to determine the short term safety and efficacy against placebo in a selected population in the USA is really relevant to the elderly, ethnically diverse population with multiple co-morbidities facing them on a Friday afternoon.

To make things even more complicated, many of the questions raised in day to day practice will never be answered by randomized controlled trials. So other methods need to be applied, all with their own challenges and potential biases. This means, like it or not, that a sound understanding of medical statistics is essential for all health professionals.

Many doctors and medical students find statistics difficult to understand, and voice the need for a concise but thorough account of the subject. They plead for the statistical analysis to draw on real life situations and to use examples that they can understand.

This book responds completely to that plea by providing an accessible format that allows individual topics to be easily found and understood. It takes the reader, not only through the theory of the underlying statistics, but also the practical steps to set up and interpret all the key research designs. The authors are an experienced academic medical statistician who has conducted many collaborative research studies and taught statistics to students and doctors (to a very high standard—I should know—she taught me), and a junior academic doctor who has published his own work. They have written a book that meets all the needs of doctors and students carrying out their own research, and for those appraising others' research.

Professor Peter Littlejohns
Clinical and Public Health Director
National Institute for Health and Clinical Excellence

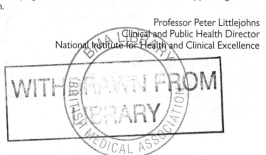

Preface

To practice evidence-based medicine, doctors need to critically appraise research evidence. The majority of medical research involves quantitative methods and so it is essential to be able to understand and interpret statistics. In addition, many doctors conduct research which requires the use of statistics throughout the research process – from design, to data collection and analysis, and to the interpretation and dissemination.

Doctors study statistics at undergraduate and postgraduate level and there is an increasing move towards teaching programmes that are based on real clinical problems and real data. However, in our experience both as teacher and former medical student, courses do not always fully equip doctors to critically appraise research evidence or to conduct research and communicate the findings. We have written this book to help bridge this gap by covering a wide span of topics from research design, through collecting and handling data, to both simple and complex statistical analyses.

We have aimed to be as comprehensive as possible in this handbook and so we have included all commonly-used statistical methods as well as more advanced methods such as multifactorial regression, mixed models, GEEs, and Bayesian models that are seen in medical papers. However, medical statistics is a broad and ever-growing discipline and so it is inevitable that some newer or less commonly-used topics have not found their way into this edition. For all methods we have provided clear guidance on when methods may be used and how the results of analyses are interpreted using examples from the medical literature and our own research. We have chosen to give formulae and worked examples for the 'simpler' methods as we know that the more mathematically minded readers may want to understand where the numbers come from. For those who do not wish to know, or who simply don't have time, these can be ignored without loss of continuity.

This book is written in the popular Oxford Handbook style with one topic per double page spread, providing easy access to discrete topics for busy doctors and students. Writing in this format has provided a challenge to us since many topics in medical statistics build on other topics and therefore assume prior knowledge. For this reason we have included many cross-references to other sections of the book so that other relevant information is clearly signposted. We have also included references for further reading where we believe that readers may wish to explore the topic in more detail. Writing any material in a punchy, brief style carries the danger of omitting material or 'dumbing it down'. We have fought hard to avoid doing this, not excluding material but making the format both accessible and thorough. We hope that you agree that we have managed to make this work.

Acknowledgements

So many people have helped us in so many ways with the design, writing and publication of this book. Unfortunately it is inevitable that in naming people we may have missed some out, but we are incredibly grateful to everyone who has helped in any way. Our first thanks go to the OUP clinical reviewers, Tom Turmeziei, Kam Cheong Wong and Ryckie Wade, who provided invaluable feedback on the manuscript, especially in the early days, which helped us to shape the book. Our statistical colleagues, Jenny Freeman and Andrew Smith, gave us very thorough reviews of the draft script and their comments have made the book so much better. We wish to thank Diane Morrison who proof-read the first draft for us to a very short deadline. Of course any errors which remain are our own.

We are very grateful to the OUP editors, Catherine Barnes, Sara Chare, Liz Reeve, and Selby Marshall for agreeing with us that this book needed to be written and for helping us to make it happen, and to Kate Wanwimolruk for guiding us through the production process. We especially want to express our appreciation to Anna Winstanley for the tremendous encouragement and enthusiastic support she has given us throughout the project, as well as her patience when we didn't always make our writing deadlines.

We want to thank colleagues at Dartmouth College New Hampshire, USA, where we both have links, especially Margaret Karagas, who hosted Janet so generously to enable her to make a start writing the book. We thank our senior academic colleagues, Paul Roderick for his encouragement and support, and Martin Bland who has always been such a help and inspiration to us both.

Finally we wish to say a huge thank you to our spouses, Eric and Becky, for all their helpful comments and suggestions during the writing and proof-reading process, but most of all for their continued confidence in us and graciousness when at times we neglected them so this book could be completed.

Contents

Detailed contents

9 Diagnostic studies   **339**

10 Other statistical methods   **353**

Symbols

❶	caution
✍	website
📖	cross reference
▶	important
∞	infinity
α	alpha
β	beta
μ	mu
χ	chi
ρ	rho
τ	tau
$\pm$	plus minus
$\times$	multiply
°	degree
$\geq$	greater than or equal to
$>$	greater than
$<$	less than
$\leq$	less than or equal to

Research design

Introduction

It is important to understand the main issues involved in study design in order to be able to critically appraise existing work and to design new studies. In this chapter we describe the main features of the design of interventional and observational studies and the differences and similarities between research and audit. We discuss when a sample size calculation is needed, describe the main principles of the calculations and outline the steps involved in preparing a study protocol. Most sections are illustrated with examples and we give particular attention to the statistical issues that arise in designing and appraising research.

Introduction to research

Engaging with research

At any one time a clinician or medical student who is engaging with quantitative research may be doing so for one or more of the following reasons:

- To critically appraise research reported by others
- To conduct primary research that aims to answer a specific question or questions, and thus generate new knowledge or extend existing knowledge
- To gain research skills and experience, often as part of an educational programme
- To test the feasibility of a particular research design or technique

The following issues are important for all of these:

- What is the study question or aim?
- What design is appropriate to answer the question(s)?
- What statistics are appropriate for the study?

Conducting and appraising primary research

Primary research requires rigorous methods so that the design, data, and analysis provide sound results that stand up to scrutiny and add to current knowledge. Similarly when critically appraising research, it is important to have a solid understanding of good research methodology.

Conducting research as part of an educational programme

When research is conducted purely for educational purposes, such as with a medical student project, the main purpose is not to generate new knowledge but instead to provide practical training in research that will equip the individual to conduct sound primary research at a later stage.

It is important that as far as possible, research projects conducted within an educational programme are carried out rigorously. However, since these research projects usually face constraints such as a narrow time frame and a limited budget, it may not be possible to fully meet the high standards set for primary research. For example, it may not be possible to recruit sufficient subjects to satisfy standard sample size calculations in the time given for a student project. If the purpose of the research is truly educational and not primarily to further knowledge, and this is made clear in any reporting, then this is not a problem.

Publishing research conducted as part of an educational programme

Although student projects are often limited in scope, they may be sufficiently novel and of a high enough standard to be published. This is to be encouraged to further experience of the publication process and to encourage high standards. For examples of student projects that have been published, see Peacock and Peacock[1] and Peacock et al.[2]

References

1 Peacock PJ, Peacock JL. Emergency call work-load, deprivation and population density: an investigation into ambulance services across England. *J Public Health (Oxf)* 2006; **28**(2):111–15.
2 Peacock PJ, Peters TJ, Peacock JL. How well do structured abstracts reflect the articles they summarize? *European Science Editing* 2009; **35**(1):3–5.

Research questions

Introduction

Research aims to establish new knowledge around a particular topic. The topic might arise out of the researcher's own experience or interest, or from that of a mentor or senior, or it may be a topic commissioned by a funding body. Sometimes a research study follows on directly from a previous study, either conducted by the researcher themselves or another researcher, and on other occasions it may be a completely new topic.

As the research idea grows, the researcher generates a **specific question** or set of questions that he/she wants to pursue. It can be quite difficult to focus down on specific questions if the topic is broad and there are many things that are interesting to explore. The scope of the study will determine how many questions can be investigated – an individual with no research funds may only be able to centre on one question, whereas one with a funded programme of research can investigate a number of related questions.

Even when a particular study investigates many questions, it is important that each question is **tightly framed** so that the right data can be collected and the appropriate analyses conducted. If questions are too vague or too general then the study will be difficult to design and may not ultimately be able to answer the real questions of interest.

Research questions

These should be:
- **Specific** with respect to time/place/subjects/condition as appropriate
- **Answerable** such that the relevant data are available or able to be collected
- **Novel** in some sense so that the study either makes a contribution to knowledge or extends existing knowledge
- **Relevant** to current medicine

Types of question

Most questions fall into one or more of the following categories:
- **Descriptive**, e.g. incidence/prevalence; trends/patterns; opinion/ knowledge; life history of disease
- **Evaluative**, e.g. efficacy/safety of treatments or preventive programmes; may be comparative
- **Explanatory**, e.g. causes of disease; mechanisms for observed processes or actions or events

Examples

- **What is the prevalence of diabetes mellitus in the population?**
  This is a simple descriptive study
- **How effective is influenza vaccination in the community-based elderly?**
  This is a comparative study, comparing individuals who had vaccines with those who did not
- **Does lowering blood pressure reduce the risk of coronary heart disease?**
  This is an evaluative study, investigating the efficacy of lowering blood pressure
- **Is prognosis following stroke dependent on age at the time of the event?**
  This is an observational study
- **Why does smoking increase the risk of heart disease?**
  This is an explanatory study investigating the mechanism behind an observed relationship
- **What evidence is there for the effectiveness of antidepressants in treating depression?**
  This study is a meta-analysis of existing interventional studies

Interventional studies

Study designs

> - **Interventional vs observational**
> - **Time-course**: prospective; retrospective; cross-sectional
> - **Source of data**: new data; routine data; patient notes; existing data, e.g. secondary data analysis, meta-analysis

Intervention studies test the effect of a treatment or programme of care. The purpose is usually to test for efficacy but in early drug trials, safety and dosage are established first.

No control group

- Preliminary drug trials investigating **safety and tolerance** are often uncontrolled and this is reasonable

Control group

- It is highly desirable to have a control or comparison group in **efficacy studies** to be able to demonstrate superiority or inferiority
- For example it may be useful to know that a new drug lowers blood pressure, but it is more important to know how it compares to medications already in common use, especially as existing drugs are likely to be cheaper

Historical controls

- Patients given a new treatment are compared with patients who have already been treated with an existing treatment regime and who at the time of testing the new treatment have already been treated, assessed, and discharged
- The comparison of the treatment group and the control group is **not concurrent** and may be problematic as other factors change over time, such as hospital staff and patient mix
- Interpretation is difficult – it is impossible to be sure that any differences observed between the new treatment group and the control group are solely due to the treatments received

Randomization between intervention and control group

- This is the best way to ensure **comparisons are concurrent and unbiased** (📖 Randomization in RCTs, p. 10)

When randomization is not possible

- It is hard to test the efficacy of a treatment that is widely used and accepted against no treatment or a placebo.
  For example, the use of adrenaline for cardiac arrest is generally accepted as effective. It would be difficult, if not impossible, to formally test this against a control treatment.

Natural experiments

- Individuals receive different interventions concurrently but in a non-randomized manner

Example 1

The effect of the fluoridation of drinking water may involve a comparison of subjects in areas where the water is subject to natural, artificial, or no fluoridation. Subjects are **not allocated** to the different types of fluoridation; this is determined by where they live.

Example 2

The effect of treatment may be compared in **patients who choose** conservative surgery for breast cancer rather than radical surgery. Patients are not randomized.

When intervention studies are unethical

- It is not ethical to experiment on humans when the intervention is likely to cause harm
- It is not ethical to test whether environmental agents cause harm, and so observational studies are used to determine effects
- Natural experiments may allow a better comparison to be made of individuals who are exposed and unexposed than a cross-sectional analysis. For example **before and after studies** have been used to compare health status before and after the introduction of the smoking ban in public places in USA and UK.[1,2] In this way a reasonable assessment of the effect of passive smoke exposure was made.

Design and analysis for non-randomized studies and natural experiments

- Collect as much data as possible on the subjects' key characteristics.
- Use statistical analysis to adjust for these differences.
- Note that, even with statistical adjustment, there may still be differences between the groups that are unknown and so comparisons may still be biased. We probably won't know.
- Interpretation of non-randomized trials is difficult and firm conclusions are hard to draw.

References

1 Eisner MD, Smith AK, Blanc PD. Bartenders' respiratory health after establishment of smoke-free bars and taverns. *JAMA* 1998; **280**(22):1909–14.
2 Allwright S, Paul G, Greiner B, Mullally BJ, Pursell L, Kelly A *et al*. Legislation for smoke-free workplaces and health of bar workers in Ireland: before and after study. *BMJ* 2005; **331**(7525):1117.

Randomized controlled trials

Introduction

A randomized controlled trial (RCT) is an intervention study in which subjects are randomly allocated to treatment options. Randomized controlled trials (RCTs) are the accepted 'gold standard' of individual research studies. They provide sound evidence about treatment efficacy which is only bettered when several RCTs are pooled in a meta-analysis.

Choice of comparison group

- The choice of the comparison group affects how we interpret evidence from a trial
- A comparison of an **active agent** with an inert substance or **placebo** is likely to give a more favourable result than comparison with another active agent
- Comparison of an active agent against placebo when an existing active agent is available is generally regarded as unethical (see the extract from the **Declaration of Helsinki, item 32** (ℜ www.wma.net)
- For example it would not be ethical to test a new anticholesterol drug against a placebo; any comparison of new therapy would have to be against the currently proven therapy, statins.

> 'The benefits, risks, burdens and effectiveness of a new intervention must be tested against those of the best current proven intervention, except in the following circumstances:
> - The use of placebo, or no treatment, is acceptable in studies where no current proven intervention exists; or
> - Where for compelling and scientifically sound methodological reasons the use of placebo is necessary to determine the efficacy or safety of an intervention and the patients who receive placebo or no treatment will not be subject to any risk of serious or irreversible harm'
>
> (Declaration of Helsinki, item 32)

Comparison with 'usual care'

When an intervention is a programme of care, for example an integrated care pathway for the management of stroke, it is common practice for the comparison group to receive the **usual care**.

Declaration of Helsinki (℘ www.wma.net)

The Declaration of Helsinki was first developed in 1964 by the World Medical Association to provide guidance about ethical principles for research involving human subjects. It has had multiple revisions since, with the latest version published in 2008. Although not legally binding of itself, many of its principles are contained in laws governing research in individual countries, and the declaration is widely accepted as an authoritative document on human research ethics.

The declaration addresses issues such as:
- Duties of those conducting research involving humans
- Importance of a **research protocol**
- Research involving **disadvantaged or vulnerable persons**
- Considering **risks and benefits**
- Importance of **informed consent**
- Maintaining **confidentiality**
- **Informing participants** of the research findings

The full 35-point declaration is available online at ℘ www.wma.net.

Randomization in RCTs

Why randomize?

- Randomization ensures that the **subjects' characteristics** do not affect which treatment they receive. The allocation to treatment is **unbiased**
- In this way, the treatment groups are **balanced** by subject characteristics in the long run and differences between the groups in the trial outcome can be attributed as being caused by the treatments alone
- This provides a **fair test of efficacy** for the treatments, which is not confounded by patient characteristics
- Randomization makes blindness possible (📖 Blinding in RCTs, p. 14)

Randomizing between treatment groups

The usual way to do random allocation is by using a **computer program** based on **random numbers**. The random allocation process may work in two different ways:

- **The program is interactive** and provides the allocation code for each patient as he/she is entered into the trial. This may be a code which refers to a treatment to maintain blindness or if the treatment cannot be blinded, for example with a technology, it will be the name of the actual intervention
- **A computer-generated list** of sequential random allocations is produced and administered by someone who is independent of the team that is recruiting patients to the trial. In this way, there is no bias in recruitment or allocation. In drug trials, the pharmacy may conduct the randomization and provide numbered containers to which it holds the code, so that the researcher and the patient can be kept blind to the actual allocation

Audit trail

It is important to have an **audit trail** of the recruitment and randomization process including **keeping a log** of the recruited patients. This information is needed for later reporting of the trial and assists with checking that the trial is being conducted according to the protocol.

Non-random allocation

❶ Alternate allocation, or a method based on patient identifiers such as hospital number or date of birth, are not random methods and are **not recommended** because they are open, and in the case of alternate allocation, predictable. These methods make blinding difficult and leave room for the researcher to change the allocation or recruit according to the treatment that is to be received (e.g. give a sicker patient the new treatment).

Stratification for prognostic factors

If there are **important prognostic factors** that need to be accounted for in a particular trial, the random allocation can be **stratified** so that the treatment groups are balanced for the prognostic factors. For example in trials of treatment for heart disease, the random allocation may be stratified by gender so that there are similar numbers of men and women receiving each treatment.

Minimization

Minimization is another method of allocating subjects to treatment groups while allowing for important prognostic factors.[1,2] The allocation takes place in a way that best maintains balance in these factors. At all stages of recruitment, the next patient is allocated to that treatment which minimizes the overall imbalance in prognostic factors. For a worked example see Altman and Bland[1] or Pocock.[2] Software to do minimization is available free from Martin Bland's website: ℘ www-users.york.ac.uk/~mb55/guide/minim.htm

Blocking

Blocking is used to ensure that the **number of subjects in each group is very similar** at any time during the trial. The random allocation is determined in discrete groups or *blocks* so that within each block there are equal numbers of subjects allocated to each treatment.

Example using blocks of size 4 and two treatments A, B

There are six possible blocks or arrangements of A and B, which give equal numbers of As and Bs:

AABB; ABAB; BBAA; BABA; ABBA; BAAB

We randomly choose blocks, so say the first two chosen blocks are:

BBAA; AABB

Then the first eight subjects will be allocated B, B, A, A, A, A, B, B

The total subjects on A and B as subjects 1 to 8 are recruited will be

(0,1), (0,2), (1,2) (2,2), (3,2), (4,2), (4,3), (4,4)

Hence, at all times, the total on A and the total on B will only differ by a maximum of 2 and so the treatment numbers will always be very similar and the numbers will be exactly balanced after every fourth subject is randomized.

Further extensions of 'blocking' are available with a mixture of different block sizes, whereby random combinations of blocks are selected.

Further reading on randomization: see articles by Altman and Bland.[3,4]

References

1 Altman DG, Bland JM. Treatment allocation by minimisation. *BMJ* 2005; **330**(7495):843.
2 Pocock SJ. *Clinical trials: a practical approach*. Chichester: Wiley, 1983.
3 Altman DG, Bland JM. Statistics notes: Treatment allocation in controlled trials: why randomise? *BMJ* 1999; **318**(7192):1209.
4 Altman DG, Bland JM. Statistics notes: How to randomise. *BMJ* 1999; **319**(7211):703–4.

Patient consent in research studies

Introduction

It is generally accepted that all subjects participating in research give their prior informed consent. The Declaration of Helsinki (item 24, ℘ www.wma.net) states the following:

> 'In medical research involving competent human subjects, each potential subject must be adequately informed of the aims, methods, sources of funding, any possible conflicts of interest, institutional affiliations of the researcher, the anticipated benefits and potential risks of the study and the discomfort it may entail, and any other relevant aspects of the study. The potential subject must be informed of the right to refuse to participate in the study or to withdraw consent to participate at any time without reprisal. Special attention should be given to the specific information needs of individual potential subjects as well as to the methods used to deliver the information. After ensuring that the potential subject has understood the information, the physician or another appropriately qualified individual must then seek the potential subject's freely-given informed consent, preferably in writing. If the consent cannot be expressed in writing, the non-written consent must be formally documented and witnessed.'

(Declaration of Helsinki, item 24)

Informed consent
- This requires giving patients detailed description of the study aims, what participation is required, and any risks they may be exposed to
- Consent must be voluntary
- Consent is confirmed in writing and a **cooling off period** is provided to allow subjects to change their minds
- Consent must be obtained for all patients recruited to an RCT
- Giving or withholding consent must not affect patient treatment or access to services
- For questionnaire surveys, consent is often implicit if the subject returns the questionnaire where it is clear in the accompanying information that participation is voluntary
- Consent may not be required if the study involves anonymised analyses of patient data only

When consent may be withheld

In some situations, obtaining patient consent to a study may be problematic.

Example 1

For example where the intervention is so desirable that patients would not want to risk being randomized to the control group. This is particularly so when it is not possible to mask the intervention such as where the intervention is a programme of care and the control treatment is 'usual care'. Subjects may not be willing to enter the trial and risk not getting the new intervention, or they may enter the trial but drop out if they are allocated to the control group.

One solution in situations like these is for the researcher to decide in advance to offer the intervention to all control group subjects after the trial has finished, assuming that the intervention proves to be effective. For example in exercise therapy trials, control group subjects may be offered the exercise regime at the end of the trial if it has been shown to work. Such an approach is stated in the Declaration of Helsinki (item 33; ℘ www.wma.net) and would need to be costed into the trial.

> 'At the conclusion of the study, patients entered into the study are enti-tled to be informed about the outcome of the study and to share any benefits that result from it, for example, access to interventions identi-fied as beneficial in the study or to other appropriate care or benefits.'
>
> (Declaration of Helsinki, item 33)

Example 2

Patients may be reluctant to agree to enter a trial of a new therapy when there is an existing treatment which is known to work. In such situations, assuming that there is equipoise, it is the responsibility of the clinician to explain the study clearly enough to allow the patient to make an informed choice of whether or not to take part.

Further discussion of patient consent is beyond the scope of this book but the General Medical Council UK website has detailed guidance (℘ www.gmc-uk.org/guidance/current/library/research.asp).

Blinding in RCTs

Concealing the allocation

- Blinding is when the treatment allocation is concealed from either the subject or assessor or both
- It is done to avoid conscious or unconscious bias in reported outcomes
- A trial is **double blind** if neither the subject nor the assessor knows which treatment is being given
- A trial is **single blind** if the treatment allocation is concealed from either the subject or the assessor but not both
- ▶ Note that **randomization makes blinding possible** and is its most important role

Examples

A subject who knows that he is receiving a new treatment for pain which he expects to be beneficial may perceive or actually feel less pain than he would do if he thought he was receiving the old treatment.

An assessor who knows that a subject is receiving the new steroid treatment for chronic obstructive pulmonary disease, which he expects to work better than the old one, may tend to round up measurements of lung function.

> If the treatment allocation is concealed, then both the patient and assessor will make **unbiased assessments** of the effects of the treatments being tested.

Placebo

- An inert treatment that is indistinguishable from the active treatment
- In drug trials it is often possible to use a placebo drug for the control which looks and tastes exactly like the active drug
- The use of a placebo makes it possible for both the subject and assessor to be blinded

When blinding is not possible

In some situations blinding is not possible, such as in trials of technologies where concealment is impossible. For example in trials comparing different types of ventilator, it is impossible to blind the clinician, and similarly in trials of surgery versus chemotherapy.

Possible solutions are the use of **sham treatments**, such as sham surgery, but this may not be ethically acceptable. Trials of the effectiveness of acupuncture have used sham acupuncture for the control group to maintain blindness[1] and trials involving injections sometimes use **saline injections** in the control group, although this may raise ethical objections.

Sometimes ingenuity can be employed to address blindness, such as in a trial of electrical stimulation in non-healing fractures, where patients in the control group also received an electric current of non-therapeutic power but sufficient to interfere with radio in the same way as the active coil did.[2]

Double placebo (double dummy)

If a trial involves two active treatments that have different modes of treatment, for example a **tablet versus a cream**, a double placebo ('double dummy'), can be used whereby each patient receives two treatments. In the example given, patients would receive either the active tablet plus a placebo cream, or a placebo tablet plus an active cream. A double dummy can also be used if the timing of treatment is different for the two drugs being tested, for example if one drug is given once a day in the morning (drug A) and the other is given twice a day, morning and evening (drug B). In this case one group of patients would receive the active drug A in the morning and placebo drug B both morning and evening and the other would receive the placebo drug A in the morning and active drug B both morning and evening.

Active placebo

Trials may use an **active placebo**, which mimics the treatment in some way to maintain blindness. For example some treatments give patients a dry mouth and so the presence or absence of this side effect may indicate to the patient which treatment they are on.

Example

In a trial of dextromethorphan and memantine to treat neuropathic pain, patients in the placebo group were given low dose lorazepam to mimic the side effects of dextromethorphan and memantine and thus help conceal the treatment allocation.[3]

References

1 Scharf HP, Mansmann U, Streitberger K, Witte S, Kramer J, Maier C *et al.* Acupuncture and Knee Osteoarthritis: A Three-Armed Randomized Trial. *Ann Intern Med* 2006; **145**(1):12–20.
2 Simonis RB, Parnell EJ, Ray PS, Peacock JL. Electrical treatment of tibial non-union: a prospective, randomised, double-blind trial. *Injury* 2003; **34**(5):357–62.
3 Sang CN, Booher S, Gilron I, Parada S, Max MB. Dextromethorphan and memantine in painful diabetic neuropathy and postherpetic neuralgia: efficacy and dose-response trials. *Anesthesiology* 2002; **96**(5):1053–61.

RCTs: parallel groups and crossover designs

Two or more parallel groups

- This is a trial with a head-to-head comparison of two or more treatments
- Subjects are allocated at random to a single treatment or a single treatment programme for the duration of the trial
- Usually, the aim is to allocate equal numbers to each trial, although unequal allocation is possible
- The **groups are independent** of each other

Crossover trials

- **This involves a single group study** where each patient receives two or more treatments in turn
- Each patient therefore acts as their own control and comparisons of treatments are made **within patients**
- The two or more treatments are given to each patient **in random order**
- Crossover trials are useful for **chronic conditions** such as pain relief in long-term illness or the control of high blood pressure where the outcome can be assessed relatively quickly
- **They may not be feasible for treatments for short-term illnesses** or acute conditions that once treated are cured, for example antibiotics for infections
- It is important to avoid the **carry-over** effect of one treatment into the period in which the next treatment is allocated. This is usually achieved by having a gap or **washout period** between treatments to prevent there being any carry-over effects of the first treatment when the next treatment starts
- The simplest design is a two treatment comparison in which each patient receives each of the two treatments in random order with a washout period of non-treatment in between
- There are some particular **statistical issues** that may arise in crossover trials which are related to the washout period and carry-over effects, and how and whether to include patients who do not complete both periods. Senn gives a full discussion of the issues and possible solutions.[1]

Example: crossover trial

A randomized, double-blind, placebo-controlled crossover study tested the effectiveness of valproic acid to relieve pain in patients with painful polyneuropathy. Thirty-one patients were randomized to receive either valproic acid (1500 mg daily) and then placebo, or placebo followed by valproic acid. Each treatment lasted for four weeks. No significant difference in total pain or individual pain rating was found between treatment periods on valproic acid and placebo (total pain (median) = 5 in the valproic acid period vs 6 in the placebo period; P = 0.24).[2]

Choice of design: parallel group or crossover?

Advantages of parallel group designs
- The comparison of the treatments takes place concurrently
- Can be used for any condition, especially an acute condition which is cured or self-limiting such as an infection
- No problem of carry-over effects

Disadvantages of parallel group designs
- The comparison is between patients and so usually needs a bigger sample size than the equivalent cross-over trial

Advantages of crossover designs
- Treatments are compared within patients and so differences between patients are accounted for explicitly
- Usually need fewer subjects than the equivalent parallel group trials
- Can be used to test treatments for chronic conditions

Disadvantages of crossover designs
- Cannot be used for many acute illnesses
- Carry-over effects need to be controlled
- Likely to take longer than the equivalent parallel designs
- Statistical analysis is more complicated if subjects do not complete all periods

References

1 Senn S. *Cross-over trials in clinical research*. Chichester: Wiley, 2002.
2 Otto M, Bach FW, Jensen TS, Sindrup SH. Valproic acid has no effect on pain in polyneuropathy: a randomized, controlled trial. *Neurology* 2004; **62**(2):285–8.

Zelen randomized consent design

Introduction

This design can be used when comparing a new treatment programme with usual care and attempts to address problems with patient consent (📖 Patient consent in research studies, p. 12).

Allocation to treatments

- Subjects are randomly allocated to treatment or usual care
- Only those subjects who are allocated to treatment are invited to participate and to give their consent
- Subjects allocated to usual care (control) are not asked to give their consent
- Among the treatment group, some subjects will refuse and so this design results in three treatment groups[1,2]

1. Usual care (allocated)
2. Intervention
3. Usual care (but allocated to intervention)

- The analysis is performed with patients analysed in the original randomized groups, i.e. 1 versus 2 + 3 (📖 Intention to treat analysis, p. 22)

Double randomized consent

- Patients are randomized to intervention or control and then their consent is sought, whichever group they are allocated to
- Patients are allowed to choose either the treatment they are allocated to or the other treatment
- The analysis is performed with patients analysed in the original randomized groups, whichever treatment they chose or received (📖 Intention to treat analysis, p. 22)

Justification

The single randomized Zelen design has been criticized as being unethical since some subjects are not informed that they are in a trial. However, it is generally agreed that some trials could not take place without the use of this design because in some situations patients would not wish to take part if they were allocated to the control group. It could be argued that this therefore justifies its use.[3]

Advantages of Zelen's single randomized design

- It avoids patient refusal at the outset due to the possibility of their being allocated to control
- It avoids later withdrawal in subjects who initially consent but then withdraw when they are allocated to the control group
- It allows a new and potentially desirable programme to be evaluated rigorously in a randomized trial

Disadvantages of Zelen's single randomized design

- Patients in the control group do not know they are in a trial, which has ethical implications
- The design leads to three groups and will lead to bias if subjects are not analysed in the group to which they were allocated irrespective off the treatment they chose or received
- Will only work if the data required are routinely collected, otherwise no data will be available for the control group
- It is less efficient statistically than a straightforward two-group design since, when subjects choose not to accept the allocated treatment, the true treatment effect is diluted

Advantages of Zelen's double randomized design

- It randomizes patients but allows them to choose which treatment they prefer
- It avoids the ethical problems of not seeking consent for patients allocated to control
- It thus allows a new and potentially desirable programme to be evaluated rigorously in a randomized trial

Disadvantages of Zelen's double randomized design

- It almost inevitably leads to severe contamination of the groups since some patients will choose the opposite treatment to which they have been allocated
- It is less efficient statistically than a straightforward two-group design since, when subjects choose not to accept the allocated treatment, the true treatment effect is diluted

References

1 Zelen M. A new design for randomized clinical trials. *N Engl J Med* 1979; **300**(22):1242–5.
2 Zelen M. Randomized consent designs for clinical trials: an update. *Stat Med* 1990; **9**(6):645–56.
3 Torgerson DJ, Roland M. Understanding controlled trials: What is Zelen's design? *BMJ* 1998; **316**(7131):606.

Superiority and equivalence trials

Superiority trials
- Seek to establish that one treatment is **better** than another
- When the trial is designed the sample size is set so that there is high statistical power to detect a clinically meaningful difference between the two treatments
- For such a trial a statistically significant result is interpreted as showing that one treatment is more effective than the other

Equivalence trials
- Seek to test if a new treatment is **similar** in effectiveness to an existing treatment
- Appropriate if the new treatment has certain benefits such as fewer side effects, being easier to use, or being cheaper
- Trial is designed to be able to demonstrate that, within given acceptable limits, the two treatments are equally effective
- **Equivalence** is a pre-set maximum difference between treatments such that, if the observed difference is less than this, the two treatments are regarded as equivalent
- The **limits of equivalence** need to be set to be appropriate clinically
- The tighter the limits of equivalence are set, the larger the sample size that will be required
- If the condition under investigation is serious then tighter limits for equivalence are likely to be needed than if the condition is less serious
- The calculated sample size tends to be bigger for equivalence trials than superiority trials

Non-inferiority trials
- Special case of the equivalence trial where the researchers only want to establish if a new treatment is no worse than an existing treatment
- In this situation the analysis is by nature one-sided (📕 Tests of statistical significance, p. 246)

Practicalities
- In general the design and implementation of equivalence trials is less straightforward than superiority trials
- If patients are lost to follow-up or fail to comply with the trial protocol, then any differences between the treatments is likely to be reduced and so equivalence may be incorrectly inferred
- It is especially important that equivalence trials need very strict management and good patient follow-up to minimize these problems
- It is often helpful to include a secondary analysis where subjects are analysed according to the treatment they actually received, 'per protocol' analysis

Examples

- Is atorvastatin more effective at reducing blood cholesterol levels than simvastatin?
  This is an example of a superiority trial
- Are angiotensin receptor blockers (e.g. valsartan) as effective at reducing blood pressure in hypertensive patients as angiotensin converting enzyme (ACE) inhibitors (e.g. ramipril)?
  This is an example of an equivalence trial

Superiority and equivalence
- It is important to distinguish between superiority and equivalence when designing a trial
- Choice depends on the purpose of the trial
- A trial designed for one purpose may not be able to adequately fulfil the other
- In general, equivalence trials tend to need larger samples
- A trial designed to test superiority is unlikely to be able to draw the firm conclusion that two treatments which are not significantly different can be regarded as equivalent

---

For further details of equivalence trials, see the books on clinical trials by Matthews[1] and Girling and colleagues.[2]

References

1 Matthews JNS. *Introduction to randomized controlled clinical trials.* 2nd ed. Boca Raton, FL: Chapman & Hall/CRC, 2006.
2 Girling DJ, Parmar MKB, Stenning SP, Stephens RJ, Stewart LA. *Clinical trials in cancer principles and practice.* Oxford: Oxford University Press, 2003.

Intention to treat analysis

Introduction

The statistical analysis of RCTs is straightforward where there are complete data. The primary analysis is a direct comparison of the treatment groups, and this is performed with subjects being included in the group to which they were originally allocated. This is known as **analysing according to the intention to treat (ITT)** and is the only way in which there can be certainty about the balance of the treatment groups with respect to characteristics of the subjects. ITT analysis therefore provides an unbiased comparison of the treatments.

Change of treatment

If patients change treatment they should still be analysed together with patients in their original, randomly allocated group, since change of treatment may be related to the treatment itself. If a patient's data are analysed as if they were in their new treatment group, the balance in patient characteristics which was present after random allocation will be lost. A **per protocol** analysis, where patients are analysed according to the treatment they have actually received, may be useful in addition to the ITT analysis if some patients have stopped or changed treatment.

Missing data

Missing data are unfortunately common in all research studies, particularly where there is follow-up. Where there are missing data it may not be possible to include a particular individual in the analysis, and clearly if there are a lot of missing data, the validity of the results is called into question.

Where possible, all subjects should be included in the analysis. In a trial with follow-up it may be possible to include subjects with no final data if they have some interim data available, either by using the interim data directly or by statistical modelling. These issues should be considered at the design stage to minimize later loss of data through careful design of outcome data and strategies to minimize loss to follow-up.

All subjects recruited should be accounted for at all stages so that a detailed account can be given of how the trial was conducted and what happened to all subjects. This is particularly important for the interpretation of the findings and so is included when the study is written up.

A fuller discussion of missing data is given elsewhere (📖 Missing data, p. 402).

Intention to treat (ITT) and missing data

- Analyse subjects in the groups they were originally allocated to even if they don't comply or change treatment
- This provides an unbiased comparison of the treatments
- Per protocol analysis may be useful but only in addition to ITT and not as the primary analysis
- Keep a record of all subjects to be able to account for their treatment and for any subjects who withdraw

---

Further reading

Fuller details of how to design and conduct RCTs are given in the books by Pocock,[1] Senn,[2] and Matthews.[3]

References

1 Pocock SJ. *Clinical trials: a practical approach.* Chichester: Wiley , 1983.

2 Senn S. *Cross-over trials in clinical research.* Chichester: Wiley, 2002.

3 Matthews JNS. *Introduction to randomized controlled clinical trials.* 2nd ed. Boca Raton, FL: Chapman & Hall/CRC, 2006.

Case–control studies

Observational studies

In observational studies the subjects receive no additional intervention beyond what would normally constitute usual care. Subjects are therefore observed in their natural state.

Case–control study

- This study investigates causes of disease, or factors associated with a condition
- It starts with the disease (or condition) of interest and selects patients with that disease for inclusion, the **'cases'**
- A comparison group without the disease is then selected, **'controls'**, and cases and controls are compared to identify possible causal factors
- Case–control studies are **usually retrospective** in that the data relating to risk factors are collected after the disease has been identified. This has consequences, which are discussed later in this section.

When to use a case–control design

- To investigate risk factors for a rare disease where a prospective study would take too long to identify sufficient cases, e.g. for Creutzfeldt–Jakob disease
- To investigate an acute outbreak in order to identify causal factors quickly – for example where an answer is needed about the causes of an outbreak food poisoning, or an outbreak of legionnaire's disease

Choice of controls

As with intervention studies, the choice of controls affects the comparison that is made. Common choices include:

- Patients in the same hospital but with unrelated diseases or conditions
- Patients one-to-one matched to controls for key prognostic factors such as age and sex
- A random sample of the population from which the cases come

Clearly the best control group is the third option, but this is rarely possible. For this reason some case–control studies include more than one control group for robustness.

Matched controls

Matching is popular but needs to be carefully specified, for example 'age matched within two years' gives the range within which matching can be made. It is not usually possible to match for many factors, as a suitable match may not exist. In a matched design, the statistical analysis should take account of the matching and factors used for matching cannot be investigated due to the design. Where one subject in a matched pair has missing data, then both subjects are omitted from the statistical analysis.

Sample size for controls

It is common to choose the sample size so that there is the same number of cases as controls. For a given total sample size this gives the greatest statistical power, i.e. the greatest possibility of detecting a true effect.

If the number of available cases is limited, then it is possible to increase the power by choosing more controls than cases However, the gain in power diminishes quickly so that it is rarely worth choosing more than 3 controls per case.[1]

Collecting data on risk factors

Since case–control studies start with cases that already have the disease, data about their exposure to possible risk factors prior to diagnosis is collected retrospectively. This is an advantage and a disadvantage. The advantage is that the exposure has already happened and so the data simply need to be collected; no follow-up period is needed. The disadvantage relates to the quality of the data. Data taken from clinical notes may contain errors that cannot be rectified or gaps that cannot be filled. Data obtained directly from subjects about their past is susceptible to recall bias because cases may have different recall of past events, usually better, than the controls. For example a case with a gastrointestinal condition may be more conscious of what they have eaten in the past than a healthy control who may have simply forgotten.

Reference

1 Taylor JM. Choosing the number of controls in a matched case–control study, some sample size, power and efficiency considerations. *Stat Med* 1986; **5**(1):29–36.

Case–control studies (continued)

Limitations of design

- The choice of control group affects the comparisons between cases and controls
- Exposure to risk factor data is usually collected retrospectively and may be incomplete, inaccurate, or biased
- If the process that leads to the identification of cases is related to a possible risk factor, interpretation of results will be difficult (ascertainment bias)

For example suppose the cases are young women with high blood pressure recruited from a contraception clinic. In this situation a possible risk factor, the oral contraceptive (OC) pill, is linked to the recruitment of cases and so OC use may be more common among cases than population controls for this reason alone.

- Time-course relationships need careful interpretation since changes in biological quantities may precede the disease or be a result of the disease itself. For example a raised serum troponin level is associated with myocardial infarction, but is only raised after the event. Therefore a case–control study may find that high troponin levels are associated with myocardial infarction but this cannot in fact be a risk factor
- Risk estimates for exposures cannot be estimated directly because the case and control groups are not representative samples of their respective target populations and so estimates of risks are biased. This has implications for the statistical analysis and the interpretation of results. Risks are usually estimated using odds and ratios of odds, and these only approximate to risks and ratios of risks when the disease under investigation is rare
- This limitation can be overcome with certain designs, for example where a case–control study is nested in a cohort study where all cases and controls are identified prospectively and a truly random sample of controls is available (🕮 Cohort studies, p. 28). In this situation, the relative risk can be calculated directly

Example of case–control study

A recent study investigated the association between genitourinary infections in the month before conception to the end of the first trimester, and gastroschisis.[1] Subjects were 505 babies with gastroschisis (the 'cases'), and 4924 healthy liveborn infants as controls.

The study reported data (Table 1.1) showing a positive relationship between exposure to genitourinary infections and gastroschisis (odds ratio = 2.02; 95% CI: 1.54 to 2.63).

Table 1.1 Genitourinary infections in the month before conception to the end of the first trimester, and gastroschisis

Exposed to infection?	Cases	Controls
Yes	81/505 (16%)	425/4924 (9%)
No	424/505 (84%)	4499/4924 (91%)

Reference

1 Feldkamp ML, Reefhuis J, Kucik J, Krikov S, Wilson A, Moore CA et al. Case–control study of self reported genitourinary infections and risk of gastroschisis: findings from the national birth defects prevention study, 1997–2003. *BMJ* 2008; **336**(7658):1420–3.

Cohort studies

Introduction

A cohort study is an observational study that aims to investigate causes of disease or factors related to a condition but, unlike a case–control study, it is longitudinal and starts with an unselected group of individuals who are followed up for a set period of time. Cohort studies are sometimes used to confirm the findings of case–control studies, such as happened when Doll and Hill observed a relationship between smoking and lung cancer in a case–control study[1] and subsequently established the longitudinal study of doctors in the UK.[2]

Design of a cohort study

- This starts with an unselected group of 'healthy' individuals
- The subjects are **followed up** to monitor the disease or condition of interest and potential risk factors
- The length of follow-up is chosen to allow sufficient subjects to get the disease and risk factors to be explored
- In the simplest case, where there is a single risk factor that is either present or absent, the incidence of disease can be related directly to the presence of the risk factor
- Usually **prospective**, with the risk factor data being recorded before the disease is confirmed
- Can be **retrospective** but requires that full risk factor data are obtained on all individuals with and without the disease of interest using **data that were recorded prospectively**

When to use a cohort study design

- When **precise estimates of risk** associated with particular factors are required, for example when a case–control study has established that an association exists but is unable to provide estimates of the risk
- When information on past risk factors in individuals with disease is unavailable or too unreliable to use
- When the **time-course** of a risk factor is of interest, for example with smoking, where cohort studies have been able to demonstrate the cumulative adverse effects of long-tem smoking and the potential benefits of quitting after smoking for different lengths of time[2]
- When resources and time are sufficient to support a lengthy study

Difficulties with cohort studies

- A large number subjects is needed to obtain enough individuals who get the disease or condition, particularly if it is uncommon
- The length of follow up may be substantial to get enough diseased individuals and so the cohort study is not feasible for rare diseases
- There is difficulty in maintaining contact with subjects, particularly if the follow-up is lengthy
- The resources required may be very high

Example of a cohort study

A cohort study examined the relationship between body mass index (BMI) and all-cause mortality in 527 265 US men and women in the National Institutes of Health–AARP cohort who were 50–71 years old at enrolment in 1995–1996.[3] BMI was calculated from self-reported weight and height.

The study found that among those who had never smoked, excess body weight during midlife was associated with a higher risk of death. Table 1.2 gives results for men who had never smoked.

Table 1.2 Relative risk of death in men aged 50–71 at enrolment by BMI

BMI at age 50	Relative risk
<18.5	1.29
18.5–20.9	1.14
21.0–23.4	1.04
23.5–24.9	**1.00**
25.0–26.4	1.05
26.5–27.9	1.31
28.0–29.9	1.49
30.0–34.9	1.96
35.0–39.9	2.46
≥40.0	3.82

All relative risks were adjusted for confounding factors (see paper for details[3]). The reference category for BMI is shown in **bold**.

References

1 Doll R, HILL AB. Smoking and carcinoma of the lung; preliminary report. *Br Med J* 1950; **2**(4682):739–48.

2 Doll R, Peto R, Boreham J, Sutherland I. Mortality in relation to smoking: 50 years' observations on male British doctors. *BMJ* 2004; **328**(7455):1519.

3 Adams KF, Schatzkin A, Harris TB, Kipnis V, Mouw T, Ballard-Barbash R et al. Overweight, obesity, and mortality in a large prospective cohort of persons 50 to 71 years old. *N Engl J Med* 2006; **355**(8):763–78.

Cohort studies (continued)

Mixed designs

Larger programmes of study may involve a mixture of designs such as cohort and case–control, a cross-sectional study being extended to become a cohort study and so on. Trial populations may be followed up after the trial part has ended, simply as a cohort of like individuals.

Cohort study with a nested case–control study

In a cohort study it may be worthwhile to identify all individuals with a disease and then retrospectively select a sample of the non-diseased individuals for comparison. This design may be desirable if:

- The resource implications of collecting data on all non-diseased individuals is too high
- All information was available but unprocessed
- Biological samples were collected but not analysed

This study is known as a **nested case–control study** and provides an efficient way of investigating particular factors once the outcomes from the cohort have been established.

Bias in risk factor data

- In a nested case–control study such as this, the risk factor data should not be as biased as it may be in a conventional case–control study, since it was collected prospectively
- There is a potential problem if there is differential loss to follow-up as this would reduce the availability of true controls and bias the comparisons

Example: UK National Child Development Study (NCDS)

Description of the study
- All babies born 3–9 March 1958 in Great Britain were studied to investigate and document perinatal mortality
- The subjects were followed into childhood and further assessments were made at ages 7, 11, 16, 23, 33, 41–42, 44–46, and 49–50
- The study aims broadened over the years to monitor physical, educational, social, and economic development in the subjects
- The recent sweeps have obtained measures of ill health and biomedical risk factors to address a range of hypotheses
- Data available from UK data archive (⅌ www.esds.ac.uk)
- While follow-up has been careful, the reduction in numbers at each sweep can be seen in Table 1.3

Table 1.3 Numbers of subjects at different follow-ups in the NCDS (longitudinal achieved sample)

1958	17,416
1965	15,051
1969	14,757
1974	13,917
1981	12,044
1991	10,986
2000	10,979
2005	9,175

Cross-sectional studies

Introduction

In a cross-sectional study a sample is chosen and data on each individual is collected at **one point in time**. Note that this may not be exactly the same time point for each subject. For example, a survey of primary care consultations may be conducted over a week – each patient will fill in the survey once but different subjects will fill out their survey on different days depending on when they came to the surgery.

When to use a cross-sectional study

- Surveys of prevalence, such as a survey to ascertain the prevalence of asthma
- Surveys of attitudes or views, such as: studies of patient satisfaction, patient/professional knowledge; studies of behaviour, such as alcohol use and sexual behaviour
- When inter-relationships between variables are of interest, for example a study to determine the characteristics of heavy drinkers, a cross-sectional study allows comparisons by sex, age, and so on

Cautions in interpreting cross-sectional study data

Temporal effects

Since the data on each individual are collected at one time point, care is needed in inferring temporal effects unless the exposure is constant, such as with a congenital or genetic factor (e.g. blood groups). For example, if a relationship is observed between a disease and blood group then we can safely assume that this is a true association since the blood group of the subjects would not be changed by the disease process. The same could not be assumed if a cross-sectional study showed an association between a disease and blood pressure since the disease might have led to the rise in blood pressure rather than the other way around.

Repeated cross-sectional studies

Sometimes cross-sectional studies are repeated at different times and/or in different places to look at the variability in findings. For example, many cross-sectional studies have estimated the prevalence of asthma in school-children. Comparisons of prevalence in different places is straightforward but comparisons of the prevalence at different times is less so because each cross-sectional survey is likely to have included a slightly different sample of children at the different time points, and so interpretation of changes must be made cautiously.

Cross-sectional studies that appear to be longitudinal

Cross-sectional studies can be misinterpreted as if they were longitudinal studies. For example, a cross-sectional study in a sample of fetuses where the gestational age of the fetuses spans a range, say 22–28 weeks. Some researchers have used data such as these to estimate growth trends. This is dubious because each fetus is measured just once and so the trend is being estimated from different fetuses. Thus differences between fetuses are likely to contribute to some of the differences observed by gestational age.

Example: cross-sectional study

A study investigated differences in cardiovascular risk in British South Asian and in white children in 10 towns.[1] The study included 73 South Asian and 1287 white children and measured fasting glucose levels as a measure of insulin resistance, plus a number of other markers of cardiovascular risk. Each child was assessed just once, thus this is a cross-sectional study.

Reference

1 Whincup PH, Gilg JA, Papacosta O, Seymour C, Miller GJ, Alberti KG et al. Early evidence of ethnic differences in cardiovascular risk: cross sectional comparison of British South Asian and white children. *BMJ* 2002; **324**(7338):635.

Case study and series

Differences in aims

A **case study** or **case report** is like a case series but it includes only one individual:
• The aim is to describe a single and unusual incident or case

A **case series** is a descriptive study involving a group of patients who all have the same disease or condition:
• The aim is to describe common and differing characteristics of a particular group of individuals

Similarities

For both a case study and a case series:
• The aim is not to draw general conclusions
• It is not a true research study
• It may provide useful indications for further research

Example: a case study

An article published in *The Lancet* described the case of an 80-year old woman who presented with episodes of unconsciousness and disorientation over several years.[1] During a subsequent episode she was found to have a blood glucose of 1.5 mmol/L (normal range 3.5–5.5 fasting). Routine blood tests were normal and a 72-hour fast produced no symptoms of hypoglycaemia (low blood sugar).

Further investigations led to the discovery of an insulin-secreting tumour in the body of the pancreas. The tumour was producing excess insulin in response to glucose, therefore causing glucose-induced hypoglycaemia.

Example: a case series

An article published in *Brain* described a series of patients with pneumococcal meningitis.[2] The paper reported the symptoms, complications, and outcome in 87 consecutive meningitis patients seen in a particular neurology department. The authors stated that their analysis can help doctors identify prognostic factors in patients, and can guide the design of future research studies.

References

1 Wiesli P, Spinas GA, Pfammatter T, Krahenbuhl L, Schmid C. Glucose-induced hypoglycaemia. *Lancet* 2002; **360**(9344):1476.
2 Kastenbauer S, Pfister HW. Pneumococcal meningitis in adults: spectrum of complications and prognostic factors in a series of 87 cases. *Brain* 2003; **126**(**Pt 5**):1015–25.

Deducing causal effects

Association and causation

Observational studies frequently reveal associations. It is important in interpreting such associations to consider if they are likely to represent actual causes.

- Causal effects can only be firmly concluded from RCTs. In other words it is only when a study has randomized subjects to treatments that researchers are able to deduce that differences observed between treatment groups are due to the treatment alone
- Observational studies often reveal relationships between a disease and a risk factor. However, we cannot be sure that the risk factor *caused* the disease. It may be that another factor that was related to both the disease and the risk factor was in fact the causal factor, and that the relationship observed was due to **confounding**
- Cigarette smoking is a common confounder since the characteristics of smokers and non-smokers differ in many ways, some of which may be related to disease simply because of their association with smoking. In such cases when smoking is controlled for in the analysis, the associations diminish or disappear

Example

A study of factors affecting birthweight observed that on average pregnant women with low blood folate levels had smaller babies. The data were analysed further and showed no evidence for this relationship in women who were non-smokers although the relationship was seen in the women who smoked. It was further discovered that women who smoked had lower mean folate levels than women who did not smoke.

Further multifactorial analysis was conducted and the effect of folate on birthweight became non-significant after controlling for smoking whereas the effect of smoking remained significant after adjusting for folate level.

It was concluded that the 'folate effect' that was observed was simply due to smoking. In other words women with low folate levels had smaller babies because of their smoking and not because of the folate levels. The folate effect was a confounder and not a directly causal effect.

The Bradford-Hill criteria for causation

The British medical statistician, Austin Bradford-Hill, published a set of criteria for causation.[1] The criteria are conditions which, if fulfilled, allow causation to be more confidently inferred from an observational study. They are:

- Strength of association
- Consistency in different studies, settings, etc.
- Specificity of association of risk factor with a particular disease
- Temporal relationship – exposure precedes disease
- Dose–response relationship
- Biological plausibility for causality
- Coherence – association is consistent with current knowledge
- Experimental evidence for causality
- Existence of analogous evidence between a similar exposure and disease

Reference

1 Hill AB. The environment and disease: association or causation? *Proc R Soc Med* 1965; **58**: 295–300.

Designing an audit

What is audit?

'Clinical audit is a quality improvement process that seeks to improve the patient care and outcomes through systematic review of care against explicit criteria and the implementation of change. Aspects of the structures, processes and outcomes of care are selected and systematically evaluated against explicit criteria. Where indicated, changes are implemented at an individual team, or service level and further monitoring is used to confirm improvement in healthcare delivery.'[1]

Audit cycle

The aim of audit is to monitor clinical practice against agreed best practice standards and to remedy problems. Where problems in practice are identified, attempts are made to resolve these and then clinical practice is re-audited against the agreed standards. This is the audit cycle (Fig. 1.1).

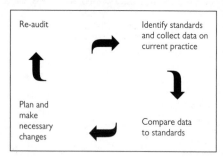

Fig. 1.1 The audit cycle.

Choosing the topic

Audits are designed to monitor and improve clinical practice and so the choice of topic is guided by indications of areas where improvement is needed in addition to local and national requirements. The following criteria help guide the choice of topics in general.

Possible topics

- Areas where a problem has been identified, e.g. an infection outbreak
- High volume practice, e.g. prescribing antibiotics in general practice
- High risk practice, e.g. major surgery
- High cost, e.g. *in vitro* fertilization
- Areas of clinical practice where guidelines or firm evidence exists, e.g. National Institute for Health and Clinical Excellence (NICE) guidelines or government targets

Aims of audit
- This defines the overall purpose and can be a question or statement
- The focus is on improvement in clinical practice
- The organization carrying out the audit should have the ability to make changes based on the findings. For example, there would be no point for a hospital to audit the number of referrals received from general practitioners (GPs) unless it could influence the practice of the GPs who were referring

Determining the standard
- This is the best currently available clinical practice based on best evidence
- It must be measurable

Data collection: retrospective
- Can be used to investigate acute events
- Useful when resources – time, cost, human resources, are limited
- Tends to use routine data, thus may provide limited information

Data collection: prospective
- Provides current data
- Allows a choice of data to be collected
- Requires forward planning
- Has resource implications – time, cost, human resources

Census or sample?
- A census is needed if outcome is critical, e.g. death rates after surgery
- A sample is okay if a snapshot will suffice
- Sample may be dependent on a fixed number or a length of time
- Sample size needs to be big enough to provide robust information for key aims of audit and use standard sample size calculations to ensure this (📖 Choosing a sample size, p. 56)
- Sampling strategy needs to be representative of the target population (📖 Sampling strategies, p. 54)
- Beware of seasonal effects when choosing a sample
- Use random samples if possible, or representative consecutive samples

Further help
Most hospitals have clinical audit departments, which can provide support for clinicians designing and conducting clinical audits.

Reference
1 Copeland G. *A practical handbook for clinical audit.* 2008. Available from: ℘ www.hqip.org.uk/clinical-audit-handbook/ (accessed 30 Dec 2009).

Data collection in audit

Data forms
- Consider how the data will be analysed when designing the form
- Design the form in advance – standard forms or example forms may be available
- If audit is new to you, discuss draft form with an experienced colleague
- Pilot the data collection on a few cases to check for feasibility and usability of the form, etc.

Outcomes measured
These may take one of several forms:
- A direct outcome, e.g. death, infection, re-admission
- A process, e.g. whether or not cholesterol was measured in patients admitted with cardiovascular disease
- A surrogate outcome, e.g. spirometry as a measure of lung function

Data analysis
In general, the same methods of statistical analysis are used for audit as for research, although complicated statistical methods may not be needed. In particular:
- Simple descriptive analyses may be sufficient to answer audit questions
- Summary statistics should always be calculated first such as percentages for frequencies and mean, standard deviation, median range for continuous data
- Graphical display may be helpful
- Where the size of an estimate is critical, it should be accompanied by a 95% confidence interval to show how precise it is (Chapter 8, p. 237)
- Comparisons of proportions or means can be done using standard significance tests as described later in this book (Tests of statistical significance, p. 246)

Examples of audit topics

- Are all hospital patients seen by a doctor every day?
- How many inpatients have acquired meticillin resistant *Staphylococcus aureus* (MRSA) in hospital?
- Is there adherence to antibiotic protocols?
- What proportion of patients in an emergency department stay longer than four hours?

Research versus audit

Introduction

The main difference between audit and research is in the aim of the study. A clinical research study aims to determine what practice is best, whereas an audit checks to see that best practice is being followed. In this way audit and research may follow each other in a cycle whereby research leads to new best practice which needs to be audited and audits lead to new questions which require investigating in research studies.

Research and knowledge

Research uses rigorous scientific methods to generate new knowledge which can be generalized to other patient groups, to other settings and so on. In medicine, research findings are used to determine best practice.

Audit and quality

Audit aims to improve patient care by reviewing clinical practice in a given setting against best practice standards and instigating change in practice as needed, to maintain or raise quality.

Common features of research and audit

- Both address a particular question related to best clinical practice
- Both consider and collect the appropriate data required to fulfill the aims of the study
- Both usually involve samples and a determination of the appropriate type and size of sample
- Both require data checking and data analysis
- Both require scientific rigour appropriate to the aims of the study

Grey areas

It is difficult to classify some studies as either wholly audit or wholly research. It is best to get local advice in such situations. Examples include:

- Patient surveys that seek views and attitudes about clinical practice
- Evaluations of a modified or new service to see if it works

Data collection: sources of data

New data

This is when data collection is designed specifically for the study and the data are newly collected.

Advantages
- Researcher has control over what data are collected, i.e. fit-for-purpose
- Current

Disadvantages
- Cost
- Time to collect and process
- Possibility of unknown quantity of missing data due to refused participation, subjects lost, etc.

Routine data

This refers to data collected for another purpose, often unrelated to research, e.g. monitoring.

Advantages
- Relatively quick to obtain, particularly if computerized
- May be already processed and/or computerized
- Usually much lower cost than primary data collection

Disadvantages
- No control over data available
- Limited control over missing data and ability to fill gaps and resolve queries
- Data may not be in required format

Patient notes

These is may be in hand-written or computerized format.

Advantages
- Relatively quick to obtain
- Usually much lower cost than primary data collection

Disadvantages
- No control over data available
- Limited control over missing records data, missing records, ability to fill gaps, resolve queries
- Hand-written notes may be unformatted, difficult to search and hard to read

Secondary data

These are data collected and recorded for another research study, and which are available for use.

Advantages
- Relatively quick to obtain
- Usually already processed so that minimal checking and data cleaning is required
- Usually much lower cost than primary data collection

Disadvantages
- No control over data available
- Limited control over missing data and ability to fill gaps and resolve queries
- Data may not be in required or desirable format
- May be out of date

Example

A study investigated the association between deprivation and use of the emergency ambulance service across England. Deprivation scores for each district in the country were obtained from the Office for National Statistics. The number of '999' calls to each ambulance service over the course of a given year were obtained from the Department of Health. Information on which districts were covered by each ambulance service in England were obtained from individual ambulance services. These data were used to investigate the relationship between deprivation and ambulance service usage. No new data was collected for the study.[1]

Reference

1 Peacock PJ, Peacock JL. Emergency call work-load, deprivation and population density: an investigation into ambulance services across England. *J Public Health (Oxf)* 2006; **28**(2):111–15.

Data collection: outcomes

General principles
- In an intervention study the main or primary outcome is critical as it is used to determine the efficacy of the treatment under investigation
- In most circumstances only one primary outcome is chosen and other important outcomes are regarded as secondary
- Sample size calculations use the primary outcome to ensure the study is big enough to detect a clinically important difference
- Choice of a single outcome is not always straightforward because a similar outcome may be measurable in more than one way, for example using capillary blood glucose readings compared with HbA1c

Composite outcomes
In some situations there are multiple ways of assessing a trial outcome, for example in trials in cardiology where possible outcomes include: subsequent cardiac event, hospitalization, death. In such cases researchers may choose a primary outcome which is a composite of two or more outcomes, such that the composite outcome is positive if one or more of the component outcomes have happened. Many composite outcomes include 'death' as one of the possible events.

Advantages
Composite outcomes have several advantages:
- They allow several outcomes to be combined in settings where different outcomes are of similar importance but reflect different clinical events, for example in a trial of treatment for gestational diabetes, the primary outcome was a composite measure of serious perinatal complications, defined as one or more of: fetal death, shoulder dystocia, bone fracture, and nerve palsy[1]
- Main advantage of using a composite outcome is the gain in statistical power – where individual events are uncommon, a large sample will be required to demonstrate conclusive differences. Using a composite will increase the event rate and allows trials to recruit a lower sample size.

Disadvantages
There are some difficulties with the choice and use of composite outcomes:
- It may be hard to determine the minimum clinical difference for the composite, this requires an estimate of the incidence of the composite itself and not just the incidence of the individual components as well as clinical judgement about what constitutes an important change in rate
- The interpretation of results may be difficult – it is important that the separate component effect sizes are each reported as well as the combined effect size, to allow clinical interpretation
- If the effect sizes (e.g. relative risks) vary among the components then overall interpretation of the findings is difficult, for example if a new treatment reduces subsequent adverse events but increases death rates[2–5]

Surrogate outcomes

In studies where the outcome of interest is very rare or requires a long follow-up period to determine it, a surrogate outcome is often used to increase statistical power and efficiency. Surrogate outcomes should be chosen and used with care:

- A surrogate outcome should be closely related to the clinical outcome of interest such as a biomarker or process variable
- Examples include CD4 count for acquired immune deficiency syndrome (AIDS) morbidity and mortality, cholesterol level for cardiovascular disease, length of stay for hospital-based treatments
- Where surrogate outcomes are only weakly associated with the clinical outcome of interest, the benefit in using them is offset by the difficulty in interpreting the results

References

1 Crowther CA, Hiller JE, Moss JR, McPhee AJ, Jeffries WS, Robinson JS. Effect of treatment of gestational diabetes mellitus on pregnancy outcomes. *N Engl J Med* 2005; **352**(24):2477–86.
2 Freemantle N, Calvert M, Wood J, Eastaugh J, Griffin C. Composite outcomes in randomized trials: greater precision but with greater uncertainty? *JAMA* 2003; **289**(19):2554–9.
3 Freemantle N, Calvert M. Composite and surrogate outcomes in randomised controlled trials. *BMJ* 2007; **334**(7597):756–7.
4 Montori VM, Permanyer-Miralda G, Ferreira-Gonzalez I, Busse JW, Pacheco-Huergo V, Bryant D et al. Validity of composite end points in clinical trials. *BMJ* 2005; **330**(7491):594–6.
5 Ross S. Composite outcomes in randomized clinical trials: arguments for and against. *Am J Obstet Gynecol* 2007; **196**(2):119e1–6.

Outcomes: continuous and categorical

Introduction

In clinical medicine and in medical research it is fairly common to categorize a biological measure into two groups, either to aid diagnosis or to classify an outcome. For example blood cholesterol level is measured as mmol per litre (mm/L) but may be classified into two groups defined as less than or equal to 5.8 mm/L ('normal') or greater than 5.8 ('high'). It is often useful to categorize a measurement in this way to guide decision-making, and/or to summarize the data but doing this leads to a loss of information which in turn has statistical consequences.

Example: what happens when we categorize data

Suppose in a study of infants their birthweights are recorded. Suppose then that the birthweight data, which are continuous, are categorized as 'low birthweight' (<2500g) or 'normal birthweight' (≥2500g). This means that each birthweight value is effectively replaced by a 0 or 1 (Table 1.4) and much data are discarded.

Table 1.4 Part of a dataset showing birthweight in grams and birthweight dichotomized as low birthweight yes/no

Subject no.	Birthweight (g)	Low birthweight (<2500: no=0, yes=1)
1	2720	0
2	4040	0
3	3590	0
4	1820	1
5	3860	0

Effects of categorization on statistical significance
- Categorizing continuous data into two groups discards much data
- For statistical tests, P value will be larger than if we had analysed the data as a continuous variable
- Thus statistical tests are less likely to find a significant difference (Table 1.5)

Example: effects of categorization on statistical significance

Table 1.5 Mean birthweight (BW) and the percentage of low birth-weight (LBW) babies (BW <2500 g) in the same study by the mothers' smoking status during pregnancy

Outcome	Non-smoker	Smoker	P value
	n = 156	n = 114	
BW mean (SD) (g)	3360 (535)	3192 (483)	0.008
LBW % (n)	4.5% (7)	7.0% (8)	0.370

- Using mean birthweight (i.e. a continuous variable), the difference between non-smokers and smokers is significant with P = 0.008
- Using birthweight in two groups, low birthweight and normal birthweight, the difference between non-smokers and smokers is not significant with P = 0.370
- In the same dataset, categorization of birthweight into two groups has discarded information and gives a **less significant (bigger) P value**
- Hence when data are categorized there is **less statistical power** to detect a difference (Sample size for comparative studies, p. 62)

Outcomes: continuous and categorical (continued)

Effects of categorization on sample size
- Categorizing continuous data into two groups discards much data
- If a continuous variable is used for analysis in a research study, a substantially smaller sample size will be needed than if the same variable is categorized into two groups

Example: effects of categorization on sample size (📖 Sample size for comparative studies, p. 62)

Table 1.6 shows the sample size needed to detect a difference using means and the corresponding difference using proportions to illustrate the effects on required sample size when a continuous variable is analysed in two groups.

The calculations use standard formulae and were done using the statistical program NQuery.[1] It is assumed that birthweight follows a Normal distribution with mean 3500 g and SD 500 g. Power is 90% and significance level is 5%.

Table 1.6 Sample size needed to detect a difference in mean birthweight (BW) between two groups and the corresponding sample size (SS) needed to detect an equivalent difference in percentage low birthweight (<2500 g, LBW)

Difference in BW	SS	Difference in % LBW	SS
50 g	2103	2.9–2.3%	13 877
100 g	527	3.6–2.3%	3561
150 g	235	4.5–2.3%	1521
200 g	133	5.5–2.3%	814
250 g	86	6.7–2.3%	503

This example illustrates that, for the same size of difference, categorization increases required sample size considerably

Other effects of categorization of continuous data
- Categorizing continuous data into two groups can lead to problems in statistical analysis and give biased estimates or conceal relationships. Further discussion is beyond the scope of this book, but Altman[2] and Senn[3] give some further details
- Note that grouping is less problematic if several groups are used. For example, in regression analyses (📖 Chapter 12, p. 393) it can be helpful to analyse age in, say, five-year groups

---

Best choice?

- Categorization of a continuous variable into two groups loses much data and should be avoided wherever possible
- Categorization of a continuous variable into several groups is less problematic as fewer data are lost. It may be useful in regression analyses where non-linear relationships are being explored

---

References

1 nQuery advisor: Sample size and power calculations. ♒ www.statsol.ie
2 Altman DG, Royston P. The cost of dichotomising continuous variables. *BMJ* 2006; **332**(7549): 1080.
3 Senn S. Disappointing dichotomies. *Pharm Stat* 2003; **2**:239–40.

Collecting additional data

Descriptive, predictive and exposure data

Similar principles apply to these as apply to the selection and recording of main outcomes

- Continuous variables are preferable from a statistical viewpoint, since they will give more precision to analyses
- If the data are obtained from notes or from direct enquiry then they should be recorded with adequate precision
- If the data will be from a self-completed questionnaire, then subjects may prefer to tick boxes rather than give exact numbers and the tension between accuracy and completeness will come into play (📖 Questions and questionnaires, p. 82)

How much data to collect?

Research studies require certain specific data which must be collected to fulfil the aims of the study, such as the primary and secondary outcomes and main factors related to them. Beyond these data there are often other data that could be collected and it is important to weigh the costs and consequences of not collecting data that will be needed later against the disadvantages of collecting too much data.

- **Too little data**: missed data, if not collected, may not be able to be collected on a later occasion and so it is important to decide what key data are needed
- **Too much data**: collecting too much data is likely to add to the time and cost to data collection and processing, and may threaten the completeness and/or quality of all of the data so that key data items are threatened. For example if a questionnaire is overly long, respondents may leave some questions out or may refuse to fill it out at all.

The study protocol

Research protocol

The protocol is a written document that summarizes the proposed study. It is useful because it focuses ideas about the research question and sets the aims in the context of work already done. It documents the design, sample size, and the planned statistical analysis, and provides a timetable for the study. It therefore provides a good working document/template for applications for ethical approval and funding.

The research protocol should include the following items:
- Title
- Abstract
- Aim of study
- Background
- Study design
- Sample size (if relevant)
- Plan of the statistical analyses
- Ethical issues (if relevant)
- Costs
- Timetable
- Staffing/resources

Clinical protocol

- Guidelines to describe good practice in different clinical situations, for example to describe how patients should be managed
- May be part of research protocol

Operational protocol

This will be more detailed than research protocol as it gives full details of how study will be carried out and the guidelines for specific situations.

Example of a published protocol

Cools et al. published a study protocol for an individual patient data meta-analysis of elective high frequency oscillatory ventilation in preterm infants with respiratory distress syndrome.[1] The protocol is too long (13 pages) to reproduce here but key sections are included. The full protocol can be obtained free from the BMC website (🔗 www.biomedcentral.com/1471-2431/9/33).

Background: This section described:
- The clinical problem and the reason why the study was needed
- The limitations of an aggregate data meta-analysis
- The benefits given by the proposed individual patient data meta-analysis

Methods and design: This section described:
- The objectives of the new study
- How the individual studies for the meta-analysis were identified and the inclusion/exclusion criteria
- Data management
- The data items obtained from the individual trialists
- The planned statistical analyses including the primary and secondary outcomes
- The planned subgroup analyses
- The planned sensitivity analyses
- Additional analyses
- Ethical considerations
- Project management including the roles of the core group, the trialist group and the advisory group
- Funding obtained and competing interests
- Publication policy

Reference

1 Cools F, Askie LM, Offringa M. Elective high-frequency oscillatory ventilation in preterm infants with respiratory distress syndrome: an individual patient data meta-analysis. *BMC Pediatr* 2009; **9**:33.

Sampling strategies

Introduction

Whenever a sample is used to provide information about a wider population, we have to consider how the sample is to be chosen. There are two key properties of samples which impinge on a study. First is the size of the sample, which affects the precision of the analyses. We will address this issue below. Second is the choice of sample, which needs to be representative of the underlying population of interest for the results to be generalisable to that population.

Convenience sample

Many studies use a sample of patients available at a particular time/place, for example patients who attend an asthma clinic may be recruited into a survey of the use of spirometers. The results of this study will apply to the population from which this sample is drawn and may not apply to other populations because patients' attendance at a clinic may be due to their response to treatment or their use of spirometers. Hence they may not be representative of all patients using spirometers.

It is important when using a convenience sample to collect and report information about the baseline characteristics of the sample so that the generalizability of this sample can be deduced.

Quota sample

In choosing a quota sample, the researcher aims to identify a representative sample by choosing subjects in proportion to their numbers in the population of interest. For example if age, marital status, sex, and employment status were important characteristics, then the researcher would select a number of subjects with each combination of these characteristics so that the overall proportions with the characteristics reflected the proportions in the population. Quota sampling is often used in market research but is less common in medical research. The difficulty with quota sampling is that subjects recruited may differ from those not-recruited in subtle ways, for example if the sample is obtained by knocking on doors or by approaching people in the street or by telephoning, certain sections of the populations will be excluded. Therefore a quota sample provides no estimate of the true response rate and may not be representative of the desired population.

Random sample (simple random sample)

A random sample is chosen so that each member of the population has an equal chance of being chosen and so the selection is completely independent of patient characteristics. In order to draw a random sample a list of the population is needed, the sampling frame. A random sample will be representative of the population from which it was chosen because the characteristics of the individuals are not considered when the selection is made. Random sampling can be done using computer programs.

Stratified sample

Stratified samples are used when fixed numbers are needed from particular sections or strata of the population in order to achieve balance across certain important factors. For example a study designed to estimate the prevalence of diabetes in different ethnic groups may choose a random sample with equal numbers of subjects in each ethnic group to provide a set of estimates with equal precision for each group. If a simple random sample is used rather than a stratified sample, then estimates for minority ethnic groups may be based on small numbers and have poor precision. In terms of efficiency, a stratified sample gives the most precise overall (weighted) estimate, where the overall estimate is weighted according to the fractions sampled in each stratum.

Cluster sample

Cluster samples may be chosen where individuals fall naturally into groups or clusters. For example, patients on a hospital wards or patients in a GP practice. If a sample is needed of these patients, it may be easier to list the clusters and then to choose a random sample of clusters, rather than to choose a random sample of the whole population. (In fact it may be impossible to list the whole population). Having chosen the clusters, the researcher can either select all subjects in the cluster or take a random sample within the cluster. Cluster sampling is less efficient statistically than simple random sampling and so needs to be accounted for in the sample size calculations and subsequent analyses (Cluster samples: units of analysis, p. 388).

Choosing a sample size

Samples and populations

For pragmatic reasons, research studies nearly always use samples from populations rather than the entire population. Sample estimates will therefore be an imperfect representation of the entire population since they are based on only a subset of the population. As stated previously, when the sample is unbiased and is large enough, then the sample will provide useful information about the population. As well as considering how representative a sample is, it is important also to consider the size of the sample. A sample may be unbiased and therefore representative, but too small to give reliable estimates.

Consequences of too small a sample: studies producing estimates

Prevalence estimates from small samples will be imprecise and therefore may be misleading. For example, suppose we wish to investigate the prevalence of a condition for which studies in other settings have reported a prevalence of 10%. A small sample of, say, 20 people, would be insufficient to produce a reliable estimate since only 2 would be expected to have the condition and a decrease or increase of 1 person would change the estimate considerably (2/20 = 10%, 1/20 = 5%, 3/20 = 15%). Such a study needs a large sample to give a stable estimate.

- When estimating quantities from a sample such as a proportion or mean, we use the 95% confidence interval to show how precise the estimate is (📖 Confidence interval for a proportion, p. 270)
- If the confidence interval is narrow, then the estimate is precise and conversely if the interval is wide then the estimate is imprecise
- Sample size calculations determine the number of subjects needed to give a sufficiently narrow confidence interval

Consequences of too small a sample: studies making comparisons

When we compare two groups we use a significance test to calculate the P value and if possible, we calculate the difference and a confidence interval for the difference. For example when we compare mean blood pressure in patients given two different treatments for hypertension we can calculate the difference in means between the two groups and a 95% confidence interval for the difference. The result of the significance test may be statistically significant or non-significant, depending on the size of the P value. The P value is affected by the sample size and if the sample is too small, there may not be enough data to draw a firm conclusion about any differences. If the sample is small then, in general, the observed difference needs to be larger to be statistically significant. As a consequence, small but important differences may be statistically non-significant in small samples. Hence, if there is a true difference between groups in the target population, the study must be big enough to give a significant result; otherwise incorrect conclusions may be drawn.

- Statistical comparisons are made using significance tests which give a
  P value (📖 P values, p. 248)
- If the sample is too small a true difference may be missed

Calculating sample size

There are formulae for calculating sample size, and the simplest and most
commonly used are given below. Computer programs can be used such as
the specialist sample size programs nQuery advisor[1] and PASS,[2] which do
a wide range of sample size calculations. Some general statistical analysis
programs such as Stata[3] cover a limited number of situations. The following books also give tables for the calculation of sample size:
- Machin D et al. *Sample size tables for clinical studies*[4]
- Chow SC et al. *Sample size calculations in clinical research*[5]

Examples

Sample size calculations for studies estimating a mean or proportion, and
for studies comparing two means or two proportions are shown in the
following sections in this chapter. Before the calculations can be done
certain information is needed. This is listed, described and discussed with
examples of sample size calculations using the programs nQuery, PASS,
and Stata.

References

1 nQuery advisor: Sample size and power calculations. 🖰 www.statsol.ie

2 PASS: Power analysis and sample size software. 🖰 www.ncss.com.

3 Stata: Data analysis and statistical software. 🖰 www.stata.com.

4 Machin D, Campbell MJ, Tang S-B, Huey S. *Sample size tables for clinical studies*. 3rd ed.
London: BMJ Books, Wiley, 2008.

5 Chow SC, Shao J, Wang H. *Sample size calculations in clinical research*. 2nd ed. Boca Raton, FL:
Chapman & Hall/CRC, 2008.

Sample size for estimation studies: means

Estimating a mean with a specified precision

The following information is required:
- The standard deviation (SD) of the measure being estimated
- The desired width of the confidence interval (d)
- The confidence level

The **standard deviation** is needed because the sample size depends partly on the variability of the measure being estimated. The greater the variability of a measure, the greater the number of subjects needed in the sample to estimate it precisely.

The standard deviation can be estimated from previously published studies on the same topic, from contact with another worker in the field or from a small pilot study.

The **desired width of the confidence interval**, d, indicates the precision of the mean and is decided by the researcher.

The **confidence level** is usually set at 95%, giving a sample confidence interval that contains the true population mean with probability 95%. Other values such as 90% or 99% can be used, but are unusual in practice.

Assuming that the confidence level is 95%, the sample size, n, is then given by:

$$n = 1.96^2 \times 4 \, SD^2/d^2$$

To change the confidence level, change the multiplier '1.96^2' as follows.

> **95% confidence level**: $n = 1.96^2 \times 4 \, SD^2/d^2$
> **90% confidence level**: $n = 1.64^2 \times 4 \, SD^2/d^2$
> **99% confidence level**: $n = 2.58^2 \times 4 \, SD^2/d^2$

Where 1.96, 1.64, and 2.58 are the two-sided 5%, 10%, and 1% points, respectively, of the Normal distribution.

Example

Suppose we wish to estimate mean systolic blood pressure in a patient group with a 10 mmHg-wide 95% confidence interval, i.e. 5 mmHg either side of the mean. Previous work suggested using a standard deviation of 11.4.

- The standard deviation (SD) of the measure being estimated = 11.4
- The desired width of the confidence interval (d) = 10
- The confidence level = 95%

$n = 1.96^2 \times 4 \, SD^2/d^2$

$n = 15.37^2 \times 11.4^2/10^2$

$n = 20$

Suppose we reduce the width of the confidence interval to 5 mmHg?

$n = 1.96^2 \times 4 \times 11.4^2/5^2$

$n = 80$

So *doubling* the precision leads to a *quadrupling* of the sample size.

Sample size for estimation studies: proportions

Estimating a proportion with a specified precision

The following information is required:
- The expected population proportion, p
- The desired width of the confidence interval (d)
- The confidence level

The **expected population proportion** is the best guess of what the value will be. This need not be accurate but an approximate figure, such as 0.02 (2%) or 0.05 (5%) or 0.10 (10%), etc. This guess can be obtained from previously published studies on the same topic, from contact with another worker in the field or from a small pilot study. The 'guess' does not need to be very accurate and in most cases, the researcher will have an idea of what the value will be. If no guess is possible then use 0.50.

It may appear counter-intuitive to need to use a 'guess' of the value of the proportion in the sample size calculations for a study to produce an estimate. However, it is needed because the variability of a proportion which is needed in the calculation depends on the proportion itself. In the case of estimating a mean, the variability (estimated by the standard deviation), is independent of the mean.

The **desired width of the confidence interval,** d, indicates the precision of the proportion and is decided by the researcher.

The **confidence level** is usually set at 95%, giving a sample confidence interval that contains the true population proportion with probability 95%.

Assuming that the confidence level is 95%, the sample size, n, is then given by:

$$n = 1.96^2 \times 4\, p(1-p)/d^2$$

Note that this formula uses the proportion and not the percentage. Although these are effectively the same, this formula can only be used with p expressed as a proportion.

To change the confidence level, change the multiplier '1.96^2' as follows:

95% confidence level: $n = 1.96^2 \times 4\, p(1-p)/d^2$
90% confidence level: $n = 1.64^2 \times 4\, p(1-p)/d^2$
99% confidence level: $n = 2.58^2 \times 4\, p(1-p)/d^2$

Example

Suppose we wish to estimate the prevalence of asthma in an adult population with the width of the 95% confidence interval 0.10, an accuracy of ± 0.05. An estimate of the prevalence of asthma is 0.10 (10%).

- The expected population proportion, p = 0.10
- The desired width of the confidence interval (d) = 0.10
- The confidence level = 95%

$n = 1.96^2 \times 4 \, p(1-p)/d^2$

$n = 15.37 \times 0.1(1-0.1)/0.10^2$

$n = 138$

If we choose to double the accuracy to give a 95% confidence interval of 0.05 width:

$n = 1.96^2 \times 4 \times 0.1 \, (1-0.1)/0.05^2$

$n = 553$

Again *doubling* the precision leads to a *quadrupling* of the sample size.

Sample size for comparative studies

Significance tests: type 1, type 2 errors

A significance test to compare two groups in a sample may lead us to an incorrect conclusion about the target population in two different ways:

- **Type 1 error:**
  We conclude that there is a difference between the groups in the target populations when in fact there is not. This is actually the significance level of the test and so when we use 0.05 or 5% as the cut-off for statistical significance, then the probability of a type 1 error is 5%. This is often denoted by 'α'.
- **Type 2 error:**
  We conclude that there is no difference between the groups in the target population when in fact a real difference of a given size does exist. The type 2 error is often denoted by 'β' and $1-\beta$ is the **power** of the study.

Note that this means that the power of a study is the ability of the study to detect a difference if one exists.

In calculating the required sample size for a study we want to minimize type 1 and type 2 errors and therefore avoid spurious statistical significance and avoid missing a real difference. The significance level is usually kept at 5%, by convention, and we set a high value of the power, of at least 80%, and preferably 90% or more.

Clinically important difference

The minimum clinically important difference is needed in the sample size calculations. This is the size of difference that the researcher considers to be so important that they would not want their study to miss it. In other words, this size of difference is considered to be clinically meaningful. If the study is too small to detect this size of difference, and it exists, the comparison will be non-significant and the study will therefore be inconclusive.

The choice of a clinically important difference is not a statistical one, but relates to the context of the study. It can be difficult to decide how big a difference would be important in a given context. The literature and/ or discussions with colleagues may help decide what size of difference is important.

Pre-determined sample size

In some situations, the sample size is fixed either due to the limited availability of subjects, or due to time or financial constraints. In such cases, sample size calculations should still be done to see how big a difference could be detected with the given sample size. If the available sample size is sufficient to achieve the aims of the study then the study can go ahead but if it cannot then it is questionable whether to proceed. It is better to know in advance if the sample size is too small and choose not to do the study than to conduct a study and then find that it is too small and turns out to be inconclusive.

Some statisticians consider that it is unethical to carry out research which is likely to be inconclusive due to small sample size as it is a waste of resources, and/or a waste of patients' time and/or can lead to a wrong interpretation that there is no real difference (i.e. a type 2 error). Others argue that small studies are justified if they add to the pool of evidence and can be combined with other small studies in a meta-analysis (📖 Chapter 13, p. 447).

Sample size for comparative studies: means

In a comparative study we choose the sample size to have a high probability of detecting a difference of a given size *if it exists* but also have a low probability of finding a significant difference *when no real difference exists*. In other words we want to have high power (and hence low type 2 error) and a low significance level (low type 1 error). The formula used for comparing means and comparing proportions balances these probabilities and allows us to calculate sample sizes given certain information.

The following information is required:
- The standard deviation (SD) of the measure being compared
- The minimum difference (d) that is clinically important
- The significance level (α)
- The power of the test ($1-\beta$)

The standard deviation is estimated from previously published studies on the same topic, from contact with another worker in the field or from a small pilot study.

The *minimum difference that is clinically important* is decided beforehand by the researcher.

The *significance level*, α is the maximum acceptable type 1 error rate and is usually set at 5%.

The *power of the test*, $1-\beta$, is the probability of getting a significant result when the true difference between the means is d and is set at 80% or more, preferably 90%.

To compare the two means we need the following number of patients in each group:

$$n = \frac{2K\ SD^2}{d^2}$$

The total sample size is 2n. K is a multiplier that depends on the significance level and power and comes from the Normal distribution. Details of the formula and the multipliers (Table 1.7) are given in Bland's Chapter 18.[1]

Example

(i) A study of the effects of smoking on birthweight should be able to show a difference between smokers and non-smokers of 200 g with high power. SD for birthweight is 500 g. We will use a significance level 5% and power 90%, giving K=10.5 from Table 1.7.

- The standard deviation (SD) of the measure being compared = 500
- The minimum difference (d) that is clinically important = 200
- The significance level (α) = 5%
- The power of the test ($1-\beta$) = 90%

$$n = \frac{2K \, SD^2}{d^2}$$

$$n = \frac{2 \times 10.5 \times 500^2}{200^2}$$

n = 131 in each group

(ii) Suppose we choose 5% significance level and 80% power. This gives K = 7.8:

$$n = \frac{2 \times 7.8 \times 500^2}{200^2}$$

n = 98 in each group

(iii) Suppose we could only recruit 50 in each group, what size difference could be detected with power 80% and significance level 5% (K = 7.8)?

$$n = \frac{2K \, SD^2}{d^2}$$

Rearrange to give:

$$d^2 = \frac{2K \, SD^2}{n}$$

$$d^2 = \frac{2 \times 7.8 \times 500^2}{50} = 78\,000$$

d = 280

Under these circumstances, the study will have high probability to detect differences of 280 g or more. An observed difference of 200 g will not be statistically significant. In this situation, it may be decided that the study is unlikely to be conclusive and is not worthwhile.

Reference

1 Bland M. *An introduction to medical statistics.* 3rd ed. Oxford: Oxford University Press, 2000.

Sample size for comparative studies: proportions

To calculate the sample size for a study comparing two proportions, the following information is required:
- The expected population proportion in group 1, P_1
- The expected population proportion in group 2, P_2
- The significance level (α)
- The power of the test ($1-\beta$)

The **expected population proportion in group 1** and the **expected population proportion in group 2** are the best estimates of what these values will be. The **difference** therefore reflects the anticipated change in the proportion which would be regarded as clinically important.

The **significance level**, α is the type 1 error and is usually set at 5%.

The **power of the test**, $1-\beta$, is the probability of getting a significant result when the true difference between the proportions is d and is set at 80% or more, preferably 90%.

$$n = \frac{K[P_1(1-P_1) + P_2(1-P_2)]}{(P_1 - P_2)^2}$$

Where n is the number in each group as before.

Example

A study is planned to compare patient outcome following the current form of surgery and a new method. It is expected that the new surgery will have less complications. The proportion of patients who develop complications after undergoing current surgery is 15% and it is expected that the new form of surgery will have a 5% complication rate.

Assuming significance level 5% and power 90%, gives $K = 10.5$ from Table 1.7.

- The expected population proportion in group 1, $P_1 = 0.15$
- The expected population proportion in group 2, $P_2 = 0.05$
- The significance level (α) = 0.05
- The power of the test (1–β) = 0.90

$$n = \frac{K[P_1(1-P_1) + P_2(1-P_2)]}{(P_1 - P_2)^2}$$

$$n = \frac{10.5 \times [0.15(1-0.15) + 0.05(1-0.05)]}{(0.15 - 0.05)^2}$$

n = 183 in each group

Table 1.7 Multipliers for studies comparing two means or two proportions

Power (1–β)	Significance level (α)		
	5%	**1%**	**0.1%**
80%	7.8	11.7	17.1
90%	10.5	14.9	20.9
95%	13.0	17.8	24.3
99%	18.4	24.1	31.6

Sample size calculations: further issues

Assumptions of sample size formulae for means and proportions

- There is no attrition, i.e. the total number of patients successfully recruited and who complete the study is equal to the number required
- For comparative studies, there are equal numbers of subjects in each group
- Samples are simple random samples; any randomization is at the individual level. Sample size calculations are different for cluster samples or cluster randomization and the usual calculations will give too few subjects (see below)
- For comparative studies, a simple comparison of two groups only will be made. Multiple regression or logistic regression (📖 Chapter 12, p. 393) is not planned
- The samples are large enough to use large sample methods for the analysis (📖 95% Confidence interval for a proportion, p. 244)

Sample size calculation in other situations

- *When attrition is expected*
  If there are likely to be losses, estimate how many and multiply up the calculated numbers to allow for them so that the total number included in the study is as planned. For example if the calculated required sample size is 80 in total and it is anticipated that 20% of those recruited will not complete, then 100 patients should be recruited to ensure that 80 will complete
- *Unequal numbers in the groups*
  Unequal numbers in the groups can be dealt with in nQuery[1] and PASS[2] for many situations, and in Stata[3] for simple cases
- *Cluster randomization*
  When individuals are allocated to treatments in groups or clusters rather than as individuals, the sample size calculations are different. The **intraclass correlation coefficient** (ICC) between the clusters is needed for the calculations in addition to the usual quantities. The ICC summarizes the correlation between clusters as a ratio of the total variation between clusters to the total variation between and within clusters. Hence the ICC summarizes the extent of the 'clustering effect'. When individuals in the same cluster are much more alike than individuals in different clusters with respect to an outcome, then the clustering effect is greater and the impact on the required sample size is correspondingly greater. In practice there can be a substantial effect on the sample size even when the ICC is quite small. For more information about cluster randomization, see Kerry and Bland[4] and Donner and Klas.[5] It is probably best to consider getting statistical advice when calculating a sample size for a cluster trial
- *Multifactorial analyses are planned*
  Here the sample size calculations are difficult. The statistical power needs to be higher than for a two-group comparison. The calculations can be done if the correlation between the variables is available, but often this is not known. In such circumstances, a rule of thumb that can

be used is to increase the sample size by 10% for every extra variable added. (Note that for a categorical variable, the number of *variables* here is the total number of categories minus 1).

- **Small sample situations**
  If the calculated sample size is small, say, fewer than 50 per group, then large sample methods may not be possible for the statistical analysis and so the sample size calculations may need adjusting. This may be handled by the sample size program but it is best to check and seek advice if in doubt.

- **Survival analysis**
  If you are comparing the proportion of deaths in two groups at a fixed point and there is no censoring, then the sample size calculations for the comparison of two proportions can be used. If a log rank test is to be used to compare the survival curves then these calculations are not suitable. nQuery[1] will do the calculations, and the formulae are given in David Collet's book in Chapter 10.[6]

- **Equivalence trials**
  Sample size calculations for equivalence trials need specialized formulae which take into account the limits of equivalence that are acceptable in the trial. These can be done in nQuery and PASS.

- **Other designs and analyses**
  The latest versions of nQuery[1] and PASS[2] will calculate sample sizes for a wide range of situations

- **Other software**
  We have only commented on software that we have used. An internet search brings up several sites with sample size software. At the time of writing, the web address referenced from the University of California San Francisco, School of Medicine, lists other free software that is available[7], although we have not tested these.

References

1 nQuery advisor: Sample size and power calculations. www.statsol.ie
2 PASS: Power analysis and sample size software. www.ncss.com.
3 Stata: Data analysis and statistical software. www.stata.com.
4 Kerry SM, Bland JM. Sample size in cluster randomisation. *BMJ* 1998; **316**(7130):549.
5 Donner A, Klar N. *Design and analysis of cluster randomization trials in health research.* London: Arnold, 2000.
6 Collett D. *Modelling survival data in medical research.* 2nd ed. Boca Raton, FL: Chapman & Hall/ CRC, 2003.
7 UCSF Biostatistics: Power and sample size programs. Available from: www.epibiostat.ucsf. edu/biostat/sampsize.html (accessed 5 Jan 2009).

Sample size: other issues

When to do replicate measurements

In some situations, measurements are hard to make or are variable and so it is best if several measurements are taken. We give some suggestions:

- For quantities that are hard to measure accurately, such as skinfold thickness, take three values and use the mean
- For quantities that depend on patient effort, e.g. peak flow rate, take three values and use the maximum
- For quantities that vary, such as blood pressure which varies across the day and is subject to 'white coat syndrome', it may be necessary to take several measurements over a period of time to get an accurate assessment
- For quantities that vary due to external factors, such as blood sugar levels which vary with food intake, alternative measures may be needed (e.g. HbA1c level as a surrogate for blood sugar).

Are sample size calculations as described here always needed?

- Not if the study is a qualitative study
- Not always for a small survey

If the study is a descriptive survey then sample size calculations may be difficult. However, it is important to ensure there are sufficient subjects to achieve the aims of the study. For example, in a survey of satisfaction in two patient groups, there will need to be adequate numbers in the two groups to be able to compare satisfaction. It is useful in such situations to list the main cross tabulations that will be needed and to ensure that total numbers will give adequate numbers in the individual table cells.

- Not always for a pilot study – see Gill Lancaster's paper[1] for a general discussion of pilot studies and Steven Julious's paper regarding sample size[2]

References

1 Lancaster GA, Dodd S, Williamson PR. Design and analysis of pilot studies: recommendations for good practice. *J Eval Clin Pract* 2004; **10**(2):307–12.
2 Julious S. Sample size of 12 per group rule of thumb for a pilot study. *Pharm Stat* 2009; **4**(4): 287–91.

Using a statistical program to do the calculations

The following examples show the same sample size calculations in nQuery,[34] in PASS,[2] and in Stata.[3] The same information was input into each program to give the required sample size per group.

The study was to compare lung function in two groups of infants. Power was set at 90% and significance level at 5%. A difference of 0.5 standard deviations was considered to be clinically worthwhile. Equal numbers were to be in each group.

Examples

nQuery[1]

nQuery is a **menu-driven program** where the user chooses commands from menus provided. The data are entered into a table on the screen and when all fields are complete, the number per group is automatically calculated. This is shown below in **bold**.

Two group t-test of equal means (unequal 'ns')

Test significance level, a	0.050
1 or 2 sided test?	2
Group 1 mean, m_1	2.600
Group 2 mean, m_2	2.100
Difference in means, $m_1 - m_2$	0.500
Common standard deviation, s	1.000
Effect size, $d = |m_1 - m_2| / s$	0.500
Power (%)	90
n_1	**86**
n_2	**86**
Ratio: n_2 / n_1	1.000
$N = n_1 + n_2$	172

PASS[2]

Like nQuery, PASS is a **menu-drive program**, The data are entered into a table on the screen and when all fields are complete, the number per group is automatically calculated. This is shown in **bold.**

Two-Sample T-Test Power Analysis
Numeric Results for Two-Sample T-Test

Null Hypothesis: Mean1=Mean2. Alternative Hypothesis: Mean1<>Mean2

The standard deviations were assumed to be known and unequal.

		Allocation						
Power	N1	N2	Ratio	Alpha	Beta	Mean1	Mean2	S1	S2
0.90	**85**	**85**	1.00	0.050	0.010	2.6	2.1	1.0	1.0

Stata[3]

Stata is a **command-driven program** which means that the actual commands need to be typed and then the calculations are done. The command is in **bold** below and the following text is the results that the program gives. The sample size per group is given as 85 per group.

.sampsi 2.6 2.1, p(0.90) sd(1)

Estimated sample size for two-sample comparison of means

Test Ho: m1 = m2, where m1 is the mean in population 1
and m2 is the mean in population 2

Assumptions:

```
        alpha =    0.0500 (two-sided)
        power =    0.9000
           m1 =    2.6
           m2 =    2.1
          sd1 =    1
          sd2 =    1
        n2/n1 =    1.00
```

Estimated required sample sizes:

```
           n1 =      85
           n2 =      85
```

Note

Two of the three programs give the sample size as 85 and the other as 86. This is because the calculations involve rounding. In practice this small difference does not matter.

References

1 nQuery advisor: Sample size and power calculations. ♾ www.statsol.ie
2 PASS: Power analysis and sample size software. ♾ www.ncss.com.
3 Stata: Data analysis and statistical software. ♾ www.stata.com.

Collecting data

Introduction

Data collection is a key part of the research process, and the collection method will impact on later statistical analysis of the data. In this chapter we give suggestions for designing good questions and questionnaires, and discuss the consequences of different question designs on the resulting statistical analyses.

Data collection forms

Introduction

When the research question and study design are settled and we have decided which data to collect, we need to design the data collection forms. These are needed to provide a written or electronic record of the data collected and to facilitate data analysis using a computer. The forms can be paper or electronic. Below we give some specific and general guidance for paper and electronic forms.

Paper forms

- Try to make them clear and easy to fill out
- Allow adequate space for inserting numbers and text
- Consider using a colour other than white for the form to make them more attractive to work with
- When more than one form is required, such as when the study involves follow-up on several occasions, it can be helpful to use a different colour for each occasion to help with tracking and filing
- Long forms can be off-putting for people filling them in so consider how to make the form as short as possible while including all necessary questions

Electronic data capture

- Make sure each original data entry form or data collection session is kept for later checking. Save any edited forms in new files
- Make sure each page of a form, or each form where there are several, can be uniquely identified with a particular subject so that they can be merged together correctly later
- Keep careful audit trails with dates and file names and back up all data
- Keep careful track of the master copy of data from where editing and/ or additional data collection is taking place
- Use filters to jump to later questions where particular questions are not applicable
- Build in checks for impossible and/or inconsistent values wherever possible to avoid data recording errors
- Consider having the coding 'programmed in' (see also 📖 Form filling and coding, p. 78)

All forms

- Give an ID number for each subject for tracking purposes
- Record the date the form was filled out and by whom, if relevant
- Include clear instructions for filling out the form and for specific questions as appropriate. Give example(s) of how to fill out the form either within the form itself or as a separate document
- In large studies, training in filling out the forms may be needed to ensure accuracy and consistency
- Design the form to minimize data recording errors, e.g. give boxes to tick where possible rather than leave the response open

- Where data types may vary from subject to subject for a particular item, ensure it is clear what is recorded, e.g. metric or imperial units may be available for height – note which is used
- Number the questions or items to be collected. Number the pages in paper forms
- Decide whether to use boxes, lines, or spaces for answers, depending on the space available and the data to be recorded
- Think about the anticipated data analysis so that data are collected in the appropriate format, e.g. if a mean will be needed for the analysis, then don't record the data in categories, record the actual value
- Have a well-organized filing system so that individual forms can be easily found if needed at a later date

Anonymity and confidentiality

- Use an ID number rather than a name as the identifier to maintain confidentiality. The actual names and corresponding numbers should be stored separately and securely
- If the study is anonymous, still include an ID for each form for tracking purposes – sometimes data analysis can throw up a query that may be resolved if the specific original form can be checked

Piloting

- It is useful to test the data collection process in a range of circumstances to make sure it will work in practice
- This usually involves trialling the data collection form on a smaller sample than intended for the study and enables problems with the data collection form to be identified and resolved prior to main data collection
- With new questions or new items to be collected, piloting helps ensure the form can accommodate all possible responses where a tick box approach is used, or simply check there is enough space where a free text answer will be given

Form filling and coding

Form filling

Data collection forms nearly always need instructions on how to fill them in. The level of detail in the instructions depends on the complexity of the form and the level of experience of the person filling in the form. Where the form or the source of data is complex, for example, when extracting data from hand-written clinical notes, then some formal training may be needed to ensure accuracy and consistency. This is especially true where more than one person will be extracting data as in a large study. Below we list the sorts of items that may need consideration:

- **Writing**: use clear writing and black pen, not pencil
- **Mistakes**: don't over-write mistakes, cross through and rewrite or use correction fluid
- **Examples**: these can be helpful to show how to fill the form in
- **Guessing**: sometimes to be helpful, data extractors fill in missing values with what they assume the data value should be. For example if patient's sex is not recorded on the source document they may attempt to guess it from the first name. This should be explicitly discouraged to avoid bias
- **Calculations**: in general don't expect the person filling out the form to do calculations as this may lead to errors, e.g. calculating a length of time between two dates. Instead, record each piece of information to allow computation of the particular value later

Coding

Coding is needed to allow non-numerical data or numerical data that has been recorded in categories to be used in statistical analysis with a computer. Coding assigns a unique number to each possible response. Some statistical packages will analyse non-numerical data but it is easier to assign a number to each category. This means that when the data are analysed and reported, the appropriate label needs to be assigned back to the numerical value to make it meaningful.

The coding scheme should be designed at the same time as the form so that it can be built into the form. This can be done by writing the code next to the box (📖 see Examples of questions with possible coding, p. 80) or by having a column on the right-hand side for the code to be written in later. It is easiest if the form is effectively self-coding to save time and avoid errors, but this may make the form too cluttered.

Choosing the codes

- Use intuitive codes if possible, e.g. use 1/0 for yes/no such that responses given as 'yes' are coded 1 and those given as 'no' are coded 0. This also has the added advantage that the variable's 0/1 values can be simply summed to give the number of positive responses
- Use codes 1, 2, 3, etc. where data fall into more than two categories
- If the first category is a 'null category' such as when recording pain as 'no pain, mild pain, moderate pain, and severe pain', it may be sensible to use the codes 0, 1, 2, 3

- It is essential to keep a record of the codes for current and later reference

❶ Although the choice of coding scheme does not affect the actual statistical analysis, an intuitive scheme will make it easier to use, and mistakes less likely to occur. One study that we know of used the codes 1 for 'yes' and 2 for 'no' in some places and 1 for 'no' and 2 for 'yes' in others. This inconsistency was confusing and could have led to errors.

Missing data

- Missing data are sometimes given a special code, such as 9 with the appropriate number of 9s that could not be a real response
- For example: for a yes/no response, 9 could indicate a missing value; for height recorded in cm, 999 could be used, as this is not a possible value
- Computer packages may use a dot (.) to denote a missing value
- It may be important to distinguish between data that are simply missing from the original source and data that the data extractor failed to record. This can be achieved using different codes
- Sometimes a response to a question may be 'not applicable', such as when asking the number of cigarettes smoked when the respondent has already answered 'no' to a question about whether they currently smoke. It may be helpful to code such responses differently, for example using 8s rather than 9s.

Examples of questions with possible coding

Does the patient currently smoke?
☐ Yes   (=1)
☐ No   (=0)

This is a single yes/no question

Patient's legal marital status
☐ Married   (=1)
☐ Single   (=2)
☐ Widowed   (=3)
☐ Divorced   (=4)
☐ Separated   (=5)

This is a single question with multiple options

Patient's self-reported pain level
☐ None   (=0)
☐ Slight pain   (=1)
☐ Moderate pain   (=2)
☐ Severe pain   (=3)

This is a single question with multiple options

Patient's current medication for pain
☐ TCA   (=0/1)
☐ Anti-epileptic   (=0/1)
☐ Topical analgesic   (=0/1)
☐ Opioid   (=0/1)
☐ NSAID   (=0/1)
☐ Other   (=0/1)

This is a multiple question for which each option is no or yes since patients may be taking more than one drug or none at all

Care in the statistical analysis: a footnote

❶ The use of numerical codes for non-numerical data may give the false impression that these data can be treated as if they were numerical data in the statistical analysis. This is not so. We could calculate mean marital status using the data coded 1–5 in the example above, but since these codes have no intrinsic meaning, this would be nonsensical.

Data quality

Introduction

▶ It is critical that data quality is monitored and that this happens as the study progresses. It may be too late if problems are only discovered at the analysis stage. If checks are made during the data collection then problems can be corrected. More frequent checks may be worthwhile at the beginning of data collection when processes may be new and staff may be less experienced. Suggestions are as follows.

Check completion rates for forms

- Are all the pages filled out? If not where is it going wrong?
- Are all the questions/sections completed? If not why not?
- Do gaps reflect truly unknown data or have some data been missed out accidentally?
- Is the writing clear?

Check accuracy

- Double-check a sub-sample to determine quality
- Consider double-checking any critical data

Actions as necessary

- Issue new instructions
- Re-train people collecting data
- Alter the forms
- Recheck after changes have been implemented
- Document the quality control process

Questions and questionnaires

Designing questions

Designing questions is an art as much as it is a science. The subject is discussed in detail in some books of research methods such as Ann Bowling's book.[1] We will give a brief summary of the main issues here.

Different types of questions can be asked in medical research: facts, opinions/views/feelings, and closed and open questions. These are described below.

Facts

- *How old are you?*
- *Do you smoke cigarettes?*

The answer to a question of fact is absolute in that there is a single true answer. Of course, subjects may not give the correct answer either deliberately or unintentionally, and we may not know this.

Some information which is clearly a fact is difficult to ascertain, such as self-reported weight, partly because people may simply not know, and partly because they may report it inaccurately. Other 'facts' such as measurements of height may be inaccurate due to measurement error. We will not deal any further with measurement error in this section.

Opinions/views/feelings

- *Was your last clinic appointment long enough?*
- *How do you rate your pain today?*
- *Were you satisfied with your recent hospital stay?*

Opinion-type questions are subjective and are therefore much more difficult to ask, and the responses are harder to interpret. Seemingly similar people may give different responses to the same question, and these responses may even vary from day to day in the same person. In addition, the response can be affected by the way in which the question is asked.

A leading question is likely to produce a different answer to a more neutrally worded question. The following two questions are trying to obtain essentially the same information but ask for it in different ways, and are likely to obtain different answers:

- *Do you have any complaints about this service?*
- *Are you satisfied with this service?*

Closed questions

These can be either facts or opinion. For example:
Do you smoke cigarettes?
☐ Yes
☐ No

This is a closed question because the possible answers are pre-specified.

Similarly with the subjective pain question:

How do you rate your pain today?
☐ No pain
☐ Mild pain
☐ Moderate pain
☐ Severe pain

All possible answers are given for the subject to choose their response. 'Don't know' is also a possible response which may be given as an option in a closed question (see 📖 Designing good questions, p. 84).

Open questions
These are questions where the response is not pre-determined by the researcher, for example:

Tell us how you feel about your recent hospital stay?

_____
_____
_____

Or as a follow-up to another question where the subject has answered 'yes' and further details are sought:

If you answered 'yes' please explain why

_____
_____
_____

❶ Answers to open questions cannot be coded as they stand. For coding to be possible, similar responses need to be grouped into sub-categories and unique codes assigned to each. The groupings chosen will be influenced by the purpose of the question within the study.

Reference
1 Bowling A. *Research methods in health: investigating health and health services.* 2nd ed. Buckingham: Open University Press, 2002.

Designing good questions

Introduction
The following sections give tips for writing questions in terms of expression/language, content, precision, and sensitivity of the subject.

Expression/language
- Use simple language and short sentences
  For example use 'start' rather than 'commence'
- When the research involves patients, use lay terms for medical conditions and treatments where this would be more easily understood
  For example use 'womb' rather than 'uterus', 'shortness of breath' rather than 'dyspnoea'
- Avoid double negatives
  For example '*Is it true that there isn't a day when you don't feel pain?*'

This is easier to understand when phrased as:
'*Is it true that you feel pain every day?*' or '*Do you feel pain every day?*'

Content
- Make sure each 'question' only asks one thing and not two or more
  For example '*Do you drink tea and coffee?*' This is two questions – the subject may drink tea and not coffee and so not know how to answer!
- Be careful that closed questions include all possible options
  For example '*How many times have you seen the GP this year?*'

  ☐ 1–2 times
  ☐ 3–4 times
  ☐ 5 or more times

  This does not include an option for those who have not visited the GP this year
- Be careful with the use of leading questions as the response will be affected by how the question is asked (📖 Questions and questionnaires, p. 82)

Precision

- Avoid subjective words such as 'usually' and 'frequently', because people will interpret them in different ways
  For example *'Do you usually eat vegetables?'*
  'Do you get frequent headaches?'

  It is better to be specific and ask a 'yes/no' (*'Do you eat vegetables'*) question and then ascertain how often if this is of interest (*'every day, every 2 days, etc*).

- Give units for measurements and allow for responses in imperial or metric where both in common use
  For example *'How much did your baby weigh at birth?*
  You can give the weight in either g or lb and oz'

  _____ g
  _____ lb _____ oz

- Consider when to allow a 'don't know' option for closed questions – sometimes the researcher wants to avoid a 'don't know', and other times it is a valid response, such as when testing knowledge.
  The following question for medical students illustrates this:

  Which one of these medications should not be taken in pregnancy?
  (i) Aspirin
  (ii) Paracetamol
  (iii) Propranolol
  (iv) Isotretinoin
  (v) Don't know

Sensitive topics

Introduction
There are different reasons why a respondent may view a particular topic as sensitive and therefore be reluctant to answer questions. For example if the topic is:
- **Personal**, for example income
- **Embarrassing**, for example sexually transmitted diseases
- **Threatening** and/or **illegal**, for example under-age alcohol use, drug use

Demographic data
Demographic questions such as income may be viewed as more sensitive than questions on other topics such as occupation. For this reason, it is worth considering putting all demographic questions at the end of the questionnaire so that any failure to complete these will not jeopardize the completion of other questions.

Gaining responses
- It can be helpful to put a sensitive topic in a list among non-sensitive topics so that it is not so blunt. For example a survey in school children may find it works to include questions on alcohol consumption among questions on consumption of soft drinks and snacks
- It can be helpful to 'give permission' for the respondent to answer positively, by acknowledging that a positive or negative response is possible. For example:

  'Some parents smack their children and some do not. Have you ever smacked your child?'

  ☐ Yes ☐ No

- Alternatively, we can use an indirect approach by stating a position on the topic and then asking the subject to give their views on this. For example:

  'Some people think that smacking children is helpful in bringing up children and others do not use smacking. What do you think? Please give your views below:'

  _____

  _____

Using randomized responses

This is a statistical technique where the respondent is able to answer a sensitive question in such a way as to preserve privacy. One version works as follows: the respondent answers a sensitive question either correctly or incorrectly with a given probability which is decided, for example, by throwing a dice where they are told to answer correctly if the dice is 1, 2, 3, or 4 and incorrectly if they get 5 or 6. The researcher does not know whether the subject has answered correctly or not but probability theory can be used to estimate the true prevalence for the sensitive question.

Another version works like this: respondents are given two questions, one the sensitive question of interest, and the other an innocuous question. Only one question is answered and only the respondent knows which. The choice is made using a probability technique again such a throwing a dice.

Further details are given in Warner,[1] Greenberg *et al.*,[2] Mangat and Singh,[3] and Franklin.[4]

Further ways to manage sensitive topics

* Ensure and guarantee anonymity (but this means that follow-up is impossible)
* Use an independent interviewer such as one who is not involved in the delivery of health care in a hospital-based study
* Use interviewers who can build rapport with the subjects and so gain their confidence
* Use online surveys where respondents feel 'safer'

Further information on researching sensitive areas can be found in the following sources:

* **Overall considerations**: Renzetti and Lee, Chapter 1[5]
* **Reducing question threat**: Foddy, Chapter 9[6]
* **Cognitive testing**: Willis, Chapter 12[7]
* **A national example**: the British National Survey of Sexual Attitudes and Lifestyles (Natsal) surveys, as described in Mitchell[8]
* **Pitfalls**: How asking even an apparently non-sensitive question can go wrong, in Barrett[9]

References

1 Warner SL. Randomised response: a survey technique for eliminating evasive answer bias. *J Am Stat Assoc* 1965; **60**(309):63–69.
2 Greenberg BG, Abdel-Latif A, Abul-Ela, Simmons WR, Horovitz DG. The unrelated question randomised response model: theoretical framework. *J Am Stat Assoc* 1969; **64**(326):520–539.
3 Mangat NS, Singh RS. An alternative randomised response. *Biometrika* 1990; **77**(2):439–442.
4 Franklin L. Randomised response technique. In: Armitage P, Colton T, editors. *Encyclopedia of biostatistics.* London: Wiley InterScience, 2005.
5 Renzetti CM, Lee RM. *Researching sensitive topics.* Newbury Park, California: Sage, 1993.
6 Foddy WH. Constructing questions for interviews and questionnaires: theory and practice in social research. Cambridge: Cambridge University Press, 1993.
7 Willis GB. *Cognitive interviewing: a tool for improving questionnaire design.* London: Sage, 2005.
8 Mitchell K, Wellings K, Elam G, Erens B, Fenton K, Johnson A. How can we facilitate reliable reporting in surveys of sexual behaviour? Evidence from qualitative research. *Cult Health Sex* 2007; **9**(5):519–531.
9 Barrett G, Wellings K. Collecting information on marital status: a methodological note. *J Epidemiol Community Health* 2002; **56**(3):175–176.

Designing questionnaires

Layout

▶ The layout is as important as the content since it affects questionnaire completion rates and therefore impacts on the overall quality of the data collected. The following are particularly important for self-complete questionnaires:

- Give clear instructions and examples of how to answer questions where appropriate
- Make it clear and uncluttered
- Make it easy to navigate with any skips clearly signposted
- Consider size and length according to who will fill this in – a smaller questionnaire is easier to handle but smaller writing is harder to read
- Indicate page turns clearly to avoid respondents missing pages
- Consider which fonts will best suit the intended readers – for example, older people are likely to find small fonts hard to read
- Piloting can help identify problems with the questionnaire design and uncover any aspects that need improving (📖 Data collection forms, p. 76)

Using an existing questionnaire

It can be better to use an existing questionnaire if there is one that has already been tried and tested. This will save time and will mean that results are comparable with those of other researchers. There is usually a small charge levied to allow an existing questionnaire to be used.

Sometimes, a study needs to modify an existing questionnaire, perhaps to add further questions or adapt it for another setting. It is important that the revised questionnaire is validated for use to ensure that it is appropriate for the new setting.

Further reading on questionnaires

For a full review of the design and use of questionnaires see McColl and colleagues' *Health Technology Assessment* monograph.[1]

Reference

1 McColl E, Jacoby A, Thomas L, Soutter J, Bamford C, Steen N *et al.* Design and use of questionnaires: a review of best practice applicable to surveys of health service staff and patients. *Health Technol Assess* 2001; **5**(31):1–256.

Example of a validated questionnaire

The Dermatology Life Quality Index (DLQI)

The questions from the DLQI are reproduced in Figure 2.1. This questionnaire is commonly used in dermatology to assess the impact of skin disease on a patient's everyday life.

There is a standardized scoring system, with 'very much' scoring 3 points, 'a lot' scoring 2, 'a little' scoring 1, and 'not at all' scoring 0. The individual scores are summed to give a total score out of 30. Since many published research studies have used the DLQI, its use in clinical practice enables clinicians to compare their own patient population with those of research studies. Further, this standardized tool enables better comparisons between different studies.

1.	Over the last week, how **itchy**, **sore**, **painful** or **stinging** has your skin been?	Very much ▫ A lot ▫ A little ▫ Not at all ▫	
2.	Over the last week, how **embarrassed** or **self conscious** have you been because of your skin?	Very much ▫ A lot ▫ A little ▫ Not at all ▫	
3.	Over the last week, how much has your skin interfered with you going **shopping** or looking after your **home** or **garden?**	Very much ▫ A lot ▫ A little ▫ Not at all ▫	Not relevant ▫
4.	Over the last week, how much has your skin influenced the **clothes** you wear?	Very much ▫ A lot ▫ A little ▫ Not at all ▫	Not relevant ▫
5.	Over the last week, how much has your skin affected any **social** or **leisure** activities?	Very much ▫ A lot ▫ A little ▫ Not at all ▫	Not relevant ▫
6.	Over the last week, how much has your skin made it difficult for you to do any **sport**?	Very much ▫ A lot ▫ A little ▫ Not at all ▫	Not relevant ▫
7.	Over the last week, has your skin prevented you from **working** or **studying**?	Yes ▫ No ▫	Not relevant ▫
	If "No", over the last week, how much has your skin been a problem at **work** or **studying**?	A lot ▫ A little ▫ Not at all ▫	
8.	Over the last week, how much has your skin created problems with your **partner** or any of your **close friends** or **relatives**?	Very much ▫ A lot ▫ A little ▫ Not at all ▫	Not relevant ▫
9.	Over the last week, how much has your skin caused any **sexual difficulties**?	Very much ▫ A lot ▫ A little ▫ Not at all ▫	Not relevant ▫
10.	Over the last week, how much of a problem has the **treatment** for your skin been, for example, by making your home messy, or by taking up time?	Very much ▫ A lot ▫ A little ▫ Not at all ▫	Not relevant ▫

Fig. 2.1 The Dermatology Life Quality Index[1].

© AY Finlay, GK Khan, April 1992.[1] Reproduced with kind permission.

Reference

1 Finlay AY, Khan GK. Dermatology Life Quality Index (DLQI) – a simple practical measure for routine clinical use. *Clin Exp Dermatol* 1994; **19**(3):210–16.

Designing a new measurement tool: psychometrics

Introduction
Sometimes researchers need to develop a new measurement or questionnaire scale, for example, to measure a trait such as emotional stability or a symptom such as breathlessness. To do this rigorously requires a thorough process. We will outline the main steps here and note the most common statistical measures used in the process. Full details of developing and using measurement scales in health can be found in Streiner and Norman[1] and a shorter account is given in Bowling.[2]

▶ The following properties of measurement scales are important:

Face and content validity
Face validity
- Is the scale measuring what it sets out to measure? This is a subjective assessment and is achieved by consensus among experts.

Content validity
- Does the scale cover all the relevant areas? This is also subjective and is achieved by consensus among experts.

Reliability and stability
Are the measurements reproducible? If we repeat the measurement will we get the same answer? This applies in the following ways:
- **Between-observers consistency:** is there agreement between different observers assessing the same individuals?
- **Within-observers consistency:** is there agreement between assessments on the same individuals by the same observer on two different occasions?
- **Test-retest consistency:** are assessments made on two separate occasions on the same individual similar?

Internal consistency: Cronbach's alpha

If a scale has several questions or items which all address the same issue then we usually expect each individual to get similar scores for those questions, i.e. we expect their responses to be internally consistent. A statistical quantity, Cronbach's alpha, is often used to assess the degree of internal consistency.

Cronbach's alpha[3,4] is calculated as an average of all correlations among the different questions in the scale. It can be interpreted as follows:

- Alpha lies between 0 and 1
- Values are usually expected to be above 0.7 and below 0.9
- Alpha below 0.7 broadly indicates poor internal consistency
- Alpha above 0.9 suggests that the items are very similar and perhaps fewer items could be used to obtain the same overall information

Note that high internal consistency is not always expected – some questionnaires, such as the General Health Questionnaire (GHQ),[5] contain a number of different health questions which might not necessarily be answered in a similar way by the same individuals, such as the questions on somatic symptoms and questions on depression.

References

1 Streiner DL, Norman GR. *Health measurement scales: a practical guide to their development and use*. 3rd ed. Oxford: Oxford University Press, 2003.
2 Bowling A. *Research methods in health: investigating health and health services*. 2nd ed. Buckingham: Open University Press, 2002.
3 Cronbach LJ. Coefficient alpha and the internal structure of tests. *Psychometrika* 1951; **16**:297–333.
4 Bland JM, Altman DG. Statistics notes: Cronbach's alpha. *BMJ* 1997; **314**(7080):572.
5 Goldberg DP, Hillier VF. A scaled version of the General Health Questionnaire. *Psychol Med* 1979; **9**(1):139–45.

Measuring reliability

Continuous data

Repeatability both within individuals and between observers can be quantified in several different ways. In many medical studies the actual size of the differences between repeated measurements is of interest and so the **Bland–Altman limits of agreement**[1] gives a useful summary of this (🕮 Bland–Altman method to measure agreement, p. 360). If a relative summary is of interest then the **coefficient of variation** (standard deviation of differences divided by the mean) may be helpful, especially if the standard deviation is proportional to the mean (Bland, Chapter 15[2]).

An **intraclass correlation coefficient** (Bland, Chapter 15[2]) is also sometimes used. This is a dimensionless quantity that can be useful to compare the repeatability of several measures, but the drawback is that gives no indication of absolute differences.

Categorical data

To assess the level of agreement for data that fall into categories, Cohen's kappa is used (see 🕮 Kappa for inter-rater agreement, p. 354).

Empirical validity

There is empirical validity when the scale measures the trait, behaviour, or symptom that it sets out to measure. The two types of empirical validity usually considered are outlined below.

Convergent/criterion/concurrent validity

This can be tested by comparing it with another similar scale, where one exists, to see if both give a similar result. For example in developing a shortened version of an existing but longer questionnaire it is important to ensure that the short version gives comparable results with the longer version.

Construct validity

To assess construct validity where there are no similar scales to compare with, the researchers apply a series of tests where the answer is known to check that the scale is behaving as expected.

Examples: testing validity

Testing concurrent validity

Researchers wanted to develop an inexpensive questionnaire that parents could fill out to assess the cognitive development of their children. This questionnaire was designed to replace a lengthy examination by a paediatrician or psychologist (Bayley Mental Development Index, MDI) in a large study where individual assessment was impracticable.

Both methods were compared in a test sample of children: the new questionnaire was given to parents, and in addition and independently, a full assessment was carried out by a trained psychologist.

When the two assessments were compared they gave sufficiently similar results for the parental questionnaire to be used in the large study.[3]

Showing construct validity

In developing a new questionnaire scale to measure respiratory symptoms we would expect that patients from a chronic obstructive pulmonary disease (COPD) clinic would score higher than patients from a fracture clinic, and that patients' scores would change before and after exercise etc.

These comparisons show that the scale is working as expected and so has construct validity.

References

1 Bland JM, Altman DG. Statistical methods for assessing agreement between two methods of clinical measurement. *Lancet* 1986; **i**(8476):307–10.

2 Bland M. *An introduction to medical statistics.* 3rd ed. Oxford: Oxford University Press, 2000.

3 Johnson S, Marlow N, Wolke D, Davidson L, Marston L, O'Hare A *et al.* Validation of a parent report measure of cognitive development in very preterm infants. *Dev Med Child Neurol* 2004; **46**(6):389–97.

Questionnaire measurement scales

Likert scales

Likert scales are widely used to record the level of agreement or disagreement with a particular statement. They are discrete scales where respondents have to tick one of a number of replies to describe their degree of agreement with a statement. Each alternative reply is a verbal label. For example:

I can get an appointment with my GP when I want it:
• Strongly disagree
• Disagree
• Neither agree nor disagree
• Agree
• Strongly agree

Likert scales are always symmetrical. They may contain an odd number of choices, five, as above, allowing the neutral option 'neither agree nor disagree'. Likert scales can also contain an even number of choices, thus without a neutral option which forces the respondent to choose to agree or disagree. For example:

GPs should provide appointments outside normal working hours:
• Strongly agree
• Agree
• Disagree
• Strongly disagree

The choice of verbal label varies; for example the middle category 'neither agree nor disagree' is sometime expressed as 'undecided'. The Likert scale has been extended to apply to other situations, for example response to pain medication or patient satisfaction:

How has your pain been since you started this drug?
• Worse
• No change
• Better

How satisfied were you with your last clinic visit?
• Very dissatisfied
• Fairly dissatisfied
• Neither dissatisfied nor satisfied
• Fairly satisfied
• Very satisfied

Scoring and statistical analysis of Likert scale data

The key characteristic of Likert scales is that the scale is symmetrical. If the scale was not symmetrical, there could be bias since respondents may be led to give replies in one particular direction.

Likert scales have categories which are conceptually evenly spaced. This leads onto how we code and analyse data from these scales. Likert scales are usually coded symmetrically, e.g.:

- Strongly disagree $= -2$
- Disagree $= -1$
- Undecided $= 0$
- Agree $= +1$
- Strongly agree $= +2$

❶ Care is needed when analysing Likert scale data even though a numerical code is assigned to the responses, since the data are ordinal and discrete. Hence an average may be misleading and so a median, or the proportion in different categories, may be used as a summary measure. It is quite common to collapse Likert scales into two or three categories such as agree versus disagree, but this has the disadvantage that data are discarded.

Where there are responses to several Likert questions, the responses are sometimes summed to give an overall score. Where this overall score has a wide range, then it may be reasonable to treat it as a continuous variable and calculate means etc., for summary and for analysis. This happens with many standard questionnaires, such as the General Health Questionnaire (GHQ28), where seven Likert questions in each of four sub-groups are summed to give an overall score.

Other response scales

It is not always appropriate to record replies on a symmetrical scale. For example when recording pain it would be appropriate to use the following categories:

- No pain
- Mild pain
- Moderate pain
- Severe pain

These may be coded 0, 1, 2, 3 and the same principles apply for data summary and analysis as for Likert scale data, in that the data are ordinal and so cannot be analysed as if they were continuous.

Visual analogue scales

Introduction

A visual analogue scale (VAS) is used to assess intensity of symptoms, pain, quality of life, etc. A VAS consists of a horizontal line of a given length, usually 100 mm (10 cm) with verbal labels ('anchors') at each end defining the extremes, for example when assessing pain: 0= 'no pain' and 100= 'worst possible pain' (Fig 2.2). Subjects mark the place along the line that best describes their response.

The length of the line to the subject's mark is used as their VAS score. Since it is a measurement, VAS scores can be treated like continuous data, although the distribution may be skewed.

Advantages of VAS

- It provides continuous data, thus means and standard deviations can be calculated and tests based on the Normal distribution are possible
- Statistical power is greater than for Likert scales and other categorical rating scales and so it is possible to detect equivalent differences with smaller samples

Disadvantages of VAS

- The VAS score data are not true measurements in that they represent a subjective assessment. For example, when grading pain, what one patient may grade as '7' may be called '4' by another. Hence the clinical interpretation of a specific value is hard to define, although attempts have been made to do this in the pain field by comparison with other data[1]
- VAS scores are often skewed and so some transformation of the data may be needed before analysis. If there are zeros, these cannot easily be transformed (📖 Transforming data, p. 330)

❶ Other points about using VAS scores

- The length of the line needs to be carefully measured for accuracy
- Beware when photocopying forms with VAS since copying may distort the length of the line and introduce bias

Numerical rating scale

This is a Likert scale that behaves much like a VAS and is sometimes used as if it was a VAS. It consists of a numerical scale like a VAS, but with verbal descriptors at the ends and the numbers marked along the line, and sometimes with additional verbal descriptors alongside them to guide the respondents. Numerical rating scale (NRS) data are therefore **discrete**, for example, consisting of the possible responses: 0, 1, 2, 3, 4, 5, 6, 7, 8, 9, 10.

Although only integer values are possible, NRS data are often treated as if they are continuous measurements. Researchers report summary statistics in terms of means and standard deviations, which seems reasonable as long as most if not all of the of the scale is used across the sample.

Choice of scale – categorical scale or VAS

Where it is feasible to use a VAS, it is preferable as it provides greater statistical power than a categorical scale, especially when the categorical scale is dichotomized.

Many studies in the pain field use several tools to assess pain and so have VAS as well as categorical scales. A difficulty can arise if statistical significance is found with the VAS but not with the categorical scale data.

A sensible approach is to use a VAS score as the primary outcome and the desired categorical scales as secondary outcomes.

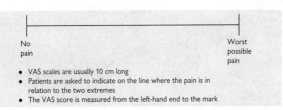

- VAS scales are usually 10 cm long
- Patients are asked to indicate on the line where the pain is in relation to the two extremes
- The VAS score is measured from the left-hand end to the mark

Fig. 2.2 Example of a VAS scale.

Reference

1 Turk DC, Dworkin RH, McDermott MP, Bellamy N, Burke LB, Chandler JM et al. Analyzing multiple endpoints in clinical trials of pain treatments: IMMPACT recommendations. Initiative on Methods, Measurement, and Pain Assessment in Clinical Trials. *Pain* 2008; **139**(3):485–93.

Handling data: what steps are important

Introduction

Correct handling of data is essential to produce valid and reliable statistics. In this chapter we discuss different methods of data entry and manipulation of datasets in computer packages. The importance of checking for errors in the data is highlighted with suggestions how to do this. Finally the role of data monitoring committees in research trials is discussed, along with the implications of ending trials early. Examples are provided throughout the chapter.

Data entry

Introduction

Data from research studies need to be coded before data are entered into a computer for statistical analysis so that all the data are numerical. This means that qualitative data, for example, data that require a 'yes' or 'no' reply, have to be converted to a number such as 1 for 'yes' and 0 for 'no' (see 📖 Form filling and coding, p. 78).

▶ It is strongly recommended that a unique numerical identifier is given to each subject, even if the research is conducted anonymously. This allows the original data collection forms and the electronic version to be matched if any queries arise later on. The identifier may be chosen so that it indicates particular sub-groups of subjects. For example, in a three-centre study with fewer than 100 subjects per centre, subjects could be numbered 101–199, 201–299, and 301–399 so that they can be easily identified or selected at a later stage.

Reducing errors

Data entry screens can be set up within some statistical or data-handling programs to mirror the data entry form and so have appropriate skips and valid ranges built in to reduce errors when data are transferred to computer.

Even with a data entry screen with skips and range checks, errors are possible. This can be further reduced by double-checking all data entered, either by entering the data twice and comparing, 'double-entry', or by hand-checking. This level of checking may not be feasible for a large dataset and in such cases it is recommended that a minimum sample of 10% is checked.

Format for data entry

Computerized datasets are often stored in a spreadsheet format with rows and columns of data. For most statistical analysis it is best to enter the data so that each row represents a different subject and each column a different variable. If possible, discuss this in advance with the person who will be analysing the data to make sure the format is suitable, and to avoid the need for data manipulation later on, which is time-consuming and can introduce errors.

▶ The following types of data need to be entered in particular ways depending on the planned analysis and statistical program to be used, making it **particularly worthwhile to allow time to talk to the data analyst/statistician beforehand**:

• Dates
• Repeated measures of the same variable in individuals
• Data which are in text format or include letters, such as a hospital number or blood group
• Variables which are summaries of other variables, such as mean blood pressure over a period of time, or maximum peak flow rate as the best of three attempts
• Composite data, such as hours and minutes – if in doubt record hours and minutes as two separate variables

Data entry (continued)

Data entry example

Table 3.1 Portion of a spreadsheet with different types of data from a neonatal study

idnum	sex	gestation	gestdays	bweight	smoking	apgar1
1	1	25+5	180	0.884	0	3
2	1	30+2	212	1.26	0	9
3	2	32+0	224	1.558	1	9
4	2	30+5	215	1.5	0	9
5	1	30+4	214	1.158	0	6

- The first row of Table 3.1 gives the variable names and each of the subsequent five rows give the data for five subjects
- Each column represents one variable
- *idnum* is the unique subject identifier
- *sex* denotes the sex of the baby and has two possible values, 1 and 2. To interpret the data we need to know the coding, i.e. to know that in this case, 1=male, 2=female
- *gestation* is the gestational age of the baby and is recorded in 'weeks + days'. This format is commonly used for descriptive purposes but is not suitable for data analysis
- *gestdays* is the gestational age in whole days and is suitable for data analysis
- *bweight* is the baby's birthweight in kg
- *smoking* is the smoking status of the mother and is recorded as 0/1 to indicate no/yes
- *apgar1* is the Apgar score at 1 minute and can take any integer value between 0 and 10
- ❶ Note that the variable names do not contain any gaps. This allows them to transfer directly into a statistical program

Notes

- If any data were missing, these could be indicated by a blank cell or preferably by a specific code such as a dot (.)
- It is important to document the coding scheme for categorical variables such as sex where it will not be obviously what the values mean
- The explanatory list above would form the basis of a **coding sheet** that provides a formal record of the codes used for each of the variables collected in the study

Summary tips for data entry into spreadsheets

- Liaise with analyst beforehand
- Use one row per subject
- Use one column per variable
- Don't leave gaps in the spreadsheet or insert comments amongst data – put any comments at the beginning or at the end
- Wherever possible avoid using non-numerical data in the cells
- Use a dot rather than a blank space to indicate any missing data unless there are specific codes for different types of missing data
- Keep a formal record of the coding used for each variable in the study

Forms that can be automatically scanned for data entry

Introduction

Specialized software programs such as Teleform are available for preparing forms which can be either filled in online or filled out on paper and then scanned automatically into a computer program (see 📖 Chapter 5, p. 155). A scanning operator is needed to oversee the process and respond to any queries that the software identifies when it cannot scan a particular field.

This form of data capture is increasingly used and has many advantages but some potential disadvantages.

Advantages

- Saves considerable time normally needed for data entry and checking
- Ideal for questions that require 'tick box' replies
- Data capture is accurate since it is automatic, unless responses are hand-written (see Disadvantages)

Disadvantages

- Specialized software has to be purchased
- Forms need to be designed and set up using the software, and the user needs to be familiar with the software
- Potentially less flexible for studies with non-tick box questions, i.e. open responses
- Hand-written numbers need to be written carefully or they can be mis-scanned, e.g. handwritten 1s and 7s can look similar so some checking may be needed

The example in Figure 3.1 shows one page from a longer data collection form used in a neonatal study. This section of the form (and the form in general), contained both 'tick box' questions and 'free-style' text questions.

Example of a questionnaire that is designed to be scanned

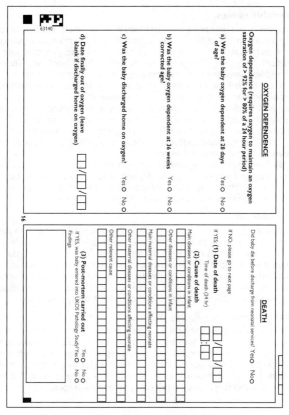

Fig. 3.1 Data collection form designed for computer scanning.

Variable names and labels

Variable names

Variable names may need to be less than nine characters. It is helpful to use intuitive names such as 'bweight' for birthweight to make data analysis and interpretation of results easier. Sometimes statistical programs automatically assign variables generic names such as 'var1' 'var2', etc. These should be changed to something meaningful as the data are entered.

It can be tricky to find unique names for each variable where multiple measurements are taken on the same variable. Prefixes or suffixes can be used to denote such repeated measurements. If there are several repeated variables, use the same 'scheme' for all to avoid confusion. For example if a suffix is used to indicate the number of the measurement, 1, 2, 3, 4 …, for example: bpd7, bpd14, etc, **or** d7bp, d14bp to denote blood pressure (BP) at 7 days and 14 days.

❶ Try to avoid mixing suffixes and prefixes as it can cause confusion. For example, if we use a suffix for BP, such as *bpd7* and a prefix for heart rate such as *d7hr* it may cause confusion later on, especially if there are a lot of variables and the analyst is searching for a particular one.

Variable labels

When using a statistical package, it is usually possible to give labels to the variables in addition to the short name, particularly when the nature of the variable is not obvious from the name itself. Although labelling takes time, it is well worth the time invested to allow you to quickly and accurately identify particular variables in the dataset itself and to be clear what variables have been used when reviewing output results. For example, *smoking* could be labelled 'Mother's smoking habit during pregnancy'.

Value labels

Similarly, when using a statistical program, it is helpful to label the values of categorical variables such as smoking '0=no' and '1=yes'. It is even more important when the variable has many possible values, and when the actual codes have no intuitive meaning. Here we give an example of some results from the statistical program Stata, both unlabelled and labelled to show how labelling makes it much easier to read the output.

Example: statistical analysis results (i) without labelling and (ii) with labelling

The variable being tabulated, 'mastatus', is the marital status in a study of pregnant women. There were five possible responses, which were coded 1, 2, 3, 4, and 5. The labelling of values is particularly needed here as the codes have no intrinsic meaning since the variable is qualitative.

Unlabelled

Mastatus	Freq.	Percent	Cum.
1	1,318	79.93	79.93
2	270	16.37	96.30
3	31	1.88	98.18
4	25	1.52	99.70
5	5	0.30	100.00
Total	1,649	100.00	

Labelled

Marital status	Freq.	Percent	Cum.
Married	1,318	79.93	79.93
Single	270	16.37	96.30
Divorced	31	1.88	98.18
Separated	25	1.52	99.70
Widowed	5	0.30	100.00
Total	1,649	100.00	

Joining datasets

Introduction

When data are entered onto a computer at different times it may be necessary to join datasets together.

▶ It is important to avoid over-writing a current dataset with a new updated version without keeping the old version as a separate file, in case the original file is needed for some reason, such as the computing process crashes and the file being updated is lost.

Appending datasets: adding new cases

For the joining process to work, the two datasets must use exactly the same variable names for the same variables and the same coding. Any spelling mistakes will prevent a successful joining. For example if one dataset used the variable name 'sex' to denote male/female and the other used the variable name 'gender', then when the datasets are merged, there will be two variables denoting male/female, and 'sex' will denote male/female for some subjects and 'gender' will denote male/female for the rest. Inconsistencies such as these can easily happen but will obviously cause problems when the data are analysed.

It is worth checking that the joining has worked as expected by checking that the total number of observations in the updated file is the sum of the two previous files, and that the total number of variables is unchanged. If there are some different variables in the two datasets to be appended, perhaps because data collection was revised part-way through, then it is also worth checking how this has been dealt with to make sure nothing has gone wrong.

Merging datasets: adding new variables

When **new data** are collected on the same individuals at a later stage (e.g. at a 1-year follow-up appointment), it may be necessary to merge datasets. In order to do this the unique subject identifier must be used to identify the records that must be matched. For the merge to work, all variable names in the two datasets must be different except for the unique identifier. For example if weight is recorded in each of the two datasets, one measured at time 1 and the other at time 2, the two variables must have different names, such as 'weight1' and 'weight2'. It is important to check how the merge has worked in terms of how many subjects have complete data and how many have data at one of the two points only.

As a further check, it may be useful to have another common variable that will not change over time in both datasets in addition to the study ID, such as the date of birth. This would need to be named, say DOB1 and DOB2 and then after the merge was done, a check could be made that DOB1=DOB2 for all individuals.

Master dataset

It is important to ensure that a unique copy of the current file, the 'master copy', is stored at all times. Where the study involves more than one investigator, everyone needs to know who has responsibility for this. It is also important to avoid having two people revising the same file at the same time.

Careful data management and good documentation are important when managing research study datasets, especially large ones, so that there is an audit trail of changes and additions that have been made.

❶ Using a spreadsheet to join datasets

Spreadsheets are useful for entering and storing data. However, care should be taken when cutting and pasting different datasets to avoid misalignment of data. For example, datasets can be merged within a spreadsheet by inserting the extra data in columns to the right of the existing data. However, this assumes that the two datasets have exactly the same number of subjects and that the two datasets have the same ordering of subjects. Similarly when **appending** by adding a new dataset as extra rows in a spreadsheet, the columns need to be in the same order in both original datasets. In addition, **sorting data in spreadsheets can go awry** if all cells are not highlighted and then only some cells are sorted, leading to mis-matched data and hence nonsense. 📖 Data checking examples, p. 118, shows an example of where spreadsheet manipulation went wrong.

Summary: joining datasets

- **Appending**: joining two datasets (or more) containing the same variables in different subjects
- **Merging**: joining two datasets containing the same subjects but different variables
- Check carefully that all data joining has worked as expected
- Keep all previous copies of datasets as back-up
- Keep a separate back-up of the current version in a different place from the main copy, e.g. on a portable storage device. Avoid keeping the main copy and the back-up together, such as in different files on the same machine, in case of loss or damage. Keep separate copies.
- Document names and the dates when data files were created
- Ensure only one person is working on the dataset at any one time
- Because joining or sorting datasets can quite easily and unknowingly go wrong, **it is best not to join or sort datasets using a spreadsheet**

Joining datasets: examples

Appending datasets (Fig. 3.2)

- Two datasets are joined
- Both have the **same four variables**, num, birthwt, gestation, headcirc but the two datasets each contain **five different cases** numbered 01–05 and 06–10
- The resulting dataset has four variables and 10 cases

num	birthwt	gestation	headcirc
01	1100	27.43	26.00
02	768	27.00	
03	1097	28.43	
04	1046	28.43	26.30
05	965	28.43	25.20

PLUS

num	birthwt	gestation	headcirc
06	990	26.29	
07	910	26.71	25.50
08	536	28.57	22.40
09	1050	28.71	25.50
10	740	27.29	27.00

GIVES

num	birthwt	gestation	headcirc
01	1100	27.43	26.00
02	768	27.00	
03	1097	28.43	
04	1046	28.43	26.30
05	965	28.43	25.20
06	990	26.29	
07	910	26.71	25.50
08	536	28.57	22.40
09	1050	28.71	25.50
10	740	27.29	27.00

Fig. 3.2 Appending datasets.

Merging datasets (Fig. 3.3)

- Two datasets are joined
- Both have the **same 10 cases**, numbered 01–10 but **different variables**: num, birthwt, gestation, headcirc num, headcirc2, weight2
  'num' is common to both datasets and is used for matching
- The datasets are joined side by side so that the cases, denoted by 'num', match
- The resulting dataset has six variables and 10 cases

num	birthwt	gestation	headcirc
01	1100	27.43	26.00
02	768	27.00	
03	1097	28.43	
04	1046	28.43	26.30
05	965	28.43	25.20
06	990	26.29	
07	910	26.71	25.50
08	536	28.57	22.40
09	1050	28.71	25.50
10	740	27.29	27.00

PLUS

num	headcirc2	weight2
01	47.1	11.70
02	48.1	11.03
03	49.0	15.84
04	50.0	13.82
05	48.0	13.11
06	48.0	14.00
07	47.2	11.40
08	47.5	9.16
09	48.0	12.96
10	48.0	10.70

GIVES

num	birthwt	gestation	headcirc	headcirc2	weight2
01	1100	27.43	26.00	47.1	11.70
02	768	27.00		48.1	11.03
03	1097	28.43		49.0	15.84
04	1046	28.43	26.30	50.0	13.82
05	965	28.43	25.20	48.0	13.11
06	990	26.29		48.0	14.00
07	910	26.71	25.50	47.2	11.40
08	536	28.57	22.40	47.5	9.16
09	1050	28.71	25.50	48.0	12.96
10	740	27.29	27.00	48.0	10.70

Fig. 3.3 Merging datasets.

Storing and transporting data

Introduction

The notes below summarize the key points to consider when storing and transporting data in paper and electronic forms.

Paper forms

- These should be file systematically to allow easy access at later date
- It is essential to ensure data are stored securely to comply with data protection requirements
- It may be appropriate to store identifying details such as names and addresses separately from the data forms to protect confidentiality, particularly when transporting data
- It is worth considering keeping a copy of forms in one location if they are being transported somewhere else in case they get damaged or lost
- If the forms or data are particularly valuable, then a copy should always be kept in a different place in case of damage or loss

Electronic files

- Identifying details such as names and addresses should always be removed when transporting electronic files by post (e.g. when mailing a CD), or when sending over a computer network
- Data files should be password protected and if possible encrypted when transporting by post, or over a computer network
- It is essential to keep more than one copy of the data in two separate locations in case of computer failure or loss. Back-ups may be created automatically, for example if an organization backs up all network files daily. It is therefore worth checking on the policy and practice in the institution where the data are stored
- It may be useful to use file names that show the version or date where files are updated during the course of a study, e.g. 'eczema data v1'

Data checking and errors

Data entry checks

If data have been manually entered, i.e. not using an automatic data capture program, then some checking for errors is needed.

- **Check early**: Where possible, it is important do some checks early on to leave time for addressing problems while the study is still in progress. Examples of problems that may be uncovered early and addressed include the following: one research assistant has illegible writing, or tends to miss out a particular question, or a particular data entry clerk makes a lot of mistakes and needs some further training. If checking is left till the end of the study, it may be too late to remedy these problems.

- **Check a random sample** of forms for data entry accuracy. If this reveals problems then further checking may be needed

- **Key variables**: If feasible, consider checking data entry forms for key variables, e.g. the primary outcome

- **Range checks**: Unless the data entry scheme has in-built range checks, tabulate all data to ensure there are no invalid values

- **Consistency**: A further check of accuracy is to make sure responses are consistent with each other within subjects, e.g. check for any impossible or unlikely combinations of responses such as a male with a pregnancy, or for outliers, such as one recording of blood pressure in a subject is very different from all of the others for the same subject

- **Original forms:** All original data forms should be kept. For studies involving patient data there may be specific requirements which determine how long the data should be kept. For example, in studies in children, data forms may need to be kept at least until the child has reached adult age, or longer if the study is ongoing. Any errors or queries identified will usually need to be checked back against the original form to identify the source of the error, i.e. data reporting or data entry.

- **Missing data**: Check where feasible that any gaps are true gaps and not missed data entry

- **Snowballing errors**: Sometimes finding one error may lead to others being uncovered. For example, if a spreadsheet was used for data entry and one entry was missed, all following entries may be in the wrong columns. Hence, always consider if the discovery of one error may imply that there are others.

- **Digit preference**: This is where a particular digit is more common than others and may indicate inaccurate reporting (e.g. people sometimes report to the nearest 10 below their true age). It may also suggest there has been mis-scanning for scanned handwritten forms. Digit preference may also simply reflect the accuracy of measurement such as blood pressure being recorded to the nearest 5 or 10 mmHg. Frequency tabulations will show if there is digit preference.

- **Scatter plots**: These can be used to identify values which are inconsistent within an individual, such as in a pregnancy study where it would be unexpected to have a pre-pregnant weight that was more than the full-term pregnancy weight. A scatter plot would show this individual as being far away from the rest of the subjects and further checks could be made to see if these values represent an error.

- **Statistical analysis**: Some data entry and/or data recording problems only come to light when the data are analysed so there may be a need to go back to the original forms later on

Correcting errors

- It is important to check the original form wherever possible to identify the source of any potential data error, such as, to determine if the error is due to a data entry error or an invalid value being recorded on the original form
- It is important not to make assumptions or guesses where data values look unusual or are missing, as this will introduce bias
- An outlying value should not be deleted simply because it is unusual. Where possible, similar data should be checked in the same individual to see if it is consistent. If a truly impossible value is found, it is important to try to locate the correct value. If this is not possible then set that value to 'missing'.
- It is important to keep a record of any changes that are made to the dataset and keep dated copies of datasets as changes are made, so that it is obvious which is the latest version. Don't overwrite datasets with edited versions as older versions may be needed later on.

Data checking: examples

Checking data using the frequency distribution

Table 3.2 Frequency distribution of the number of days a baby was ventilated ('DOV') in 78 babies

DOV	Freq.	Percent	Cum.
0	24	30.77	30.77
1	6	7.69	38.46
2	6	7.69	46.15
3	6	7.69	53.85
4	2	2.56	56.41
5	4	5.13	61.54
6	3	3.85	65.38
7	2	2.56	67.95
8	1	1.28	69.23
9	1	1.28	70.51
11	2	2.56	73.08
14	1	1.28	74.36
15	1	1.28	75.64
16	2	2.56	78.21
19	2	2.56	80.77
22	1	1.28	82.05
29	1	1.28	83.33
30	1	1.28	84.62
38	2	2.56	87.18
40	2	2.56	89.74
41	2	2.56	92.31
43	1	1.28	93.59
46	1	1.28	94.87
49	1	1.28	96.15
53	1	1.28	97.44
68	1	1.28	98.72
161	1	1.28	100.00
Total	78	100.00	

Table 3.2 shows that the highest value for 'DOV', **161** was much greater than the other values and was therefore checked to see if it was an error. It was found to be correct.

Checking for consistency

Table 3.3 shows a portion of data in a study measuring respiratory parameters at two time points in a group of babies: tidal volume (tv1 and tv2) and Hering–Breuer inflation reflex (hb1 and hb2). From looking at the data, it was clear that the values of tv2 and hb2 for baby number 2 (shaded) were markedly different to the same baby's values for tv1 and hb1, as well as being different to the values of tv2 and hb2 for the other babies in the study group. (Not all data are shown here.)

It emerged that two columns had been accidentally transposed to cause this error. This was easily corrected for statistical analysis.

Table 3.3 Part of a dataset from a study measuring respiratory parameters at two time points in infants

subject	tv1	hb1	tv2	hb2
1	5.86	68.94	4.85	186.54
1	5.04	27.98	5.80	75.08
1	6.09	8.22	4.64	132.56
1	6.08	76.36	4.70	60.85
1	4.37	367.56	4.78	84.09
2	7.45	68.00	62.20	7.53
2	8.78	103.27	42.43	6.01
2	9.73	58.84	89.87	5.13
2	7.66	51.76		
3	5.69	43.68	6.77	155.56
3	5.91	31.67	6.87	39.10
3	9.10	52.91	7.09	165.40
3	5.83	22.86	6.02	27.91
3	6.40	115.19	5.01	98.11
3	7.27	34.28	6.81	156.06
3	3.80	65.02		

Data checking: examples (continued)

Checking using a histogram

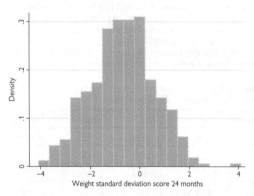

Fig. 3.4 Histogram of weight standard deviation score at 2 years in 374 infants.

Plots can be useful for checking larger datasets. Figure 3.4 shows the distribution of weight standard deviation score. The value at the very right-hand end of the distribution is some way from the rest of the distribution and is more than 4 standard deviations above the mean. This is very high and needed to be checked. It was found to be correct.

Checking using a scatter plot

Figure 3.5 illustrates how a scatter plot can also check for inconsistencies in variables that are related to each other. The data are weight standard deviation score and height standard deviation score (SDS) in infants and these would be expected to be closely correlated. The outlying value for weight SDS is clear as it is well away from the other points but as stated above, it was found to be correct.

This example illustrates the usefulness of using a scatter plot to check for outlying values but also provide a warning that some apparently outlying values are in fact correct.

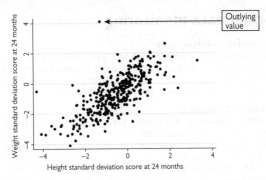

Fig. 3.5 Scatter plot of weight and height standard deviation score at 2 years in 374 infants.

Formal data monitoring

Randomized clinical trials

Studies testing new treatments in patients increasingly convene a formal data monitoring committee (DMC), which is independent of the trial steering group and has a specific remit relating to safety and adverse events, and the continuation or early stopping of the trial.

Function of the DMC

The DMC usually takes responsibility for the following items, as appropriate to the actual trial in question:

* Monitoring the safety of the treatment under trial in terms of minor and major adverse events
* Checking for any evidence of clear superiority or inferiority of the treatments
* Monitoring recruitment rates
* Monitoring the balance in key prognostic variables to check the integrity of the randomization process
* Monitoring adherence to trial protocol(s)
* Monitoring data collection and trial conduct
* Monitoring the data accrual
* Monitoring planned sample size calculations
* Assessing the importance of any new external evidence to the trial

The DMC normally reports directly to the trial steering group and can make recommendations regarding:

* Continuation of the trial in the light of observed adverse events
* Continuation of the trial if clear superiority or inferiority is demonstrated
* Continuation of the trial if a firm outcome is very unlikely given the data so far
* Issues relating to the data collection process or trial conduct in as much as it affects safety or the assessment of efficacy

Constitution of the DMC

The DMC usually comprises a small group of experts including at least one clinician with expertise in the specialty of the trial and at least one statistician. Typically a DMC will have two or three clinicians and a statistician, and one of these will be the chair of the group. The DMC meetings are attended by the trial statistician and, by agreement, also by the principal investigator.

Meetings

The DMC usually meets at the outset of the trial and then at pre-specified intervals during it, such as once a year for a lengthy trial. At the meetings the DMC discusses data provided by the trial statistician. Sometimes an analysis of the primary outcome is conducted at pre-determined points to see if there is any reason to stop the trial. There is debate as to whether interim trial data should be provided with the treatment allocation revealed or whether they are presented 'blind' as, for example, 'group A' and 'group B'. In some trials the DMC need to know which group is which to be able to determine the clinical importance of particular adverse events. In other settings the DMC may agree that it does not need to have unblinded data. In all cases, it is important that the trial team, including the principal investigator, remains blind to the allocations while the trial is in progress. The exception to this is the trial statistician who conducts the data analysis and may need to be unblinded. The UK *Health Technology Assessment* document gives a fuller discussion of the issues.[1]

DMC charter

It is helpful for the DMC to draw up a charter at the outset to set out its precise role and function and to specify how the DMC will operate. The DAMOCLES guidelines for DMCs[2] provide helpful guidance on these issues and a template for a charter.

Data quality issues

In monitoring the data collection and inspecting baseline and interim data, the DMC can highlight potential data quality problems such as the completeness of the data indicated by totals less than the maximum number of subjects.

For example, in a cancer therapy trial, the DMC noted missing data on lung function tests at baseline, which affected their ability to monitor adverse effects of treatment on the patients' lung functions after treatment.

Statistical analysis plan

The trial steering group in conjunction with the sponsor is responsible for designing the trial and therefore the statistical aspects, but the DMC will often review this document before the trial starts.

References

1 Grant AM, Altman DG, Babiker AB, Campbell MK, Clemens FJ, Darbyshire JH *et al.* Issues in data monitoring and interim analysis of trials. *Health Technol Assess* 2005; **9**(7):1-iv.
2 DAMOCLES Study group. A proposed charter for clinical trial data monitoring committees: helping them to do their job well. *Lancet* 2005; **365**(9460):711–22.

Statistical issues in data monitoring

Early stopping

The DMC may recommend that the trial is completely or partially stopped at an interim point for any of the following reasons:

- Either the treatment or control under investigation shows clear benefit for the primary outcome
- Safety concerns have been observed with one or more secondary outcomes
- There is only a small chance of the trial going on to show benefit (futility)
- There is evidence for clear harm in either one arm of the trial or in a sub-group
- There is external evidence that changes the original assumption of equipoise, i.e. no known preference, in treatment effectiveness

Stopping rules

There are several different approaches to determining if and when a trial should be stopped. The approaches are a mixture of a firm decision rule based on the data such as a P value, and judgement, such as a prior belief about the efficacy of the treatment being tested. The main approaches used can be summarized as follows:

- **Group sequential**: A limited number of interim analyses are done at pre-set times. For example Pocock's method uses the same cut-off for all interim analyses and the O'Brien–Fleming method uses a more conservative cut-off early in the trial which is less conservative as the trial continues
- **Continuous procedures**: These allow inspection of the data any time. Examples include the triangular test, the alpha spending approach and the repeated confidence interval method
- **Likelihood methods**: These are less formal approaches whereby the DMC will only recommend that the trial is stopped if there is both proof beyond reasonable doubt that one treatment is indicated for all or some patients, and the evidence is strong enough to be convincing to clinicians (Haybittle–Peto rule)
- **Bayesian approach**: This is an extension of the likelihood approach where the information is supplemented by including belief about the treatment effect from information external to the trial itself

There is general consensus that statistical techniques can only be used as a guide to the DMC, and that the whole context of the trial must contribute to the decision making.

Consequences of early stopping

Trials are only stopped early when it is considered that the evidence for either benefit or harm is overwhelmingly strong. In such cases, the effect size will inevitably be larger than anticipated at the outset of the trial in order to trigger the early stop.

Hence effect estimates from trials stopped early tend to be more extreme than would be the case if these trials had continued to the end, and so estimates of the efficacy or harm of a particular treatment may be exaggerated. This phenomenon has been demonstrated in recent reviews.[1,2] Work is ongoing to address these challenges, such as that by Pocock.[3]

Sample size

Sometimes it becomes apparent part way through a trial that the assumptions made in the original sample size calculations are not correct. For example, where the primary outcome is a continuous variable, an estimate of the standard deviation (SD) is needed to calculate the required sample size. When the data are summarized during the trial, it may become apparent that the observed SD is different from that expected. This has implications for the statistical power. If the observed SD is smaller than expected then it may be reasonable to reduce the sample size but if it is bigger then it may be necessary to increase it.

Alternatively, if recruitment is less than planned then the trial steering group may ask the DMC if it considers it acceptable to check the summary data (all groups together) to allow it to re-do the sample size calculations in the light of the observed data and thus determine if the projected recruitment will be sufficient.

Published guidance

The trial steering group will often seek the opinion of the DMC with these sorts of statistical issues to get an independent but informed view.

National documents with guidance for data monitoring committees have been published by Grant et al.[4] and the US Department of Health and Human Services.[5] A full review of statistical approaches to data monitoring with many useful references is given in Appendix I of the UK *Health Technology Assessment* document.[4]

References

1 Montori VM, Devereaux PJ, Adhikari NK, Burns KE, Eggert CH, Briel M et al. Randomized trials stopped early for benefit: a systematic review. *JAMA* 2005; **294**(17):2203–2209.

2 Bassler D, Montori VM, Briel M, Glasziou P, Guyatt G. Early stopping of randomized clinical trials for overt efficacy is problematic. *J Clin Epidemiol* 2008; **61**(3):241–246.

3 Pocock SJ. Current controversies in data monitoring for clinical trials. *Clin Trials* 2006; **3**(6): 513–521.

4 Grant AM, Altman DG, Babiker AB, Campbell MK, Clemens FJ, Darbyshire JH et al. Issues in data monitoring and interim analysis of trials. *Health Technol Assess* 2005; **9**(7):1-iv.

5 US Department of Health and Human Services. Guidance for clinical trial sponsors: establishment and operation of clinical trial data monitoring committees. 2006 Available from: ℘ www.fda.gov/downloads/RegulatoryInformation/Guidances/UCM127073.pdf (accessed 5 Jan 2009).

Presenting research findings

Introduction

The findings of research studies are usually disseminated beyond the research team. Research findings can be presented in a variety of written, graphical, or oral forms. It is vital that statistics are clearly and accurately presented to enable the reader to interpret correctly the research findings. In this chapter we discuss the different formats for disseminating research findings, the different sections of a research paper or report, and describe the best ways to present statistical results. Examples are given throughout.

Communicating statistics

Introduction

Research findings are usually communicated to people beyond the research team for several reasons:

- For interim or final review
- For comparison or amalgamation with other work
- For dissemination as new evidence

It is important that the statistical aspects are communicated clearly and accurately. There needs to be sufficient detail to convey the findings but not so much that the key results or issues become clouded. The main results presented should match the main aims of the research and/or answer the main question or questions posed. This is important even if the answer is negative or inconclusive, such as when a new treatment is not shown to be effective or no difference between two groups is observed.

Unplanned sub-group analyses should be clearly signposted as post-hoc to avoid over-emphasizing their value. This is important even if the sub-group results turn out to be more 'interesting' that those results relating to the primary aim.

Presenting study results

- The data presented and the interpretation should be directly related to the main research question
- The interpretation of the data should be methodologically sound and impartial
- The conclusions should accurately reflect the data presented

Formats for presenting

- Journal article (paper)
- Thesis or dissertation
- Report
- Conference abstract

The main features of the statistics included are similar for all types of presentation.

- Results
- Discussion

Characteristics of an article

Producing journal articles

Introduction

The most common method of disseminating research findings is through journal publications. Most original research projects will result in one or more journal 'publications'. Journal articles are usually quite short, but they are not necessarily quick or easy to write.

▶ It is important to understand the general format of an article and the specific statistical issues relating to each section. Although journals have their own specific requirements for how articles should be presented, the general structure is similar for most journals reporting health research. The main body of an article usually follows the IMRaD format (Introduction, Methods, Results and Discussion), and is accompanied by an abstract or summary.

Sections of an article

- **Abstract** – this is a brief summary of the whole article, usually around 250–300 words
- **Introduction** – this gives the background to the study, including information on previous research and why the current study has been conducted
- **Methods** – this describes how the study was carried out, including details of statistical techniques used
- **Results** – this presents the findings of the study, often including tables and/or graphs which display the results
- **Discussion** – this brings together the findings of the study and puts them in context with other research work, sometimes making suggestions for a change in practice or for further research

Statistics in articles

Statistics are included in every section of the paper, with each section requiring different information. A summary of which information to present in each section is given here. Each section is discussed in more detail on the following pages, with examples. Although geared towards journal articles, the general principles apply to the presentation of research findings in any format, such as reports, dissertations or theses.

Further details on presenting research findings can also be found in *Presenting medical statistics from proposal to publication* by Peacock and Kerry, which shows how to present statistics at all stages of a research study.[1] General guidance on writing journal articles can be found in *How to write a paper*, edited by Hall.[2]

Statistical items included in research articles

- **Introduction:**
  - The purpose of the study and hypothesis to be tested
- **Methods:**
  - The study design, including the choice and size of sample
  - The data collected, including any specific questionnaires or measurements
  - The statistical methods, including the statistical program used
- **Results:**
  - The results in a numerical format and, where relevant, also in graphs
- **Discussion:**
  - A commentary on the results highlighting key findings
  - The interpretation of the findings
  - A discussion of the findings in the light of:
    - The choice of sample (generalizability)
    - The sample size (statistical power, precision of estimates)
  - Any limitations, such as missing data

References

1 Peacock J, Kerry SM. *Presenting medical statistics from proposal to publication*. Oxford: Oxford University Press, 2006.
2 Hall GM. *How to write a paper*. 4th ed. Malden, MA: Blackwell. BMJ Books, 2008.

Research articles: abstracts

Abstracts may appear to be easy to write since they are very short documents, limited to perhaps 150, 250, or 500 words and often required to be written in a structured format. It is therefore perhaps surprising that they are sometimes poorly written, too bland, contain inaccuracies, and/or are simply misleading.[1] The reasons for poor quality abstracts are complex; abstracts are often written at the end of a long process of data collection, analysis, and writing up, when time is short and researchers are weary. Furthermore, statistical issues such as the over-emphasis of post-hoc analyses or sub-group analyses, can lead to an abstract that is not a fair representation of the research conducted.

▶ If it is summarizing a longer report or paper, then **it is important that the abstract is consistent with the body of text** and that it gives a balanced summary of the work. We live in an age where many readers will only have time to read the abstract, either because they are filtering a large body of research to identify what is relevant to them, or simply because they are short of time. Also, many journals provide only abstracts free of charge online. Hence **it is critical that abstracts are well-written, accurate and unbiased**. Sometimes, sub-group analyses are reported in abstracts as if they were the primary analysis. This is misleading, especially if the primary analysis is not reported. **To maximize its usefulness, a summary or abstract should include estimates and confidence intervals for the main findings and not simply present P values.**

Key points for presenting the statistics in abstracts
- Report the numbers of subjects and the location of the study where applicable
- Don't just give P values – give some descriptive data as well
- Give the main outcome with estimates and 95% confidence intervals where possible, whether the finding is statistically significant or not
- Make sure that the data presented in the abstract are consistent with the data in the body of the text
- Don't report unplanned sub-group analyses in the abstract
- Report conclusions that are consistent with the data presented
- Avoid bland conclusions that could be stated without the study being carried out, such as 'there may be a relationship between …'
- Be careful when making speculative statements in the abstract. If the results give rise to a new hypothesis, state this clearly.

Example of a structured abstract[2]

Reproduced from *BMJ*, Cuthbertson *et al*, **339**, b3723 © 2009 with permission from the BMJ Publishing Group Ltd.

Objectives: To test the hypothesis that nurse led follow-up programmes are effective and cost effective in improving quality of life after discharge from intensive care.

Design: A pragmatic, non-blinded, multicentre, randomised controlled trial.

Setting: Three UK hospitals (two teaching hospitals and one district general hospital).

Participants: 286 patients aged 18 years or more were recruited after discharge from intensive care between September 2006 and October 2007.

Intervention: Nurse led intensive care follow-up programmes versus standard care.

Main outcome measure(s): Health related quality of life (measured with the SF-36 questionnaire) at 12 months after randomisation. A cost effectiveness analysis was also performed.

Results: 286 patients were recruited and 192 completed one year follow-up. At 12 months, there was no evidence of a difference in the SF-36 physical component score (mean 42.0 (SD 10.6) v 40.8 (SD 11.9), effect size 1.1 (95% CI: −1.9 to 4.2), P=0.46) or the SF-36 mental component score (effect size: 0.4 (95% CI: −3.0 to 3.7), P=0.83). There were no statistically significant differences in secondary outcomes or subgroup analyses. Follow-up programmes were significantly more costly than standard care and are unlikely to be considered cost effective.

Conclusions: A nurse led intensive care follow-up programme showed no evidence of being effective or cost effective in improving patients' quality of life in the year after discharge from intensive care. Further work should focus on the roles of early physical rehabilitation, delirium, cognitive dysfunction, and relatives in recovery from critical illness. Intensive care units should review their follow-up programmes in light of these results.

Comment on abstract

This abstract includes the number of subjects recruited and followed up, the main outcome in each of the two groups and the difference with a 95% confidence interval and P value. These results agreed with those presented in the main body of the paper although the number followed up to 12 months was not explicitly stated in the paper.

References

1 Peacock PJ, Peters TJ, Peacock JL. How well do structured abstracts reflect the articles they summarize? *European Science Editing* 2009; **35**(1):3–5.

2 Cuthbertson BH, Rattray J, Campbell MK, Gager M, Roughton S, Smith A et al. The PRaCTICaL study of nurse led, intensive care follow-up programmes for improving long term outcomes from critical illness: a pragmatic randomised controlled trial. *BMJ* 2009; **339**:b3723.

Research articles: introduction and methods sections

Introduction section

The introduction section gives the background to the current study and often includes details of previous research work in the subject area. It is helpful to understand the statistical methods and findings of other research that is referred to, in order to describe previous work fairly and accurately. When citing other papers, it is advisable to obtain and read the paper referred to, rather than relying on second-hand reports as there is always a danger of 'Chinese whispers' leading to inaccurate reporting.

The extract below illustrates the reporting of findings from other studies within the introduction section.

Extract from the *Introduction* of a research paper[1]

'Department of Health (DH) statistics show that demand for emergency ambulance services has been increasing steeply in recent years. However, little has been published about factors linked to high service demand or about variations in demand across the country. Carlisle et al. found that the use of general practice and hospital accident and emergency services varied with deprivation, but their study did not examine ambulance services and only looked at one city, Nottingham. Wass and Zoltie reported that increased use of accident and emergency departments is disproportionately high among elderly patients.'

Methods section

The methods section should describe how the study was conducted. Ideally this should be in sufficient detail to enable another researcher to replicate the study, however, word limits on research papers often make this a difficult task. Nevertheless, it is important to include the following:
- The setting or area where the study was conducted
- The date(s) that the study sample was first obtained
- The subjects included in the study, including any exclusion criteria
  Note the 'subjects' are not always people, but may be an event such as an emergency ambulance call (see 📖 Example, p. 135)
- The study design (see 📖 Chapter 1, p. 1)
- Details of the measurements used
- The source of any non-original data
- The sample size, including a justification (📖 Sample size for comparative studies, p. 62)
- The statistical methods, including any computer software used

Presenting sample size calculations

Example 1: 'The target sample size of the study was 800 babies. Assuming power of 0.9 and two-sided significance level 0.05, this was sufficient to detect a difference of 11 percentage points in the primary outcome between treatment groups overall.'

Example 2: 'With a sample size of 100 infants a difference of 0.56 standard deviations in pulmonary function could be detected between the two groups, with 80% power and 5% (two-sided) significance level.'

Example of a Methods section in a research paper[2]

'All emergency 999 calls responded to by the London Ambulance Service (LAS) during the same week in 1989, 1996, and 1999 were studied (week 16: 24–30 April 1989, 29 April–5 May 1996, and 26 April–2 May 1999). This week was chosen as having a low probability of extreme weather conditions and to avoid school and public holidays, both of which may affect the nature and volume of 999 calls. Where there were multiple calls relating to the same response, only the first call was included. Data for 1989 had to be manually extracted from microfiche copies of the original individual records and entered onto a database. Data for 1996 and 1999 were already held in electronic form, having been taken from routine data forms (LA4s) by the LAS Management Information department. The following data were retrieved for each call: time and date, patient age, and patient sex.

Virtually all calls were made for a single patient, allowing us to calculate call rates using the resident population for Greater London. A very small proportion of calls (1989: n = 2 (0.03%); 1996: n = 62 (0.6%); 1999: n = 73 (0.6%)) were for more than one patient. In this case only details of the first patient were available. The changes in call responses over time were calculated as rate ratios with corresponding 95% confidence intervals. The earliest year, 1989, was used as the baseline so that changes in 1996 and 1999 were each compared with 1989. For a small percentage of calls (8% in 1989; 4% in 1996; 7% in 1999), the ambulance crew had been unable to obtain the patient's age and so simply provided a category—baby, child, adult, elderly. Where this occurred we estimated the age to fit the age distribution of the original data. This allowed us to maximise the use of the data available.

Trends in proportions of call responses from 1989 to 1999 were investigated using the χ^2 test for trend. The relations between call rates and the age/sex profile of the patient were analysed using negative binomial regression. All analyses were performed using Stata version 7.

References

1 Hall GM. *How to write a paper*. 4th ed. Malden, MA: Blackwell. BMJ Books, 2008.
2 Peacock PJ, Peacock JL. Emergency call work-load, deprivation and population density: an investigation into ambulance services across England. *J Public Health (Oxf)* 2006; **28**(2):111–15.

Research articles: results section

The results section gives the findings of the research study and is usually the section of the paper which includes the most statistical information. This section should include the following:

- **Details of the study population**: including numbers of subjects who did not complete the study, or who were excluded from the analysis for any reason. Flowcharts are a useful way of presenting these data (see Fig. 4.1)
- **Baseline characteristics for the study population**: if there are two or more groups, as in a randomized trial, then baseline data should be presented for each group
- **Main results from statistical analyses**: these are often best presented in tables and graphs (📖 Presenting statistics: tables and graphs, p. 146), with main findings presented in the text. See also 📖 Presenting statistics: managing computer output, p. 140, and Presenting statistics: P values and confidence intervals, p. 144, for how to present numerical data

❶ Space limitations for medical journals can sometimes make it difficult to include all the statistical information that we would ideally like to. More recently, online publishing has enabled additional information to be made available on journal websites, to supplement the data in the printed journal version.

Examples

Example 1: 'The 20 studies reviewed were all two-parallel-group randomized trials, two of which were equivalence trials. Of the 18 superiority trials, six (33%) reported evidence for a difference between groups in the primary outcome. Nineteen papers were first reports of trials and one was a follow-up.'
- This is an extract describing the study population from a study investigating the quality of abstracts in journal articles.[1] Note in this example the 'subjects' are not patients but journal articles

Example 2: 'Between September 2005 and October 2007, we randomly assigned 391 couples to immobilisation in a supine position for 15 minutes (199 couples; intervention group) or immediate mobilisation (192 couples; control group). The baseline characteristics were comparable in the two groups'.

Reproduced from *BMJ*, Custers *et al*, **339**, b4080 © 2009 with permission from the BMJ Publishing Group Ltd.
- This extract describes the study population from a randomized trial. In this study, further details about the baseline characteristics for the two groups were provided online on the journal's website[2]

Figure 4.1 shows a flowchart from a study which shows the numbers randomized to each group and the numbers with follow-up data.

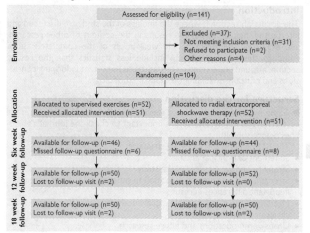

Fig. 4.1 Example of flowchart showing the time-flow of patients recruited, randomized, and followed-up[3].

Reproduced from *BMJ*, Engebretsen *et al.* **339**, b3360 © 2009 with permission from the BMJ Publishing Group Ltd.

References

1 Peacock PJ, Peters TJ, Peacock JL. How well do structured abstracts reflect the articles they summarize? *European Science Editing* 2009; **35**(1):3–5.
2 Custers IM, Flierman PA, Maas P, Cox T, Van Dessel TJHM, Gerards MH *et al.* Immobilisation versus immediate mobilisation after intrauterine insemination: randomised controlled trial. *BMJ* 2009; **339**:b4080.
3 Engebretsen K, Grotle M, Bautz-Holter E, Sandvik L, Juel NG, Ekeberg OM *et al.* Radial extracorporeal shockwave treatment compared with supervised exercises in patients with subacromial pain syndrome: single blind randomised study. *BMJ* 2009; **339**:b3360.

Research articles: discussion section

Introduction

The discussion section is where the findings of the study are discussed and interpreted, helping to put the results in the context of other research, and evaluating the strengths and weaknesses of the completed study. Although this section tends to include less statistics than the results section, a sound understanding of statistics is important in forming conclusions and critically evaluating the study methodology.

Structure for the discussion

▶ Some medical journals have a specific structure for the discussion for researchers to follow, and so it is important to check the journal's guidelines before submitting.

The *BMJ* requires the following structure:
- Statement of principal findings
- Strengths and weaknesses of the study
- Strengths and weaknesses in relation to other studies, discussing important differences in results
- Meaning of the study: possible explanations and implications for clinicians and policymakers
- Unanswered questions and future research
  (✍ http://resources.bmj.com/bmj/authors/types-of-article/research)

Statistics in the discussion section

The examples below illustrate the inclusion and interpretation of statistics within the discussion section of papers.

Example 1: 'Our data extend findings from previous studies of the relationship between early identification of hearing impairment and later outcomes. Adjusted mean vocabulary scores of children with hearing impairment, assessed at the age of 5 years, were higher in children enrolled before 11 months of age in an early intervention program in Nebraska than in those enrolled at 11 to 23 months of age (by 0.69 SD) or at 24 to 35 months of age (by 0.99 SD).'[1]

- In this extract statistical information is presented to contrast study findings from previous work

Example 2: 'Our results confirm that the risk in users of combined oral contraceptives depends on the dose of oestrogen, type of progestogen, and length of use. Reducing the dose of oestrogen from 50 μg to 30–40 μg non-significantly reduced the risk of venous thromboembolism by 17–32%. Reducing the dose from 30–40 μg to 20 μg in users of oral contraceptives containing desogestrel or gestodene significantly reduced the risk of venous thromboembolism by 18% (95% confidence interval 7% to 27%), after adjustment for duration of use of oral contraceptives. Without this adjustment the association was confounded and not significant. Together with the lack of power this may explain why few studies have been able to show this dose-response relation. The dose-response relation between oral contraceptive use and venous thromboembolism strengthens the evidence that the statistical associations reflect a causal relation.'[2]

Reproduced from *BMJ*, Lidegaard *et al*, **339**, b2890 © 2009 with permission from the BMJ Publishing Group Ltd.

- In this extract the authors show that, after controlling statistically for the confounding effect of duration of pill use, reducing the dose in users of oral contraceptives was associated with a significantly lower risk of venous thromboembolism

References

1 Kennedy CR, McCann DC, Campbell MJ, Law CM, Mullee M, Petrou S et al. Language ability after early detection of permanent childhood hearing impairment. *N Engl J Med* 2006; **354**(20):2131–41.

2 Lidegaard O, Lokkegaard E, Svendsen AL, Agger C. Hormonal contraception and risk of venous thromboembolism: national follow-up study. *BMJ* 2009; **339**:b2890.

Presenting statistics: managing computer output

Computer output

It is common practice to use a computer program to perform statistical analyses. These often produce more results than are needed and so the relevant results need to be extracted and put into a new document in a new format for presentation. Even if the computer only gives the relevant results, these may not be suitable for presentation because they are usually given to too many decimal places.

Reporting statistical analyses

The following points are particularly important in reporting statistical analyses from statistical programs:

- Don't put unedited computer output into a research document
- Extract the relevant data only and re-format as needed
- Ensure that the data presented are relevant and appropriate for the given context
- Double-check the numbers after they have been extracted to make sure they are correct

SPSS and Stata

Peacock and Kerry's book *Presenting medical statistics from proposal to publication*[1] shows how to carry out many statistical analyses using the statistical programs **SPSS and Stata**, and also shows which parts of the output are relevant in particular situations and how these extracts can be turned into tables and text suitable for a paper or report.

The data in the example on 📖 p. 141 are from a study comparing fruit and vegetable consumption in smokers and non-smokers. The researchers used a Mann Whitney U test (equivalent to the 📖 Wilcoxon two-sample signed rank test, p. 303) to analyse the data using SPSS. The computer output from a statistical test is shown with an arrow indicating the P value that can be reported. The text below the computer output illustrates how the results could be reported in a paper.

Many more examples for both SPSS and Stata are given in *Presenting medical statistics*, and each example also gives the commands needed to perform the particular analysis in the statistical program. More details about statistical programs in general are given in 📖 Chapter 5, p. 155.

Example of SPSS output indicating the relevant statistics to report for a Mann Whitney U test[1]

SPSS output

Ranks

	smokeas	N	Mean Rank	Sum of Ranks
frandveg	0	180	146.34	26342.00
	1	91	115.54	10514.00
	Total	271		

Test statistics (a)

	frandveg	
Mann-Whitney U	6328.000	
Wilcoxon W	10514.000	P value
Z	-3.089	
Asymp. Sig. (2-tailed)	.002	

a Grouping Variable: smokeas

Notes on the variables
- *smokeas* Is the variable defining smoking habit as smoker yes(1) or no (0)
- *frandveg* is the number of portions of fruit and vegetables consumed each day

Presenting the results
Methods section
The fruit and vegetable scores from smokers and non-smokers were compared using a Mann-Whitney U test. The data are presented as medians and interquartile range (IQR).

Results section
The median (IQR) number of portions of fruit and vegetable eaten per day at baseline among smokers was 3 (2, 4) and 3.75 (2, 5) among non-smokers. Smokers reported significantly lower consumption than non-smokers (P=0.002).

Reference
1 Peacock J, Kerry SM. *Presenting medical statistics from proposal to publication*. Oxford: Oxford University Press, 2006.

Presenting statistics: numerical results

Rounding

Computers usually give results to many decimal places and these should be rounded for presentation to make them easier to read and to avoid implying a falsely high level of precision. The following suggestions make numbers **easy to read and absorb** but also **include all relevant information**.

- Present means, standard deviations, and standard errors to one more decimal place than the individual data values
- Give proportions to two significant figures. State the actual number as well unless it is obvious.
- Present a proportion as a percentage if the proportion is small. Very small proportions may be easier to read if given as rates per 1000 or per 10 000, etc.
- Present percentages as two significant figures but give the actual numbers as well, unless they are obvious
- ❶ Beware of presenting percentages for very small samples as they may be misleading. Simply give the numbers alone.

Examples: means and standard deviations

Mean and standard deviation (SD) for blood pressure (systolic/diastolic) in 1753 pregnant women was given by a statistical program as:

Systolic: mean=112.0553, SD=11.17655
Diastolic: mean=67.3725, SD=8.088683

These can be rounded and reported as:

Systolic: mean (SD)= 112.1 (11.2)
Diastolic: mean (SD)= 67.4 (8.1)

Examples: proportions and percentages

i) Proportion of smokers in a sample is 484/1503 = 0.3220226
This can be reported as a percentage with the numbers in brackets:
Percentage of smokers = 32% (484/1503)

ii) Proportion of stillbirths in England and Wales 2004

= 3532/643253
= 0.0054908

Such proportions are usually reported as rates per 1000 total births:
= 5.49 per 1000 (easier to understand than 0.549%, especially when comparing several figures, e.g. for different years)

Presenting statistics: P values and confidence intervals

P values

It is not always obvious how to present P values obtained from significance tests. Statistical programs give P values to many decimal places and these are not needed for reporting. The P value is sometimes reduced to a yes/no, binary response of not significant versus statistically significant, which may be adequate if the estimate and a 95% confidence interval is also given, but in general it does not provide sufficient information. For example if two P values are close to the 0.05 boundary, one just above and one just below (e.g. 0.04 and 0.06), the interpretation of the two should not be very different. If we reduce these P values to a binary response and say that one is significant and the other is not, without qualifying that statement, we risk misrepresenting the evidence provided by the tests.

Another common practice is to give the actual P value if the test is statistically significant (i.e. if P<0.05) but to simply report the test as 'not significant' or as 'NS' if it is not significant (i.e. if P≥0.05). This again is not helpful as the *size* of the P value indicates the amount of evidence for a real difference or real effect and presenting it as it is gives the reader the opportunity to see all of this evidence, whether it is significant or not.

P values are probabilities, presented as proportions, and so it is unnecessary to report many decimal places as this obscures the meaning. It is common to see statistical significance reported as stars: * for P<0.05, ** for P<0.01, and *** for P<0.001. Stars are not needed if the actual P values are given, but they can be useful if space is limited, for example in a large table, and where confidence intervals are given as well, or in an oral presentation.

In general the following is recommended for P values:
- Give the actual P value wherever possible
- Rounding: two significant figures is usually enough

Confidence intervals

These should be given wherever possible to indicate the precision of estimates.
- Report the interval to one more decimal place than the original data as for means, standard deviations, standard errors
- Report the limits as 'x, y' or 'x to y' rather than 'x–y' or 'x–y', as a hyphen or 'n dash' could be mistaken for a minus sign

Examples: P values

The following are P values as given by a statistics program. They can be rounded and reported as shown:

0.8113 → 0.81
0.1666 → 0.17
0.0952 → 0.10
0.0402 → 0.040
0.0133 → 0.013

0.0000 → report as P<0.0001 (as P can never truly equal 0)
1.0000 → report as P>0.999 (as P can never truly equal 1)

Examples: confidence intervals

The following examples show estimates and confidence intervals for different estimates:
• Prevalence (95% CI):   0.80 (0.78 to 0.82) or 80% (78% to 82%)
• Mean difference (95% CI):   0.36 (−0.40 to 1.12)
• Odds ratio (95% CI):   1.52 (1.01 to 2.28)
• Correlation (95% CI):   0.68 (0.52 to 0.79)

(❶ Reporting the mean difference (95% CI) as 0.36 (−0.40–1.12) would be confusing to read, hence it is better to 'to' or a comma)

Presenting statistics: tables and graphs

Introduction
Tables and graphs are a useful way of presenting the results of statistical analyses. When used in written reports, a table or graph should stand alone so that a reader does not need to read the text of the report or article to be able to understand it.

General guidelines
• Give a meaningful title that explains what data are included
• State the number of subjects or data points
• Label the rows and columns (tables) or axes (graphs) clearly
• State any units used, e.g. systolic blood pressure (mmHg)
• Refer to the table or graph in the text of written reports

Example of table from research article

Table 4.1 Risk and relative risk of hospital admission before age 2 in 540 infants who were born extremely preterm by randomized mode of ventilation at birth: HFOV (high frequency oscillating ventilation), CV (conventional ventilation)[1]

Outcome	HFOV	CV	Relative risk* (95% CI)[†]
Respiratory admission ever	118/276 (43%)	112/264 (42%)	1.01 (0.83 to 1.23)
Respiratory admission	24/157 (15%)	27/179 (15%)	1.01 (0.61 to 1.68)
Surgical admission ever	59/276 (21%)	59/264 (22%)	0.96 (0.70 to 1.32)
ICU admission ever	23/276 (8%)	25/264 (9%)	0.88 (0.51 to 1.51)

* Relative risk is the ratio of the risk of admission ever in the two groups, HFOV/CV.
[†] 95% confidence interval.

• Table 4.1 has a clear title, numbers, and percentages are given, and relative risks are given with 95% confidence intervals
• A footnote explains which way round the relative risk was calculated

Common errors

❶ Avoid graphs with missing zeros or stretched scales, which can exaggerate relationships (see Fig. 4.2).

Example of stretching the scale

Figure 4.2 shows data on stillbirth rates that increased from 1985 to 1990. By stretching the scale (second graph), the effect looks more dramatic.

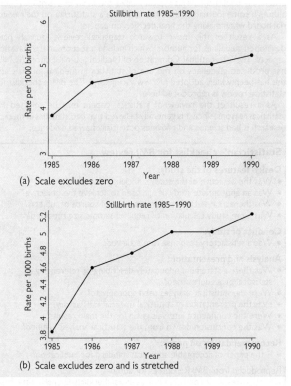

Fig. 4.2a,b Stillbirth trends over time presented with two different scales, causing the observed increase over time to look greater in the second graph.

References

1 Marlow N, Greenough A, Peacock JL, Marston L, Limb ES, Johnson AH et al. Randomised trial of high frequency oscillatory ventilation or conventional ventilation in babies of gestational age 28 weeks or less: respiratory and neurological outcomes at 2 years. Arch Dis Child Fetal Neonatal Ed 2006; **91**(5):F320-6.

Statistics and the publication process

Introduction

Many journals in medicine and health research now include statistical review as part of the peer-review process in response to the increased use of statistics in these disciplines. Statistical review usually takes place at the end of the review process when a paper has been identified as potentially publishable. This typically takes the form of a written report, although some journals such as the *BMJ* have a statistician on their editorial board when making the final decision on papers.

As a result of this move towards statistical review, journals have developed guidelines for authors, which include a section on the statistical aspects. The International Committee of Medical Journal Editors (ICMJE) has produced guidelines on the use of statistics in medical journals and this has been widely adopted (✆ www.icmje.org). The *BMJ*'s checklist for statistical review is reproduced here.

As a result of the review of statistics, papers may be rejected for statistical reasons, since it is generally believed that bad statistics in medical research is bad science and provides potentially flawed evidence.

Statistician's checklist for *BMJ* review

Design features of the study:
- Was the objective of the study sufficiently described?
- Was an appropriate study design used to achieve the objective?
- Was there a satisfactory statement given of source of subjects?
- Was a pre-study calculation of required sample size reported?

Conduct of study:
- Was a satisfactory response rate achieved?

Analysis and presentation:
- Was there a statement adequately describing or referencing all statistical procedures used?
- Were the statistical analyses used appropriate?
- Was the presentation of statistical material satisfactory?
- Were the confidence intervals given for the main results?
- Was the conclusion drawn from the statistical analysis justified?

Recommendation on paper:
- Is the paper of acceptable statistical standard for publication?

Reproduced from *BMJ* Resources for authors
(✆ http://resources.bmj.com/bmj/authors/checklists-forms/statisticians-checklist).

Reporting guidelines for specific studies

There are now reporting guidelines for several types of study, and these give helpful guidance about presenting the statistics. These are discussed in more detail in the section 📖 Research articles: guidelines, p. 150).

Research articles: guidelines

Introduction

The CONSORT (**Con**solidated **S**tandards **of R**eporting **T**rials) group was established in 1993 to try to improve the quality of reporting of clinical trials. The group produced the CONSORT statement, which is a checklist of items to include in articles reporting the outcome of randomized controlled trials (RCTs). The CONSORT statement is reproduced below. In recent years more guidelines have been developed for other study designs. Some of these are listed in the next section, 📖 Research articles: guidelines (continued), p. 152, with web addresses for further information. Many medical journals now require authors to confirm prior to submission that their article complies with the appropriate guideline.

CONSORT guidelines for reporting trials

Title and abstract:
- How participants were allocated to interventions (e.g., 'random allocation', 'randomized', or 'randomly assigned')

Introduction:
- Scientific background and explanation of rationale

Methods:
- Eligibility criteria for participants and the settings and locations where the data were collected
- Precise details of the interventions intended for each group and how and when they were actually administered
- Specific objectives and hypotheses
- Clearly defined primary and secondary outcome measures and, when applicable, any methods used to enhance the quality of measurements (e.g., multiple observations, training of assessors)
- How sample size was determined and, when applicable, explanation of any interim analyses and stopping rules
- Method used to generate the random allocation sequence, including details of any restrictions (e.g., blocking, stratification)
- Method used to implement the random allocation sequence (e.g., numbered containers or central telephone), clarifying whether the sequence was concealed until interventions were assigned
- Who generated the allocation sequence, who enrolled participants, and who assigned participants to their groups
- Whether or not participants, those administering the interventions, and those assessing the outcomes were blinded to group assignment. If done, how the success of blinding was evaluated
- Statistical methods used to compare groups for primary outcome(s); methods for additional analyses, such as subgroup analyses and adjusted analyses

Results:

- Flow of participants through each stage (a diagram is strongly recommended). Specifically, for each group report the numbers of participants randomly assigned, receiving intended treatment, completing the study protocol, and analyzed for the primary outcome. Describe protocol deviations from study as planned, together with reasons
- Dates defining the periods of recruitment and follow-up
- Baseline demographic and clinical characteristics of each group
- Number of participants (denominator) in each group included in each analysis and whether the analysis was by 'intention-to-treat'. State the results in absolute numbers when feasible (e.g., 10/20, not 50%)
- For each primary and secondary outcome, a summary of results for each group, and the estimated effect size and its precision (e.g., 95% confidence interval)
- Address multiplicity by reporting any other analyses performed, including subgroup analyses and adjusted analyses, indicating those pre-specified and those exploratory
- All important adverse events or side effects in each intervention group

Discussion:

- Interpretation of the results, taking into account study hypotheses, sources of potential bias or imprecision and the dangers associated with multiplicity of analyses and outcomes
- Generalizability (external validity) of the trial findings
- General interpretation of the results in the context of current evidence

Reproduced from Moher *et al.* 2001 ©; licensee BioMed Central Ltd. ♒ www.biomedcentral.com/1471-2288/1/2.

See also ♒ www.consort-statement.org.

Postscript

As this book is going to press, CONSORT have produced updated guidelines – see ♒ www.consort-statement.org for the most up-to date guidelines.

Research articles: guidelines (continued)

Equator network

The Equator network (Enhancing the QUAlity and Transparency Of health Research) is 'an international initiative that seeks to enhance reliability and value of medical research literature by promoting transparent and accurate reporting of research studies.' (🕮 www.equator-network.org)

The Network brings together a wide range of resources relating to health research. Up-to-date lists and links can be found on the website, and some of those available at the time of writing are as follows:

TREND: non-randomized controlled trials
🕮 www.trend-statement.org
STARD: studies of diagnostic accuracy
🕮 www.stard-statement.org
PRISMA: systematic reviews and meta-analyses (replaces QUOROM)
🕮 www.prisma-statement.org/
STROBE: observational studies in epidemiology
🕮 www.strobe-statement.org
MOOSE: meta-analyses of observational studies in epidemiology
🕮 www.consort-statement.org/mod_product/uploads/MOOSE%20
Statement%202000.pdf

Statistical problems in medical papers

Common causes for rejection

Statistical review is wider in scope than might perhaps be expected. A statistician will look for omissions and/or errors in design, analysis, presentation, and interpretation since any of these might invalidate the results (📖 see Statistics and the publication process, p. 148 for the *BMJ* guidelines). Common statistical reasons for rejecting a paper include the following:

- The study is too small to be able to show a difference or a relationship
- The sample is unrepresentative, perhaps due to a low response rate
- There is bias in the assessment or measurement
- There is bias in comparisons
- A non-significant result has been wrongly interpreted as if it meant 'there is no difference'
- No estimates of sizes of the effects and/or confidence intervals are given
- There are unplanned sub-group analyses ('data dredging')
- There are problems with the statistical analysis method(s) used
- An observed association has been interpreted as if it were causal (not considering potential confounding factors)
- The conclusions are not supported by the evidence provided
- There is poor presentation that obscures the important findings

Responding to statistical comments on a paper

A reviewer may raise questions about the statistics for any or several of the reasons given in the list above. In responding it is worth considering whether the statistics are in fact correct but insufficient detail or data have been given to make that clear. Alternatively, it may be that the methods used are not appropriate and that the analysis needs to be repeated using a more suitable method.

If uncertain about statistical comments on a paper, it is worth talking to a statistician, who might be able to provide advice on how to respond.

Choosing and using statistical software for analysing data

Introduction

In this chapter we will describe the main features of statistics packages, what they do, and what they do not do. We will describe how we as users interact with packages, how we transfer data between packages, and how to decide which package to use. There are many statistical analysis computer packages and programs on the market and this chapter will not provide a review of what is available. Instead we will discuss the main issues that drive the choice of package to use. To illustrate, we will briefly describe a few packages that we know well.

Statistical software packages

What is a statistical package?

A statistical analysis package is a suite of computer programs that can be used to carry out manipulations of data and perform statistical analyses. Most of them have a user-friendly interface and do not require the user to be an expert in statistical programming. Many statistical packages are produced by commercial companies and can be purchased from suppliers or bought online. There are increasing numbers of programs and packages available free on the Internet, although the onus is on the user to check that they come from a reputable source, as they may not have been checked to the same extent as commercial programs.

What do statistical packages do?

In general a statistical package can facilitate one or more of the following:
- Data entry
- Data management
- Data analysis
- Data presentation, such as producing graphics

Some large packages, such as SAS,[1] do all of these.

There is an increasing number of statistical packages designed specifically for certain specialized topics and analyses, such as PASS[2] and nQuery Advisor,[3] which are used only for calculating the required sample size for a study.

How packages work

Most statistical packages in common use among medical researchers are either menu-driven or command-driven.

Menu-driven packages provide options for the user to select, in menus that are usually hierarchical in design. This has the advantage that the user does not have to remember commands or computer syntax. However, menu-driven programs can be slow if there are no shortcuts through the menu system and it may be difficult to find the right menu and/or set of options to be able to carry out a particular analysis.

Command-driven packages work by the user entering a particular command, which will execute the required process or statistical method. This method is usually quicker than using menus, but it does require the user to remember and enter the actual commands. If the syntax is entered incorrectly, for example with a typo, the command will not run. With command-driven programs, or where a menu-driven program produces a copy of the commands as a **syntax file**, an analysis can be set up once and then used for repeated implementation if you need to do the same set of analyses several times.

Active and batch mode

Packages for use on personal computers mostly run immediately and work in active 'online' mode. That is, the results come back immediately after each command is entered or menu selected. Some larger computations are run 'off-line'; that is, a set of commands is submitted together and the results for all of them are returned at some future point. Packages used over networks may run online or off-line.

Operating systems

Statistical packages run under a variety of operating systems, such as Microsoft Windows or Apple Mac for personal computers, Unix, Linux, or BSD for networks. The major commercial packages tend to have versions available for several operating systems, whereas smaller packages tend to be less flexible and some free software only runs under Windows.

Costs

Some statistical packages run under a licensing arrangement whereas others are sold with perpetual licences. For most commercial packages, updated versions are regularly supplied by the vendor to allow new statistical procedures to be incorporated or existing procedures to be extended. These are usually cheaper for existing customers. Some software is available on an institutional licence. Prices for individual and licence copies may be a little less for academic institutions than commercial institutions, and greater discounts may be available for students. An increasing number of statistical packages can be bought on the Internet and some allow you to download the full version and try it out for free for a few days.

Scope of packages

The scope varies hugely, with some packages providing a very wide range of utilities. Some, such as SPSS,[4] are sold as a basic package with a number of specialized add-ons. Other packages, such as Stata,[5] have user-written procedures that are available free online to licence holders. Stata also has several different versions which are priced according to the size of the dataset that the package will analyse.

References

1 SAS: Statistical Analysis System. Available from: ℘ www.sas.com
2 PASS: Power analysis and sample size software. Available from: ℘ www.ncss.com
3 nQuery Advisor: Sample size and power calculations. Available from: ℘ www.statsol.ie
4 SPSS: Statistical Package for the Social Sciences. IBM SPSS. Available from: ℘ www.spss.com
5 Stata: Data analysis and statistical software. Available from: ℘ www.stata.com.

Choosing a package

Introduction

There are a number of things to consider when choosing a statistical package. These are outlined below:

- **Cost:**
  Do you have the resources to buy a package? What is your budget? Are you looking for a free package?

- **Support:**
  Do you need technical support? Do you have colleagues who already use a particular package and can provide support? Do the authors or marketers of the package provide support if you encounter problems when using it?

- **Your institution:**
  If you belong to an institution, does it support any particular packages? Does it have any site licences or purchasing agreements?

- **Usability:**
  How user-friendly do you want the package to be? Do you want a menu-driven package or a command-driven one? Do you want to be able to write your own programs within the package to do specific analyses?

- **Data management:**
  Do you want the package to manage data, for example merging, appending, sub-setting datasets, etc., or do you simply want to analyse the data in the package?

- **Type of analyses:**
  Do you only want to be able to perform simple analyses, or both simple descriptive analyses and complex analyses? Do you need confidence intervals? (Some packages routinely give confidence intervals for estimates whereas others do not).

- **Specialized methods:**
  Do you need to use any specialized methods, such as weighted survey analyses or meta-analyses? (These may require a separate package or a separate add-on to an existing package).

- **Graphics:**
  Do you want to produce high quality graphics? (Many packages produce good graphics but only a few claim to produce state-of-the-art graphs).

- **Size of datasets:**
  Do you need to process very big datasets with either a large number of cases or a large number of variables or both? (Packages tend to have an upper limit for the amount of data that they can process. This may depend on the package or on the computer used, or both. Some packages sell different versions, which can process different amounts of data with the larger versions costing more).

- **Transferring between packages:**
  Do you need to be able to transfer data files between packages? Is this easy to do?

- **Testing:**
  Have you tested the package or seen it being used? Are you confident it will do what you want it to do?
- **Operating system:**
  Are you using this on a personal computer or a network? Which operating system will you be using?
- **Licence versus perpetual copy:**
  Do you want a perpetual licence or will a time-limited licence meet your needs?
- **Upgrades:**
  If you are using more complex statistical methods, will you want a package that receives regular upgrades?
- **Discounted versions:**
  Does the package offer any discounts that you can take advantage of, such as a reduced rate for full-time students, or a reduced rate for academic institutions?

Using a package

Introduction

Statistical packages are wonderful tools that enable us to perform complex calculations easily. They facilitate statistical analyses that would previously have been impossible to do by hand or with a calculator, and for which the details may be technically challenging.

There is, however, a real danger of inadvertently conducting inappropriate analyses, since these packages make it possible to use statistical methods we may not fully understand. It is also very easy to 'surf' a statistical package and a dataset in the same way as we might surf the Internet, and end up using many tests and methods which may or may not be sensible. This can result in a vast set of results that have no logical thread and are impenetrable. Many of us have succumbed to this danger at times since the computer is so intoxicating.

For these reasons some general advice on using statistical packages follows, which will help avoid these pitfalls and improve the quality of your statistical analyses.

Plan the analysis

It is always good statistical practice to plan the analysis beforehand. This applies globally to a whole project and also to individual analyses within a project. Planning helps to keep us on track and avoid unnecessary analyses or data dredging that can lead us to make wrong inferences. It is also important to check that the statistical analyses planned are appropriate, that any distributional assumptions are met and the analyses answer the questions that are intended. The statistical package may still perform analyses which are invalid because the sample size, or distributional model, or design assumptions do not hold. Hence we need to be careful.

Keep a log of the analysis

When performing a statistical analysis, it is important to keep a record of the following:

- The date of the analysis
- The dataset that has been used with filename, where it is stored and the date of this version
- The commands or set of commands used to do the analyses and get the results
- The results as given by the package
- Any editing of the data that has taken place

Most statistics packages will have an option to record a log file of the routines carried out and results produced, even in menu-driven software such as SPSS.

Extracting the relevant results

Many packages produce lots of output, some of which is relevant for a given situation and some of which is not. It is necessary to know what is appropriate so that we can present the results later in a concise format. It is best not to simply cut and paste results from a statistical package and present this to colleagues, particularly in a formal document. The relevant results from the computer need to be extracted and put into a new format to highlight the key findings. It is particularly important to report the numbers of observations included in each analysis. Peacock and Kerry[1] give many examples of how to do this in two commonly used statistical packages, SPSS and Stata.

Missing data

All research has some degree of missing data and it is important to be aware of how the package handles it. For example, missing data are sometimes denoted by a blank cell or a dot (.) in a data spreadsheet (💷 Form filling and coding, p. 78). Different statistical methods have specific ways of dealing with missing data and it is important to be aware of this. For example, multiple regression usually requires data to be present on all variables included in an analysis and so the number of subjects included in a multiple regression analysis may be much less than the total sample size if many subjects have one or more missing values for some variables. Also different multiple regression analyses may have different patterns of missing data and so may be based on different sets of individuals (💷 Missing data, p. 402).

Graphics

Nowadays packages tend to be quite flexible in how they allow graphs to be exported to other applications, but it is worth checking how easy this will be. It may be necessary to export data into a separate graphics package to improve the quality of the graphs.

Format

We need to make sure that the data are in the format that the package accepts and to ensure that, for particular analyses, variables are coded appropriately. For example, for some analyses of binary outcomes the package may expect the binary data to be coded 0 or 1 to denote 'no' or 'yes'.

Books

There are many books that show how to use particular packages, especially the common ones, such as SPSS,[2] SAS,[3] and Stata.[5] These can be helpful in getting to grips with a package but they are not always a good source of information about the actual statistical methods.

References

1 Peacock J, Kerry SM. *Presenting medical statistics from proposal to publication.* Oxford: Oxford University Press, 2006.
2 SPSS: Statistical Package for the Social Sciences. IBM SPSS. Available from: 🖱 www.spss.com
3 SAS: Statistical Analysis System. Available from: 🖱 www.sas.com
4 Stata: Data analysis and statistical software. Available from: 🖱 www.stata.com.

Examples of using statistical packages

Chi-squared test

The examples that follow show the computer output results from a chi-squared test done in three commercial statistical packages: SPSS,[1] Stata,[2] and SAS.[3] The two variables are smoking (0=no, 1=yes) and low birthweight (0=no, 1=yes). The test examines whether there is any evidence for a relationship between smoking during pregnancy and low birthweight. For explanation of the chi-squared test, see 📖 Chi-squared test, p. 262.

SPSS

Crosstabs

smoking * lowbw Crosstabulation

			lowbw		Total
			no	yes	
smoking	No	Count	979	40	1019
		% within smoking	96.1%	3.9%	100.0%
	Yes	Count	454	30	484
		% within smoking	93.8%	6.2%	100.0%
Total		Count	1433	70	1503
		% within smoking	95.3%	4.7%	100.0%

Chi-Square Tests

	Value	df	Asymp Sig. (2-sided)	Exact Sig. (2-sided)	Exact Sig. (1-sided)
Pearson Chi-Square	3.818(b)	1	.051		
Continuity Correction(a)	3.320	1	.068		
Likelihood Ratio	3.651	1	.056		
Fisher's Exact Test				.066	.036
N of Valid Cases	1503				

ᵃ Computed only for a 2x2 table

ᵇ 0 cells (.0%) have expected count less than 5. The minimum expected count is 22.54.

SPSS results

This SPSS output gives row percentages for the table and gives P values for four slightly different versions of the chi-squared test. All give similar P values. Note that for Fisher's exact test, the two-sided P value is the one to use. SPSS also states the number of cells with expected values less than five so that the user can see if the test is valid (see 📖 Chi-squared test, p. 262, for more on this).

Stata

Key
frequency
row percentage
column percentage

	smoker		
lowbw	0	1	Total
0	979	454	1,433
	68.32	31.68	100.00
	96.07	93.80	95.34
1	40	30	70
	57.14	42.86	100.00
	3.93	6.20	4.66
Total	1,019	484	1,503
	67.80	32.20	100.00
	100.00	100.00	100.00

Pearson chi2 (1) = 3.8177	Pr =	0.051
likelihood-ratio chi2 (1) = 3.6505	Pr =	0.056
Cramér's V = 0.0504		
gamma = 0.2359	ASE =	0.117
Kendall's tau-b = 0.0504	ASE =	0.027

Stata results

These are set out differently from the SPSS output and are in plain text format. This analysis has also given several versions of the chi-squared test. The values are the same as given by SPSS. Stata does not give information about 'expected' values (see 📖 Chi-squared test, p. 262).

References

1 SPSS: Statistical Package for the Social Sciences. IBM SPSS. Available from: 🔖 www.spss.com.
2 Stata: Data analysis and statistical software. Available from: 🔖 www.stata.com.
3 SAS: Statistical Analysis System. Available from: 🔖 www.sas.com.

Examples of using statistical packages (continued)

SAS

TABLE OF SMOKER BY LOWBW

LOWBW	SMOKER		
Frequency			
Percent			
Row Pct			
Col Pct	0	1	Total
0	979	454	1,433
	65.14	30.21	95.34
	68.32	31.68	
	96.07	93.80	
1	40	30	70
	2.66	2.00	4.66
	57.14	42.86	
	3.93	6.20	
Total	1,019	484	1,503
	67.80	32.20	100.00

Frequency Missing = 10

STATISTICS FOR TABLE OF LOWBW BY SMOKER

Statistic	DF	Value	Prob
Chi-Square	1	3.818	0.051
Likelihood Ratio Chi-Square	1	3.651	0.056
Mantel-Haenszel Chi-Square	1	3.815	0.068
Phi Coefficient		0.050	
Contingency Coefficient		0.050	
Cramer's V		0.050	
Effective Sample Size = 1503			
Frequency Missing = 10			

SAS output
This is similar to the Stata output. SAS additionally states the number of observations used in the analysis and the number of subjects with missing data.

Comparisons between outputs

All three give the same test statistics and P values for the main chi-squared test. Varying additional tests statistics are given. The layout is slightly different in the three packages.

For all three sets of results, the output is not suitable for reporting as it is. All three packages, and most packages in practice, give more information than is needed for reporting. The appropriate results should be extracted and reported either in text, or if part of a set of analyses, in a table (see example below, and also Peacock and Kerry[1]).

These three packages have been shown as they are familiar to us and to illustrate what you might see when you use a package. There are many other packages which can also be used (see 📖 Common packages, p. 170).

Example: presenting results from a chi-squared test

Table 5.1 provides a template for presenting the results of the chi-squared test shown in the section 📖 Examples of using statistical packages, p. 162. In this example, the results could be combined with those for other risk factors for low birthweight, such as alcohol and illicit drugs (data not shown here). Underneath the table is an example of the accompanying text that could appear in a document reporting the results.

Table 5.1 Risk factors for low birthweight

	Birthweight		
Risk factor during pregnancy	**Normal (n=1433)**	**Low (<2500g) (n=70)**	**P-value for chi-squared test**
Smoking	31.7% (454/1433)	42.9% (30/70)	0.051
Alcohol			
Illicit drug use			

Description

There was a higher prevalence of smoking during pregnancy among mothers with low birthweight babies, compared with those with normal weight babies. This difference was of borderline statistical significance (P=0.051, Table 5.1).

References

1 Peacock J, Kerry SM. *Presenting medical statistics from proposal to publication*. Oxford: Oxford University Press, 2006.

Using spreadsheets for analysis

Spreadsheets can be used for data entry and data analysis by means of their in-built routines. The statistical methods available are limited but there are also add-ons available for purchase online that will extend the scope of the spreadsheet. These can be found by searching on the Internet.

We show below the results of doing the chi-squared analysis shown in the section 📖 Examples of using statistical packages, p. 162, for SPSS, Stata and SAS, using Excel with two different add-ons, XLSTAT[1] and Analyse-it.[2] These analyses were both done using the 30-day free trial versions of the packages.

XLSTAT

Test of independence between the rows and the columns (Chi-square):

Chi-square (Observed value)	3.818
Chi-square (Critical value)	3.841
DF	1
p-value	0.051
alpha	0.05

Test interpretation:

H0: The rows and the columns of the table are independent.

Ha: There is a link between the rows and the columns of the table.

As the computed p-value is greater than the significance level alpha=0.05, one should accept the null hypothesis H0.

The risk to reject the null hypothesis H0 while it is true is 5.07%.

Comment on XLSTAT output

The test statistic and P value were, as expected, the same as for the other three packages shown in the section 📖 Examples of using statistical packages, p. 162.

The output included an interpretation that fits with the usual significant/ not significant interpretation of a P value and which talks in terms of accepting or rejecting the null hypothesis. In medical statistics we do not usually use this interpretation since it implies that if P is greater than 0.05, then the null hypothesis is true. In fact, a P value greater than 0.05 simply means is that there is insufficient evidence that an association exists (i.e. there is insufficient evidence to reject the null hypothesis). In this case P is only just greater than 0.05 (0.051) and so a more measured conclusion is appropriate. See Altman and Bland[3] for further discussion of 'non-significant' findings.

Analyse-it

The same analysis was repeated using Analyse-it.[2] The output has been re-formatted from that produced by the package to allow it to fit here. The package has a report facility but this was not available in the free evaluation version.

		SMOKING		
n	1503			
LOWBW		no	yes	Total
no	979		454	1433
	(971.5)		(461.5)	
yes	40		30	70
	(47.5)		(22.5)	
Total	1019		484	1503
Pearson's X^2 statistic	3.82			
DF	1			
p	0.0507			

Comment on Analyse-it output

The test statistic and P value were the same as found in the other packages. The additional feature is that this package gives 'expected' values in brackets in the table, although there is no legend to say that this is what they are (📖 Chi-squared test, p. 262).

General comments

Both packages were easy to download and use for a chi-squared test but a full review has not been undertaken for either add-in. Since these and other similar add-in packages can be tried for free, it is easy to do your own evaluation before buying.

References

1 XLSTAT: Data analysis and statistical solution for Microsoft Excel. Available from: ℘ www. xlstat.com.

2 Analyse-it: Statistical analysis software for MS Excel. Available from: ℘ www.analyse-it.com

3 Altman DG, Bland JM. Absence of evidence is not evidence of absence. *BMJ* 1995; **311**(7003):485.

Transferring data between packages

Introduction

We sometimes need to transfer data files between packages or between computers, for example, because data are entered in one package and will be analysed in another or because some analyses need to be done in one package and some in another. It is worth thinking about this at the outset to reduce the possibility of things going wrong. Statistical packages often store the data as a **coded file** that cannot be directly transferred from one program to another and so another approach is needed.

Ways of transferring data

- By **creating an export version** of the data within the package which can be directly imported into another package. Not all packages can do this.
- Via a **spreadsheet**: some packages hold their data internally in a spreadsheet and data can be cut and pasted from one spreadsheet to another, although this is not recommended (☐ Joining datasets, p. 110)
- Via a **data transfer program** such as Stat/Transfer,[1] which will take coded files from a range of packages and transfer them directly into the right format for another package. Using a transfer program will usually mean that variable names and labels are also transferred. Other methods listed above may not do this.

Potential problems

- **Missing data:** how are these handled in the transfer? Has it worked properly?
- **Data format:** have text data transferred properly and are they in the right format, for example are data in string format still in string format? Have numerical data transferred correctly and are they in the right format?
- **Versions of programs:** problems of compatibility can occur when transferring data files between different versions of the same package. Data files created with later versions of a package may not be readable in earlier versions.

Checking

It is best to check carefully that the transfer has been successful, and that values and formats have not changed, particularly if doing a particular transfer for the first time. Check all the data if possible or a representative sample.

Reference

1 Stat/Transfer: Data conversion software utility. Available from: 🖰 www.stattransfer.com.

Common packages

Comments and disclaimer

- There is always a danger when providing any such list that it will miss key items and/or it will be immediately out of date. Table 5.2 is not an exhaustive list of statistical packages, and references are not given.
- Most packages have a website, which can be found using a simple Internet search. More packages, particularly free ones, and specialized packages can be found in the same way.
- This is not a review of statistical packages – we have not used all of the packages listed but believe them to be in common use
- Many commercial packages allow a free trial version to be downloaded from the Internet. It is worth trying out different ones.

Table 5.2 Commonly used statistical packages

Package name	Comment	Commercial or Free
Analyse-it	Add-on to MS Excel	C
CIA	Confidence interval analysis available with book '*statistics with confidence*', Altman *et al.*[1]	C
Epi-info	Produced by CDC Atlanta	F
Excel	Spreadsheet	C
GenStat	General statistics package	C
MedCalc	For biomedical sciences	C
Minitab	General statistics package	C
MLwiN	For fitting multi-level models	C
NCSS	General statistics package	C
NQuery Advisor	For sample size calculations	C
OpenEpi	Companion to EpiInfo (CDC Atlanta)	F
PASS	For sample size calculations	C
R	Programming language for statistics	F
SAS	General statistics package	C
SigmaPlot	For graphics	C
SigmaStat	For group analysis	C
SPC XL	Add-on to MS Excel	C
S-Plus	General statistics package	C
SPSS	General statistics package	C
Stat/Transfer	Transfer data between packages	C
Stata	General statistics package	C
STATISTICA	General statistics package	C
StatsDirect	General statistical package	C
Statxact	Exact analyses; useful for small samples	C
StudySize	For sample size calculations	C
SUDAAN	Add-on to SPSS/SAS for survey analysis	C
Systat	General statistics package	C
Unistat	General statistical package & MS Excel add-in	C
WinBUGS	For Bayesian analysis	F
XLSTAT	Add-on to MS Excel	C

Reference

1 Altman DG, Machin D, Bryant TN, Gardner MJ. *Statistics with confidence: confidence intervals and statistical guidelines.* London: BMJ Books, 2000.

Summarizing data

Introduction

In this chapter we describe types of quantitative and categorical data and show how these different types of data can be summarized numerically and in graphs. We give worked examples of how to calculate mean, median, standard deviation, and interquartile range, and give examples of displaying data in graphs.

Why summarize data?

Introduction

There are several different reasons why we may wish to summarize data:

- For data quality monitoring – checking the data as they are collected
- For data checking – checking the data that have been collected and/or entered onto a computer – this process is sometimes called 'data cleaning'
- To report the basic features of the sample in a study – baseline data
- As a precursor to more complex methods of statistical analysis

Data quality monitoring

The aim of this is to check that the **data are complete** as collection takes place so that any problems can be addressed before it is too late (📖 Data quality, p. 81). Often all that is needed is a count of the data items for each variable or question to check for any missing items. For example a particular question in a self-completed questionnaire may frequently be missed because it is on another page. This can be picked up early by simply counting the number of replies to each question.

Data checking and data cleaning

The aim of this is to make sure that the **data are correct** on the computer record. Errors can arise if a research subject mis-reports information or the researcher mis-records that information. Further errors may be introduced when the data are transferred onto a computer. Some errors can be identified by simple range checks – computing the minimum and maximum values for a particular response. This will highlight values outside the expected range but errors that are still within range will not be found in this way. Other errors can be identified by simple cross-tabulations, which may highlight inconsistent combinations, such as in a study that is recording smoking habits a subject is recorded as a non-smoker but has given the number of cigarettes smoked (📖 Data checking examples, p. 118).

Baseline data in a study

Simple descriptive data is informative in supplying the backcloth against which more analytical findings can be interpreted: for example, the numbers of subjects in various demographic categories, or mean values for key variables such as the main diagnosis. This enables the researchers and readers to interpret the findings and determine the context in which the results could be more generally applied. For example, the results of a study conducted in one country may apply in another country if both countries have similar baseline characteristics.

Before doing a complex analysis

It is relatively easy to do quite complex statistical analyses using a computer program but in order to interpret the results in a meaningful way, and be sure that they are appropriate methods to use in the first place, descriptive summary data are needed. For example, before doing any sort of regression analysis with several variables, simple descriptive analyses are needed for the variables involved to determine the individual inter-relationships.

Summary points

Summary statistics:
- Allow us to look at the data carefully
- Are useful at all stages of a study
- Help improve the quality of the data by highlighting possible errors
- Provide a backcloth against which later analyses can be interpreted and thus allow researchers to draw more meaningful conclusions

---

Types of data

Quantitative and categorical data

In order to know what sort of statistical analysis is appropriate, it is important to know what type of data we are handling. There are several ways of classifying data, which are discussed in this chapter, but the simplest is to consider data as either **quantitative** or **categorical** (see 📖 Quantitative data, p. 178, and Categorical data, p. 180).

❶ Note that categorical data are sometimes known as 'qualitative' data. This term is rather ambiguous as it can be confused with those data collected from a **qualitative study**, such as text obtained from in-depth interviews. Data from purely qualitative studies are analysed using non-statistical methods and are not considered in this book.

A variable

A variable is a quantity that is measured or observed in an individual and which varies from person to person.

For example, blood pressure is a variable because blood pressure varies from person to person. Another example is blood group, which also varies from person to person. A further example is gender, where people can be classified as either male or female. We use the term 'variable' in statistics to refer to any such quantity.

Note that variables can be derived when the research subject is an organizational unit rather than a person, such as when studying the use of operating theatres in a set of hospitals and calculating the proportion of time that they are in use in each hospital. The concept of variables is discussed further in Chapter 7 (📖 Independence: data and variables, p. 204).

Statistic

A statistic is any quantity that is calculated from a set of data.

For example mean blood pressure calculated in a group of subjects is a statistic. Another example is the proportion of people who are overweight in a sample. A statistic summarizes the data in some sense.

There are many different statistics that can be calculated from data and the choice of which to use is driven partly by the type of data and partly by the purpose of the study. In many cases several statistics will be calculated from the same set of data. A simple example of this is if we calculate both the minimum and maximum age of subjects in a study – these are two different statistics, both of which are useful summary measures.

Quantitative data

Definition

Quantitative data are data that can be **measured numerically** and may be continuous or discrete.

- **Continuous data** lie on a continuum and so can take any value between two limits. The only limitation is that imposed by the accuracy of the method of measurement so that some continuous data may be recorded as integers, although that is an approximation to the true value
- **Discrete data** do not lie on a continuum and can only take certain values, usually **count**s (integers)

Examples

- Weight is a **continuous** variable because it is **measured** using weighing scales. A person's weight lies on a continuum and the only limitation is the accuracy of the scales
- The number of previous pregnancies in a pregnant woman is **discrete** data since it is **counted** and only whole numbers are possible
  Quantitative data can be further classified as being on an 'interval scale' or on a 'ratio scale'.

Interval scales

On an **interval** scale, differences between values at different points of the scale have the same meaning. For example if a man who weighs 12 stone gains weight and becomes 12½ stone, his weight gain is the same as that of a woman who goes from 9 stone to 9½ stone – both the man and the woman gain half a stone (7 pounds) and the meaning is exactly the same, even though their starting weights were different.

Ratio scales

Data can be regarded as on a **ratio** scale if the ratio of two measurements has a meaning. For example we can say that twice as many people in one group had a particular characteristic compared with another group and this has a sensible meaning. Similarly we could say that one person's weight loss was twice that of another and this would also have an interpretable meaning.

In contrast, temperature is not ratio data because we cannot say that one temperature is twice as hot as another. To demonstrate this consider if we looked at 30°C which is 'twice' 15°C. But if we convert it to Fahrenheit, 30°C=86°F and 15°C=59°F. So, in degrees Fahrenheit the temperature is not doubled. This is of course because of the arbitrary zero on the scale for temperature. Note that even using a temperature scale based on 'absolute zero' the concept of a doubling of temperature would still be nonsensical in everyday use.

Ordinal data

Quantitative data are always **ordinal** – the data values can be arranged in a numerical order from the smallest to the largest. Questionnaire scale data are often ordinal and are often counts, such as when adding the number of positive responses to a set of questions to get a total score. Categorical data may also have an inherent ordering and so be ordinal, such as stage of disease.

Notes

- Interval scale data are always ordinal. Ratio scale data are always interval scale data and therefore must also be ordinal
- In practice, **continuous data may look discrete** because of the way they are measured and/or reported. For example gestational age of babies is often reported in whole weeks, such as 38 weeks, and so appears to be discrete. It is however continuous because it could be reported to a greater degree of accuracy, for example as a decimal, such as 38.5 weeks
- ❶ **All continuous measurements are limited by the accuracy of the instrument** used to measure them, and many quantities such as age and height are reported in whole numbers for convenience

Categorical data

Definition

Categorical data are data where individuals fall into a number of **separate categories or classes**. For example:

- Gender: male or female = two classes
- Disease status: alive or dead = two classes
- Stage of cancer: I, II, III, or IV = four classes
- Marital status: married, single, divorced, widowed, or legally separated = five classes

Ordering

Different categories of categorical data may be assigned a number for coding purposes (Form filling and coding, p. 78), and if there are several categories, there may be an implied ordering, such as with stage of cancer where stage I is the least advanced and stage IV the most advanced. This means that such data are **ordinal but not interval** because the 'distance' between adjacent categories has no real measurement attached to it. The 'gap' between stages I and II disease is not necessarily the same as the 'gap' between stages III and IV. Apparently similar gaps between categories may not have the same clinical meaning. Similarly, calculating a mean stage of cancer for a group of individuals would be nonsensical.

Where categorical data are coded with numerical codes, it might appear that there is an ordering but this may not necessarily be so. It is important to **distinguish between ordered and non-ordered data** because it affects the analysis. For example, marital status as given above might be coded 1, 2, 3, 4, and 5, but is not ordered data – we cannot say that 'single' comes before 'divorced' or that 'widowed' comes before 'legally separated' in any meaningful sense.

Dichotomous data

This is where there are **only two classes** and all individuals fall into one or other of the classes. These data are also known as **binary data**.

Categorizing continuous data

It is possible to reclassify continuous data into groups, perhaps for ease of reporting. For example it is common to report birthweight in bands, giving the numbers of babies who fall into each birthweight band.

Example: categorizing birthweight
<2500 g
2500–2999 g
3000–3499 g
3500–3999 g
4000–4499 g
≥4500 g

Consequences of categorizing continuous data

- ❶ **Dichotomizing** (re-categorizing data into two groups) is **potentially very problematic** because a great deal of information is discarded and statistical power is lost in the analysis (📖 Outcomes: continuous and categorical, p. 46). In addition, the nature of any relationships may be masked. For example, if the relationship was curved, this may be weaker if the data were categorized and if the relationship was U-shaped, categorization may totally obscure it.
- If continuous data are **reclassified into several groups, the effect on statistical power is less** than when dichotomizing. Grouping causes no problem if the reclassification is done simply to present summary statistics but the original data are used in the analysis.
- Sometimes it can be useful to reclassify continuous data into several groups when we are examining a **non-linear relationship**. The analysis may be more straightforward and more meaningful if the data are grouped.

Summarizing quantitative data

Continuous data
Continuous data can be summarized in several different ways and many of these are either a measure of the **centre of the data distribution** or a **measure of the variability of the data**.

Measures of the centre of the data
- Mean
- Median

Measures of variability
- Standard deviation (variance)
- Range (minimum, maximum)
- Interquartile range

Mean
This is the simple average of all the data: the sum of all values divided by the total number of values. This mean is known as the **arithmetic mean**. Two other types of mean, the geometric mean and the harmonic mean, are described in the section 📖 Geometric mean, harmonic mean, mode, p. 188.

Median
This is the **middle value** when the data are arranged in ascending order of size. If there are an odd number of values in the sample then the median will be the value with the same number of values both bigger than it and smaller than it. If there is an even number of values, there will be two middle values and the median will be the mean of the two.

Standard deviation
This indicates **how dispersed the data are** and is a measure of the average difference between the mean and each data value. It is calculated by taking the square root of the variance. The **variance** is calculated by summing the squared differences between the overall mean and each value and then dividing by the number of values minus one. The sample standard deviation is often abbreviated to '**SD**' or '**S**'.
- The advantage of the **standard deviation** over the variance is that it is in the **same units as the original data** and so is easier to interpret
- ❶ Note that a different denominator is used when the whole population variance is calculated; we divide by n. Since **we virtually always have a sample, the SD is obtained by dividing by $n-1$ because it can be shown to give a more accurate estimate of the population standard deviation**

Range
This is the difference between the smallest and largest value and is usually expressed as the **minimum and maximum**. Sometimes the actual difference between the two extremes is presented, but this is not a good idea as it does not show the extremes.

Interquartile range

This is the range of values that includes the **middle 50% of values** and is bounded by the **lower and upper quartile**. The lower quartile is found by ranking the data as for the median and then taking the value below which 25% of the data sit. The upper quartile is the value above which the top 25% of data points sit.

Percentiles (centiles) in general

The median and quartiles are examples of percentiles – points which divide the distribution of the data into set percentages above or below a certain value. The median is the 50th centile, the lower quartile is the 25th and the upper quartile is the 75th. Although these are the most common centiles that we calculate, any percentile can be calculated from continuous data. For some data, a different percentile may provide a useful summary. For example, child growth charts show several different centiles (calculated from the general population) to allow detection of children with poor growth. The formula is given below (📖 Calculation of median, interquartile range, p. 186, has worked examples):

---

1. When $q(n+1)$ is an integer where q is a decimal between 0 and 1, from a data set with n values, the qth centile is:

$x_{q(n+1)}$ ie the $q(n+1)$th value of x

2. When $q(n+1)$ is not an integer then if k is the integer part of $q(n+1)$, the centile must lie between the kth and $(k+1)$th values, x_k and x_{k+1}. The qth centile will then be:

$x_k + (x_{k+1} - x_k)(q(n+1) - k)$

Calculation of mean, SD

The data: heights of 106 women in cm

156	161	172	162	167	158	163	160	155
160	165	173	152	168	160	161	169	158
161	172	160	167	164	151	166	172	
167	153	177	166	161	176	164	167	
166	156	156	155	166	166	162	161	
165	165	161	148	149	158	163	177	
167	169	156	159	160	160	158	160	
163	162	170	142	157	156	162	170	
157	167	162	160	164	167	147	158	
177	154	169	161	157	160	163	157	
156	159	159	160	172	173	166	167	
168	154	165	167	175	167	163	164	
165	170	177	159	161	170	163	164	

Algebraic notation

- Greek symbols are used as shorthand in mathematics and statistics to make it easier to give general formulae for statistical quantities
- The **sigma** symbol Σ is used to define a **sum** of a number of items which are identified by subscripts such as x_1, x_2, x_3 and so on and in general x_i

- Hence $\sum\limits_{i=1}^{n} x_i$ indicates the sum of all xs from x_1, x_2, x_3 to x_n

  i.e. $x_1 + x_2 + x_3 + \ldots + x_n$
- $\bar{x}$ denotes the **mean** of the variable x. It is spoken as '**x bar**'.

The calculations

Mean: $\dfrac{\left(\sum\limits_{i=1}^{n} X_i\right)}{n}$

$= (156 + 160 + 161 + \ldots + 155 + 158)/106$

$= 162.764$ (to 3 decimal places)

$= 162.8$ cm (to 1 decimal place, sufficient accuracy for reporting)

Variance (to get standard deviation) $\left\{\dfrac{\sum\limits_{i=1}^{n}(X_i - \overline{X})^2}{n-1}\right\}$

$\dfrac{(156 - 162.764)^2 + (160 - 162.764)^2 + (161 - 162.764)^2 + \ldots + (158 - 162.764)^2}{105}$

$= \dfrac{4735.104}{105}$

$= 45.095 \text{ cm}^2$

Standard deviation

$\sqrt{45.095}$

$= 6.7$ cm to 1 decimal place

Calculation of median, interquartile range

The data
These are as given in 📖 Calculation of mean, SD, p. 184.

Median and quartiles
- First tabulate the data in order of size:

Height	Frequency	Cumulative frequency
142	1	1
147	1	2
148	1	3
149	1	4
151	1	5
152	1	6
153	1	7
154	2	9
155	2	11
156	6	17
157	4	21
158	5	26
159	4	30
160	10	40
161	8	48
162	5	53
163	6	59
164	5	64
165	5	69
166	6	75
167	10	85
168	2	87
169	3	90
170	4	94

Height	Frequency	Cumulative frequency
172	4	98
173	2	100
175	1	101
176	1	102
177	4	106

- The median is the half-way point, which is between the 53rd and 54th value
- These are 162 and 163 and so the median is (162+163)/2 = 162.5 cm
- The lower quartile (LQ) is calculated using the formula given previously: $q(n+1)$ =0.25 × 107 = 26.75 so LQ lies between 26th and 27th values, 158 and 159
  LQ= 158 + (159–158) × 0.75 = 158.75 cm
- The upper quartile (UQ) is calculated using the same formula: $q(n+1)$=0.75 × 107=80.25 so UQ lies between 80th and 81st values, both 167
  UQ is therefore 167 cm
- The interquartile range is therefore 159 to 167 (rounded)

Geometric mean, harmonic mean, mode

Introduction

The mean that we calculated previously (Summarizing quantitative data, p. 182) is the arithmetic mean and is most commonly used. This gives a measure of the middle of the distribution when the data follow a reasonably symmetrical distribution, but when the data are skewed it will not represent the middle. Most non-symmetrical data distributions have a positive skew, that is, the tail of the distribution is longer on the right-hand side. In such cases the arithmetic mean will be disproportionately inflated by the small number of high values in the upper tail of the distribution and so the geometric mean may be preferred.

Geometric mean

This is **calculated using log-transformed data** – each data value is replaced by its logarithm to base e. The arithmetic mean is then calculated on the new log-transformed scale and this is back-transformed using the exponential transformation to give a mean that is in the same units as the original data.

Harmonic mean

The harmonic mean is also based on transformed data values and is the back-transformation of the **arithmetic mean of the reciprocal of the data** (1/value). It can be used when the data are highly positively skewed, but it is not commonly seen in practice.

Mode

The mode is the value which has the greatest frequency. It has limited usefulness for continuous data but is useful for categorical data where it indicates the most common category.

Example

Figure 6.1 shows a histogram of alcohol data, which are also shown in Graphs, scatter plots and shapes of distributions, p. 198. The distribution is positively skewed. These data are used to illustrate the calculation of geometric and harmonic means.

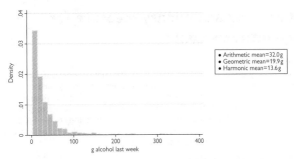

Fig. 6.1 A skewed distribution: alcohol intake in 854 pregnant women.

Calculation of geometric and harmonic means

As this is a large dataset, we only show a few values before and after transformation of the data to illustrate the calculations:

Alcohol (g)	Log$_e$(alcohol)	1/alcohol
3	1.0986	0.3333
20	2.9957	0.0500
25	3.2189	0.0400
102	4.6250	0.0098

To calculate the geometric mean:

$$\frac{1.0986 + 2.9957 + 3.2189 + 4.6250 + \ldots}{854}$$

$$= \frac{2552.285}{854} = 2.9886$$

Geometric mean = exp(2.9886) = 19.9 g(to 1 decimal place)

To calculate the harmonic mean:

$$\frac{0.3333 + 0.0500 + 0.0400 + 0.0098 + \ldots}{854}$$

$$= \frac{62.6304}{854} = 0.0733$$

Harmonic mean $= \dfrac{1}{0.0733} = 13.6$ g (to 1 decimal place)

Note that the geometric mean is smaller than the arithmetic mean and is close to the median value, 20 g. The harmonic mean is smaller still.

Choosing a summary measure for quantitative data

Introduction

It is usually useful to present more than one summary measure for a set of data and we give some suggestions as to what summary measures will be useful in different situations. **If the data are going to be analysed later using methods based on means then it makes sense to present means rather than medians.** If the data are skewed they may need to be transformed before analysis and so it is best to present summaries based on the transformed data, such as geometric means.

Centre of distribution

- Continuous data with symmetrical distribution – use arithmetic mean
- Continuous data with positively skewed distribution – consider geometric or harmonic mean but be aware that these do not allow zero values. See notes on transformations (📖 Transforming data, p. 330) for more on this topic.
- Continuous data with skewed distribution – consider median
- Discrete data – present median unless the range of data is large enough to make the calculation of a mean sensible
  For example, the number of children in a family is discrete and although sometimes the mean number is calculated ('2.4 children'), it may be difficult to interpret.

Spread of distribution

- Continuous data – use standard deviation (see notes 2 and 3 below)
- Continuous data with skew – consider using interquartile range (see notes 2 and 3)
- Continuous data – the range (min to max) is often useful if there is room to present this in addition to the standard deviation

Notes

1 For very skewed data rather than reporting the median, it may be helpful to present a different percentile (i.e. not the 50th), which better reflects the shape of the distribution. This may be particularly useful when comparing two groups where the medians are the same but the outer tails of the distributions are different.

2 Some researchers are reluctant to present the standard deviation when the data are skewed and so present the median and range and/ or quartiles. If analyses are planned which are based on means then it makes sense to be consistent and give standard deviations. Further, the useful relationship that approximately 95% of the data lie between mean ± 2 standard deviations, holds even for skewed data (see Bland, Chapter 4[1]).

3 If data are transformed, the standard deviation cannot be back-transformed correctly and so for transformed data a standard deviation cannot be given. In this case the untransformed standard deviation can be given or another measure of spread. This is discussed further in Chapter 8 (📖 Transforming data, p. 330).

4 For discrete data with a narrow range, such as stage of cancer, it may be better to present the actual frequency distribution to give a fair summary of the data, rather than calculate a mean or dichotomize it.

5 It is good practice to report the actual number of data values as well as the summary values since in general we have more confidence in greater numbers.

Reference

1 Bland M. *An introduction to medical statistics.* 3rd ed. Oxford: Oxford University Press, 2000.

Summarizing categorical data

Unordered categories (nominal data)

These can be summarized using the **frequencies in each category together with either the overall proportions or percentages**. The choice of whether to use proportions or percentages is a personal one although percentages are more commonly seen. The complete set of frequencies is the **frequency distribution**. An example is given in Table 6.1.

Table 6.1 Type of housing in a sample of women

Housing	No. (%)
Owner	899 (62)
Council rent	258 (18)
Private rent	175 (12)
With parents	72 (5.0)
Other	39 (2.7)
Total	1443

Ordered categories (ordinal data)

These can also be summarized by frequencies and percentages as above but in addition we can calculate **cumulative frequencies** and **percentages**. This can be useful to show the percentage below a certain cut-off. An example is given in Table 6.2, which shows the occupational classification in 1436 women. Note that the percentages do not quite add to 100% due to rounding.

Table 6.2 Occupational classification in 1436 women

Occupational classification	Frequency	%	Cumulative frequency	%
Professional	115	8.0	115	8.0
Managerial	390	27	505	35
Skilled non-manual	148	10	653	45
Skilled manual	578	40	1231	85
Semi-skilled manual	143	10	1374	95
Unskilled	62	4.3	1436	100
Total	1436			

The cumulative percentage is quite useful and here can highlight the percentage of women in non-manual occupations: 45%.

Cross tabulations

It is often useful to tabulate one categorical variable against another to show the proportions or percentages of the categories of one variable by the other (for example, see Table 6.3).

Table 6.3 Incidences of different types of cancer in England by gender[1]

Cancer type	Male	Female	Total
Lung	18 105 (59%)	12 354 (41%)	30 459 (100%)
Breast	0 (0%)	36 939 (100%)	36 939 (100%)
Prostate	29 406 (100%)	0 (0%)	29 406 (100%)
Colorectal	16 103 (54%)	13 448 (46%)	29 551 (100%)
Other	54 191 (51%)	53 075 (49%)	107 266 (100%)
Total	117 805 (50%)	115 816 (50%)	233 621 (100%)

Notes

- When categorical data are coded for data analysis with numerical codes these **cannot be considered quantitative data** and so care is needed to analyse such data appropriately

  For example, if we had allocated the codes 1, 2, 3, 4, and 5 to the five categories of the housing data shown previously, we could calculate 'mean housing' using these numbers but it would of course be completely meaningless. Similarly male and female are often coded 1 and 2, respectively, but again a 'mean gender' would make no sense.

- Where ordered categorical data have numerical codes, these may be used under some circumstances to **test a trend in the data** but care is needed not to over-interpret the ordering and to gauge an appropriate numbering that reflects the 'gap' between categories

Reference

1 Department of Health. *Health profile of England 2007. Section 2 - Snapshot of Health and Well-being in England, 8.* London, Crown Publications, 2008.

Graphs: histogram, stem and leaf plot

Histogram

This is a diagram which shows the distribution of the data by plotting the data in rectangles known as '**bins**' corresponding to categories along the horizontal (x) axis. The rectangles have heights or areas that are proportional to the frequencies in these categories. The vertical (y) scale is the frequency per interval (see Fig. 6.2 for an example).

Note that if the widths of the bins are the same then the height of each rectangle is proportional to its frequency, but if they are not the area indicates the frequency. It is best where possible to keep the width the same for all bins.

Example

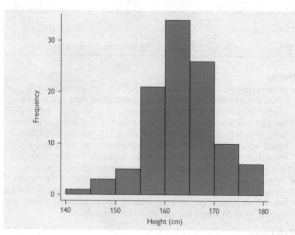

Fig. 6.2 Histogram showing distribution of height in 106 women.

Stem and leaf plot

A stem and leaf plot is a graph that shows the main features of a set of data. In the stem and leaf plot the numbers themselves are used to demonstrate the shape of the distribution. The **'leaf' is the final digit** of each height and the **'stem' is all the other numbers**. It may be used instead of a histogram for small datasets or alongside to show patterns of occurrence for certain numbers (see Fig. 6.3).

Example

Figure 6.3 shows a stem and leaf plot for the height data which were displayed opposite as a histogram. The first row of the plot below represents the value 142 cm, the second represents 147, 148, and 149 cm and so on. The plot provides a useful summary of data structure while at the same time showing other characteristics such as a tendency for certain trailing digits to be more common than others (so called **digit preference**). We can see here that 154 cm and 155 cm both occur twice, 156 cm occurs six times, and so on. In some datasets where observers are reporting measurements to the nearest 5 or 10, there will be an excess of these trailing digits. That does not appear to be the case in these data but is a common feature of blood pressure data.

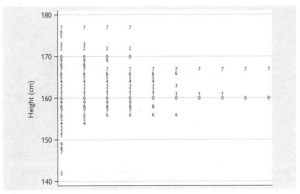

Fig. 6.3 Stem and leaf plot of height in 106 women.

Graphs: box and whisker plot, dot plot

Box and whisker plot

A box and whisker plot contains five pieces of summary information about the data:

- Median = horizontal line in box
- Upper quartile = top edge of the box
- Lower quartile = lower edge of box
- Maximum = top of 'whisker'
- Minimum = bottom of 'whisker'

Example

Figure 6.4 shows the height data from Figure 6.2 split according to occupation. It illustrates how useful a box and whisker plot can be to display data in groups. Note that an outlier is indicated by a separate circle outside the plot. This is a height of 142 cm which is quite small, but was found to be a correct value and not an error.

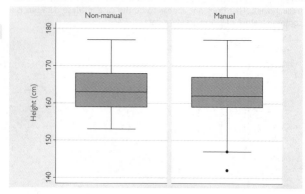

Fig. 6.4 Box and whisker plot showing the distribution of height by occupation in 106 women (37 non-manual, 69 manual occupations).

Dot plot

A dot plot is an alternative way of displaying the distribution of a set of data and is particularly useful for small datasets where a histogram may be uneven. It is also useful for showing the distributions in two or more groups side by side. Each value is plotted on the y-axis while the x-axis denotes the group.

Example

Figure 6.5 shows the distribution of height by occupation again. The dot plot provides an alternative to the box and whisker plot (Fig. 6.4) and has the advantage that the actual data points are shown. The disadvantage is that summary statistics are not shown as in the box and whisker plot.

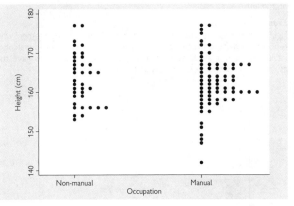

Fig. 6.5 Dot plots showing the distribution of height by occupation in 106 women (37 non-manual, 69 manual occupations).

Graphs: shapes of distributions

Importance of shape

▶ By looking at the shape of a distribution we can learn a lot about a set of data in terms of its central values, its extreme values, and where the bulk of the data lie.

Positively skewed data

Many variables follow reasonably symmetrical distributions, such as adult height (📖 Fig. 6.2, p. 194), but some variables commonly encountered in medical statistics are skewed. Most of these skewed variables have a positive skew, in that the tail on the right-hand side is longer than the tail on the left.

Example

Figure 6.6 shows the distribution of alcohol intake among women who reported drinking in pregnancy. Most women reported no or low alcohol intake and only a small number reported drinking a lot. This gave the asymmetrical distribution that seen in the figure.

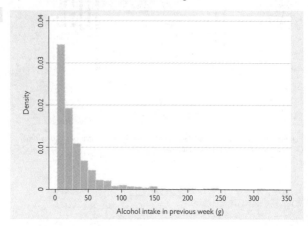

Fig. 6.6 A positively skewed distribution: alcohol intake in pregnancy.

Other examples of medical data with a positive skew includes many blood indices such as cholesterol, and weight, and blood pressure, where a few individuals have very high values, stretching the right-hand tail.

Negatively skewed data

It is unusual to see negatively skewed data in medical research where the longer tail is on the left, but gestational age is one such variable (see Fig. 6.7). Gestational age has this shape since the preterm births stretch out the lower left-hand tail, and there is a 'ceiling' effect at the upper end due to the limiting size of the mother/fetus and clinical practice of induction beyond 40 weeks.

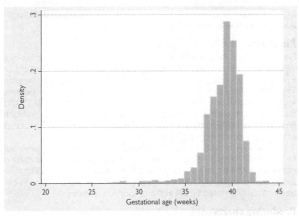

Fig. 6.7 A negatively skewed distribution: gestational age of 1513 babies.

Babies' birthweight also has a similar negative skewed distribution when all live births at all gestations are included. But if preterm births are excluded, then the birthweight distribution is reasonably close to a Normal distribution.

Graphs: bar chart, pie chart

Displaying categorical data

Graphs can be used to provide visual summaries of categorical data. The two most commonly used are bar charts and pie charts.

Bar charts

In a bar chart, each category is given its own bar along the horizontal (x) axis. The height of each bar is proportional to the frequency of observations. An example is given in Figure 6.8.

Pie charts

Pie charts show the distribution of individuals in different categories of a variable where every individual belongs to one and only one category. In a pie chart, each category is given an area (or slice) of the graph (the pie). The area of each slice is proportional to the frequency of observations within that category and is calculated by dividing the whole pie, 360°, into slices. Pie charts enable comparison of proportions in different population groups, for example, comparing self-rated health status in Bristol with that of the population at large (Fig. 6.9).

Pie charts are only useful where there are three or more categories but become hard to read if there are more than 10 categories. A pie chart is not needed where there are only two groups, such as when reporting the proportion of males and females in a single sample – this information can be more usefully stated simply as the proportion of males.

Producing charts

Both bar and pie charts can be easily produced using software packages. Many packages will also produce three-dimensional (3D) graphs. We do not recommend using these for simple graphs as they can distract from the data summary. With pie charts, '3D' imaging can produce a misleading graph as the area of the slice is no longer proportional to the number of observations in that category. With bar charts it is harder to deduce the frequency when the bar is shown in 3D. However, 3D graphs can be very useful to show complex mathematical relationships.

Examples

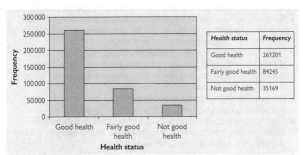

Fig. 6.8 Bar chart showing self-reported health in the 2001 census by people living in Bristol, England (Office for National Statistics. Census 2001 data. Available from: ✍ http://neighbourhood.statistics.gov.uk/).

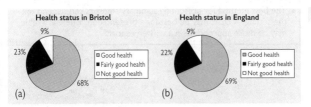

Fig. 6.9a,b Pie charts showing self-reported health in Bristol, and in England as a whole from the 2001 census.

Notes

- The two pie charts shown side by side demonstrate the very similar distributions of responses in the two groups. This is a useful format for displaying data in oral presentations. For reports, this information could be shown in a table and this would allow more information to be given. It can be helpful to show some data alongside the graph as we have in the first bar chart.
- For further information on displaying data, see the excellent book by Freeman and colleagues, *How to display data*,[1] and examples in Peacock and Kerry, Chapter 5.[2]

References

1 Freeman JV, Walters SJ, Campbell MJ. How to display data. *BMJ* Books, Blackwell Publishing, 2008.
2 Peacock J, Kerry SM. *Presenting medical statistics from proposal to publication.* Oxford: Oxford University Press, 2006.

Summary

- Summarizing data can be helpful in checking data quality as well as in presenting findings to others. Simple summaries can help detect errors in raw data which would alter findings.
- When performing complex statistical analyses, basic summaries should be performed first, as errors may not be so easily spotted during advanced tests. In addition, later results are easier to interpret alongside basic summary data.
- Data can be classified into different types, and the methods for summarizing data vary depending on the type of data
- Commonly used summary statistics for quantitative data include mean, median, standard deviation, range, and interquartile range. For skewed data, other statistics may be required.
- Categorical data can be graphically presented using histograms, box plots, stem and leaf plots, and dot plots. These can all be easily produced with statistical computer packages.
- Categorical data may be graphically presented using bar charts and pie charts
- The best method for presenting summary statistics can depend on the setting. A chart may be best for a presentation, whereas a table may be more appropriate in a written report.

Probability and distributions

Introduction

Probability and probability distributions play a central part in medical statistics. In this chapter we define what we mean by probability and describe the rules by which probabilities are combined. We then describe how the use of probability leads to the concept of a probability distribution and show how these distributions are used in medical statistics. We give examples of the use of key distributions: the Normal distribution, the Binomial distribution and the Poisson distribution.

Independence: data and variables

Introduction

We have previously defined a 'variable' as a quantity that is measured or observed in an individual subject and which varies from subject to subject (📖 Types of data, p. 176). For this reason, in statistics we sometimes call these '**random variables**'. We have shown in Chapter 6 how to summarize variables using various summary statistics, such as means and proportion; the choice of statistic depends on the type of data and the purpose of the data summary.

Independent data

The notion of data points being independent or not is important in medical statistics. Many statistical procedures assume that the data points in a sample are independent of each other. If two values are independent then this means that knowing something about one value tells us nothing about the other. In some situations it is straightforward to determine whether or not data are independent but in others it is not so easy.

Examples

1. We have a set of height measurements on a sample of children attending a hospital clinic. These heights will be **independent** of each other, assuming the children are not related to each other.
2. We have a series of height measurements over 5 years on the same sample of children. *Within each child*, the measurements will **not be independent** of each other because knowing one measurement for a particular child will give us some information about another measurement on the same child: any two measurements in a child will be closely related to each other.
3. We have a set of heights of mothers of all children born in a particular maternity unit over 5 years. These data may not be totally independent if some women had more than one pregnancy during the time period and were included more than once.

Independence matters

❶ The concept of independence is not just esoteric – **if we treat data as if they are independent when they are not we may make incorrect statistical inferences**.

In example 3, if shorter women tended to have more babies than taller women, then the overall mean height based on the mothers of all babies would be smaller than it should be because some shorter women would be included more than once. In general it is important to take any data dependence into account when designing and analysing data.

Examples of designs with intrinsic non-independence

- **Serial measures** within individuals, for example, growth studies where we have regular measurements of height and weight in a group of children over time. In such cases **we must take the non-independence into**

account when we analyse these data (📖 Serial (longitudinal) data, p. 378)

• **Clustered studies** where individuals fall naturally into groups or clusters, such as all patients in a particular general practice where the general practice is the cluster. An example is a cluster trial where clusters of individuals are randomly allocated to treatments so that everyone in a cluster receives the same treatment. ▶ **It is essential to take the 'clustering' into account in such studies** (📖 Cluster samples, pp. 388–392)

Independent variables

Two *variables* measured within a sample of individuals may be related to each other and so are not independent. In fact it is **often the case that variables are related to each other and we use this in medical research to test hypotheses and determine risk factors for disease**.

Suppose we wish to determine if one variable, the amount of exercise an individual takes, is related to their weight. If exercise and weight are found to be related, i.e. not independent, we may decide to investigate whether increasing the amount of exercise taken might reduce weight.

❶ Note that when doing a regression analysis, the terms '**dependent**' and '**independent**' variables are sometimes used in a different sense to describe the **outcome** and **explanatory variables** used in a statistical model (📖 Simple linear regression, p. 296).

Probability: definitions

Why probability is important in medical statistics

The theory of statistics is based on probability theory which was originally used to investigate patterns in gambling games using cards and dice. The theory of statistics underpins medical statistics and probability theory enables us to answer questions in medical research.

Samples and populations

In medical research we often use a sample of individuals rather than the entire population of interest because it is too expensive or is simply not possible to include the whole population. When we do this we use results from the **sample** to draw conclusions about the whole **population.**

Example

Suppose in a clinical trial we find that a sample of patients allocated to a new drug do better on average than those allocated to an old one:
• Is this a real effect?
• Is the observed difference simply due to random variation?
• In other words, to what extent is the observed effect likely to be typical of what would happen in other patient groups?
   Whenever we use a sample to infer something about a population, there is always a **degree of uncertainty** attached to the findings. Probability theory is used to measure this uncertainty and to help to draw conclusions from the sample study (📖 Samples and populations, p. 240).

Definition of probability (frequency definition)
• The proportion of times an event happens in the long run which can be estimated from a proportion calculated in a sample

For example, the proportion of stillbirths out of total births in England and Wales in 2006 was 3602/673 203 = 0.0054. Since this was a census and therefore a large sample, we can use this as an estimate of the probability that a baby born in England and Wales will be stillborn.[1]

Jargon

In statistics we talk about each occurrence of the event of interest as the **event**. So in the example of the probability of a stillbirth, the event is a stillbirth.

The probability of an event is sometimes called the **probability of success** and the total number of 'tries' in which the event could happen is known as the **sample size, _n_** (sometimes called the **number of trials**). So for the stillbirth data, the sample size is the total number of live births and stillbirths (673 203 in the example).

An alternative definition of probability

In the definition just given, probability is interpreted as a relative frequency. The advantage of this is that is usually enables us to estimate probabilities in an objective way. However, this is not always possible and there is a different interpretation of probability as a **degree of belief**. This is more **subjective**, but it is what we commonly do in everyday life: the statement 'I think it's as likely as not to rain today' implies a 50:50 chance of rain which, if based on observing the current weather, is a subjective judgement.

In some situations we do have some prior knowledge about the likelihood of an event and, as long as it can be quantified, it is possible to combine the prior belief with frequency data to give an updated and arguably better estimate of the probability.

This way of thinking can be illustrated when we apply **Bayes' theorem** to diagnostic data and use the prevalence and sensitivity to give the positive predictive value (📖 Bayes' theorem, p. 234; likelihood ratios, pretest odds, post test odds, p. 346). Further application using distributions of degrees of belief to modify data gives rise to the body of statistical methods known as **Bayesian statistics** (📖 Chapter 14 p. 477).

Reference

1 Office for National Statistics. Birth statistics 2006 series FM1 No 35. 2007. Available from: 🕮 www.statistics.gov.uk/STATBASE/Product.asp?vlnk=5768 (accessed 6 Jan 2009).

Probability: properties

Three basic rules of probabilities

1. A probability must lie between 0 and 1 inclusive
2. If two events are mutually exclusive so that they cannot both happen, the probability of either happening is the sum of the individual probabilities
3. If two events are independent then the probability of both occurring is the product of the individual probabilities

---

Interpretation of the properties

1. If a probability is 0 then the event **never happens**.
   If it is 1, the event **always happens**.
2. If two events are **mutually exclusive** then only one can happen.
   For example death and survival are mutually exclusive – a patient cannot both survive and die at the same time.
3. If two events are independent then the fact that one has happened does not affect the chance of the other event happening.
   For example the probability that a pregnant woman gives birth to twins (event 1) and the probability of a white Christmas (event 2). These two events are unconnected since the probability of giving birth to twins is not related to the weather at Christmas.

Examples using coin tossing

Tossing coins is often used to illustrate probability and we will do the same here. We will use the shorthand notation Pr(H) to denote the probability of a head and Pr(T) as the probability of a tail.

Tossing one coin

If we toss a fair coin then it can either come up heads (H) or tails (T). If we toss the same coin several times we will get some heads and some tails. If we toss it many times we will get a similar number of heads as tails, because it is a fair coin.

Hence we can say that the probability of a head is ½ or 0.5,

i.e. Pr(H) = Pr(T) = 0.5

Tossing two coins

If we toss two coins there are four possible outcomes: HH, HT, TH, and TT. The four possible outcomes are all equally likely so the probability is ¼ (or 0.25) for each. Each toss of the coin is independent and so the outcome for the first coin toss does not affect the outcome for the second coin toss. Hence we can use the rules of probability stated above to calculate the following:

Pr(HH) = Pr(H and H) = Pr(H) Pr(H) using rule 3

$$= ½ \times ½ = ¼$$

Now what is the probability of getting one head? There are two different ways of getting one head, either TH or HT, each happening with probability ¼. So using rule 2 (as TH and HT are mutually exclusive):

Pr(1 Head) = Pr(TH or HT) = Pr(TH) + Pr(HT)

$$= ¼ + ¼ = ½$$

Probability distributions

Introduction

A probability distribution is a set of exclusive events that includes all events that can happen. The sum of probabilities is therefore equal to 1 and the set of all possible probabilities make up a **probability distribution**.

From first coin tossing example

When we toss one coin (📖 Tossing one coin, p. 209), we get either H with probability ½ or T with probability ½.

Suppose X is the number of heads in one toss of a coin. X can take the value 0 or 1 and $Pr(X=0) = ½$, $Pr(X=1) = ½$.

This is a simple probability distribution and can be depicted on a graph (Fig. 7.1).

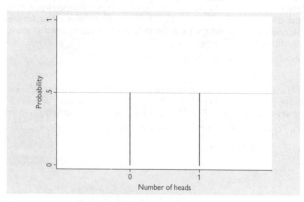

Fig. 7.1 Distribution of the number of heads in one toss of a coin.

From the second coin tossing example

If we toss two coins (📖 Tossing two coins, p. 209), there are four possible outcomes, HH, HT, TH, and TT, each occurring with probability ¼.

If Y is the number of heads, then:

$Pr(Y=0) = ¼$
$Pr(Y=1) = ¼ + ¼ = ½$
$Pr(Y=2) = ¼$

This too is a probability distribution which can be depicted as shown in Figure 7.2.

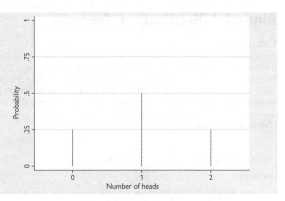

Fig. 7.2 Distribution of the number of heads in two tosses of a coin.

Note that this **probability distribution** is discrete since the number of heads is a count. Each possible value of the number of heads is associated with a particular probability, and is shown as a **vertical line**. As the number of coin tosses increases, there are more lines and the binomial distribution begins to take a stronger shape as can be seen in Figure 7.3 for the distribution of the number of heads out of four coin tosses where there are 16 possible arrangements.

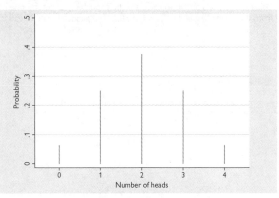

Fig. 7.3 Distribution of the number of heads in four tosses of a coin.

Binomial distribution: formula

Calculations

As the number of coin tosses increases it becomes difficult to list all the possible arrangements and so instead we can use a formula for the Binomial distribution, given below. This allows us to calculate the probability of any particular value of the number of successes (events) as long as we know the **probability of success** and the **total sample size**, n.

Binomial formula

$$\Pr(r \text{ events out of } n) = \frac{n!}{(n-r)!\,r!} p^r (1-p)^{n-r}$$

Where:

n is the sample size (i.e. number of coin tosses, number of people studied etc), r is the number of successes, p is the probability of success

n! is n (n–1) (n–2) ... 2 1 (e.g. 6! = 6×5×4×3×2×1 = 720, 📖 Example: the two parts of the formula, p. 215)

To show that the formula 'works', it is used for the coin tossing example with two coins (Example 1) and then in a more practical example (Example 2).

Example 1: tossing two coins

Using the formula above to calculate the probability of getting one head from two coins tosses: $n=2$, $r=1$, $p=0.5$. The probability of 1 head is:

$$= \frac{2!}{(2-1)!\,1!} 0.5^1 (1-0.5)^{2-1}$$

$$= \frac{2 \ 1}{1 \ 1} 0.5 \ 0.5$$

$$= 2 \times 0.25 = 0.5 \text{ as before when calculating by hand}$$

Example 2: probability of surviving

Suppose the probability of surviving from a particular disease is 0.9 and there are 20 patients. The number surviving will follow a Binomial distribution with $p=0.9$ and $n=20$. What is the probability that no more than 1 patient dies?

This will occur if **either none die (all survive) or only one dies (19 survive)**. This can be calculated as follows:

Probability all survive is $Pr(r=20)$, calculated using the Binomial formula:

$$= \frac{20!}{(20-20)!\,20!}\,0.9^{20}(1-0.9)^{20-20}$$

$$= \frac{20!}{0!\,20!}\,0.9^{20}0.1^{0}$$

$$= 0.9^{20} = 0.12$$

Now we can calculate the probability that 19 survive, $Pr(r=19)$:

$$= \frac{20!}{(20-19)!\,19!}\,0.9^{19}(1-0.9)^{20-19}$$

$$= \frac{20!}{1!\,19!}\,0.9^{19}0.1^{1}$$

$$= 20 \times 0.9^{19} \times 0.1 = 0.27$$

If no more than 1 dies then either all 20 survive or 19 survive. The probability of this is found by **adding** the two separate probabilities:

$Pr(20\ survive) + Pr(19\ survive)$

$= 0.12 + 0.27 = 0.39$

Note that $0! = 1$ (📖 Binomial distribution: derivation, p. 214)

Binomial distribution: derivation

Where the formula comes from

There are two parts to the formula:

(i) The first part:

$$\frac{n!}{r!(n-r)!}$$

This is a standard formula for the number of arrangements of r things out of n.

(ii) The second part

$$p^r(1-p)^{n-r}$$

This is the probability for each individual arrangement of r successes and $n-r$ failures.

Hence the total probability is this probability multiplied by the number of arrangements.

Values of p

In the coin tossing example (📖 Example 1, p. 212), p was 0.5 because we assumed that heads and tails were equally likely. But any value of p between 0 and 1 can be used in the formula as 📖 Example 2, p. 213, showed with a survival probability of 0.9.

Note that no matter what the value of p, the total probability of r successes out of n is the always the same as the probability of $n-r$ failures.

Factorials $n!$

The mathematical expression $n!$ is called 'factorial n' and is the product of all integers between 1 and n.

So $5! = 5 \times 4 \times 3 \times 2 \times 1$

1! is clearly equal to one. Mathematicians make an exception for 0! by defining it as one, so 0! =1.

Example: the two parts of the formula

When tossing two coins we saw that there were two possible ways of getting one head – HT or TH

Using the formula, where $n=2$, $r=1$ we get the same answer:

$$\frac{2!}{1!(2-1)!} = \frac{2 \times 1}{1 \times 1} = 2$$

As we were able to list all four possible combinations of H and T, we could deduce the probability of any one combination as ¼ and so we calculated that the probability of one head was $2 \times ¼ = ½$.

We see that the formula gives the same answer for the probability of any one arrangement of one head:

$0.5^1 \times (1-0.5)^{2-1} = 0.5 \times 0.5 = 0.25$ or ¼

Poisson distribution

Introduction
The Poisson distribution is used widely in statistics for **count data** and is therefore a **discrete distribution**. It is used to describe the distribution of counts of events, such as when specific events happen randomly in time or when small particles are distributed randomly in space. It assumes that the underlying rate is constant.

Example

New cases of disease often happen randomly and the Poisson distribution can be used to compare the counts in a period of time in two or more groups, or to model risk factors for the disease (see 📖 Example of use of Poisson distribution, p. 219, for an example where the risk for lung cancer was modelled using the Poisson distribution).

Formula

If the mean number of events that happen in a single period of time is m then the probability of r events in a single period of time is:

$$Pr(r \text{ events in a single period of time }) = \frac{e^{-m}m^r}{r!}$$

where e^{-m} is the exponential function

Examples of calculations with m=2

- $Pr(0 \text{ events}) = \dfrac{e^{-2}2^0}{0!} = e^{-2} = 0.135$ (to 3 decimal places)

- $Pr(1 \text{ event}) = \dfrac{e^{-2}2^1}{1!} = e^{-2} \times 2 = 0.271$ (to 3 decimal places)

The Poisson distribution with different means
As with the Binomial distribution, the Poisson distribution takes a different shape with different values of its parameter, the mean number of events. We illustrate this in Figure 7.4 with three Poisson distributions with means 1, 5, and 25.

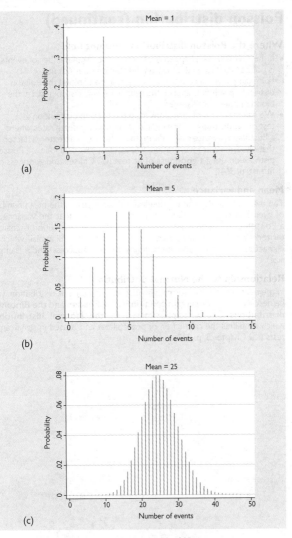

Fig. 7.4a–c Poisson distributions with means 1, 5, and 25.

Poisson distribution (continued)

Where the Poisson distribution does not hold

- If the events do not happen randomly or the mean number of events is not constant, then the Poisson distribution does not fit.
  For example when counting cells in a volume of blood the Poisson distribution will only apply if the cells are evenly distributed, i.e. the blood sample is well stirred
- We can make use of deviations from the Poisson distribution as a test of **randomness.** For example, in monitoring death rates where a fluctuation in rates may indicate the influence of an external factor that needs further investigation. We can test that data follow a Poisson distribution using a **goodness of fit test** (📖 Chi-squared goodness of fit test, p. 364).

Mean and variance

The mean of the Poisson distribution is denoted by m, the mean number of events in single unit time or space. It turns out that the variance of a Poisson distribution is also m. Thus the Poisson distribution is characterized by only one parameter, the mean, unlike the Binomial, which is characterized by two parameters: p (probability of success) and n (sample size).

Relationship to the Normal distribution

In the next section the Normal distribution, a continuous distribution, will be described. **Under certain conditions, the Poisson and the Binomial distributions can be approximated by the Normal distribution**, which simplifies the calculation of probabilities and is used in significance tests (📖 Chapter 8, p. 237).

Example of use of Poisson distribution

A multiethnic cohort study in California and Hawaii, USA, investigated differences in the risk of lung cancer associated with cigarette smoking among 183 813 African American, Japanese American, Latino, Native Hawaiian, and white men and women.[1]

The study assumed that lung cancer rates followed a Poisson distribution. The authors fitted a Poisson regression model in order to estimate the risk of lung cancer among subjects who had never smoked, former smokers, and current smokers, taking into account age, duration and quantity of smoking, sex, ethnic group, occupation, education, and diet.

The results showed that there were statistically significant differences in lung cancer risk by ethnic group among lighter smokers (<30 cigarettes per day) with higher risk among the African American and Native Hawaiian cohorts. There was no evidence for ethnic differences for those smoking more than 30 cigarettes per day.

(For more details on Poisson regression see 📖 Poisson regression, p. 432).

Reference

1 Haiman CA, Stram DO, Wilkens LR, Pike MC, Kolonel LN, Henderson BE *et al.* Ethnic and racial differences in the smoking-related risk of lung cancer. *N Engl J Med* 2006; **354**(4):333–42.

Continuous probability distributions

Introduction

The Binomial and Poisson distributions are discrete distributions followed by discrete variables that can only take a limited set of values. **Continuous probability distributions** are distributions that can take any value between given limits. If we consider a histogram of a continuous variable then we can imagine making the intervals, 'bins', on the x-axis smaller and smaller. The histogram of the data would then begin to look like a **smooth curve** – the probability density (see Fig. 7.5).

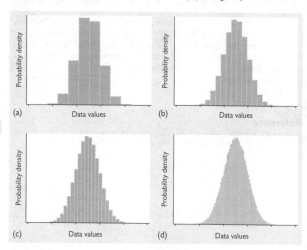

Fig. 7.5a–d Histograms with 10, 20, 30, 100 bins.

Interpreting a continuous probability distribution

- There are an infinite number of possible values for a continuous variable and the probability of any specific value is zero
- The height of the frequency curve cannot then be taken as the probability of a particular value
- Probabilities are determined by measuring the **area under the curve** between two values
- Since the whole curve represents all possible values, the total area under the curve equals one
- For example, the area to the left of the mean for a symmetrical distribution is 0.5, i.e. the probability of a value less than the mean is 0.5

Normal distribution

Introduction

The Normal distribution is a continuous probability distribution that has a symmetrical bell-shape (See Fig. 7.6). The Normal distribution is characterized by the following mathematical function:

$$y = \frac{1}{\sqrt{2\pi}} exp\left(\frac{-x^2}{2}\right)$$

where x is the co-ordinate on the x-axis and y is the probability density. However, the formula is not needed in everyday use since tables or computers are available for calculations (□ Normal distribution: calculating probabilities, p. 224). The important things to know about a Normal distribution are its mean and standard deviation which uniquely characterize it.

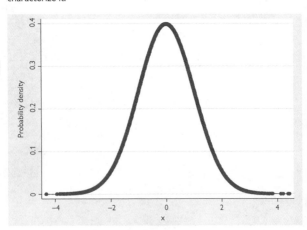

Fig. 7.6 The Standard Normal distribution.

Different Normal distributions

There are an infinite number of possible Normal distributions depending on the mean and standard deviation in a specific situation. However, any Normal distribution can be converted into a standard format, the Standard Normal distribution, which has mean=0 and standard deviation=1 as shown below.

Converting to the Standard Normal distribution

- Any position along the x-axis can be expressed as a number of standard deviations (+ or −) from the mean. This distance is the **Standard Normal deviate** (**SND**) or **Normal score**.
- Any Normal distribution can be therefore converted to the Standard Normal distribution by subtracting the mean from each observation and dividing by the standard deviation, ie

---

Standard Normal deviate (Normal score)

$$\frac{x - \overline{x}}{SD}$$

where x is the observation, $\overline{x}$ is the mean and SD is the standard deviation

---

Normally distributed variables

- Many biomedical variables are Normally distributed, such as height and peak flow rate
- However, some common variables are not Normal, such as weight, serum cholesterol and blood pressure, which are skew

Normal distribution: calculating probabilities

Introduction

Probabilities are obtained by calculating the area under the Normal distribution curve between two values. This requires the use of calculus and can be done using a statistical package or a special table, such as Table 7.1. To calculate probabilities we need to know the mean and standard deviation of the Normal distribution that we are using.

Tables of the Standard Normal distribution

Table 7.1 gives the probability for a value less than x for values of x from -3 to $+3$. So we can see, for example, that the probability that a value less than 0 is 0.5, and the probability that a value less than -2.0 is 0.023. This table assumes that we are using a Standard Normal Distribution, i.e. mean=0 and SD=1. It is the area to the left of x as shown shaded in Figure 7.7.

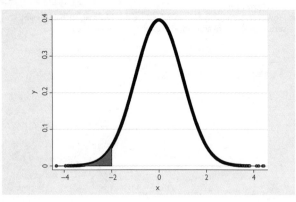

Fig. 7.7 The Standard Normal distribution showing the area in the tail.

Table 7.1 Probabilities for the Standard Normal distribution

X	Probability	x	Probability
−3.0	0.001	0.1	0.540
−2.9	0.002	0.2	0.579
−2.8	0.003	0.3	0.618
−2.7	0.003	0.4	0.655
−2.6	0.005	0.5	0.691
−2.5	0.006	0.6	0.726
−2.4	0.008	0.7	0.758
−2.3	0.011	0.8	0.788
−2.2	0.014	0.9	0.816
−2.1	0.018	1.0	0.841
−2.0	0.023	1.1	0.864
−1.9	0.029	1.2	0.885
−1.8	0.036	1.3	0.903
−1.7	0.045	1.4	0.919
−1.6	0.055	1.5	0.933
−1.5	0.067	1.6	0.945
−1.4	0.081	1.7	0.955
−1.3	0.097	1.8	0.964
−1.2	0.115	1.9	0.971
−1.1	0.136	2.0	0.977
−1.0	0.159	2.1	0.982
−0.9	0.184	2.2	0.986
−0.8	0.212	2.3	0.989
−0.7	0.242	2.4	0.992
−0.6	0.274	2.5	0.994
−0.5	0.309	2.6	0.995
−0.4	0.345	2.7	0.997
−0.3	0.382	2.8	0.997
−0.2	0.421	2.9	0.998
−0.1	0.460	3.0	0.999
0.0	0.500		

Using the table

- The table is symmetrical due to the symmetry of the distribution
- To find the probability of a value lying between two points a and b, where $b>a$, we find $Pr(x<b) − Pr(x<a)$, e.g., probability that x lies between 1.5 and 2.0 is given by:
  $Pr(x<2.0) − Pr(x<1.5) = 0.977 − 0.933 = 0.044$

Normal distribution: percentage points

The Normal distribution is also tabulated using percentage points. The **one-sided p percentage point** of the distribution is the value x such that there is a probability $p\%$ of an observation greater than or equal to x. Similarly, the **two-sided p percentage point** is the value x such that there is a probability $p\%$ of an observation being greater than or equal to x or less than or equal to $-x$. Table 7.2 shows these percentage points.

Table 7.2 Percentage points of the Standard Normal distribution

One-sided		Two-sided	
Percentage	x	Percentage	x
50	0.00		
25	0.67	50	0.67
10	1.28		
5	1.64	10	1.64
2.5	1.96	5	1.96
1	2.33		
0.5	2.58	1	2.58
0.1	3.09		
0.05	3.29	0.1	3.29

Example

The histogram in Figure 7.8 shows the distribution of birthweight among 1400 women who gave birth to term babies. The sample mean was 3397 g and the standard deviation was 445 g. The figure also shows the corresponding Normal curve, i.e. the Normal distribution with the same mean and standard deviation as this set of data. Since the Normal curve is a close fit to the data, it is reasonable to assume that the data follow a Normal distribution and use the Normal distribution to calculate some useful quantities.

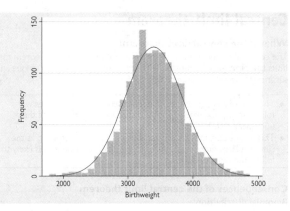

Fig. 7.8 Histogram of the data with corresponding Normal curve.

Calculations

1. Probability of a birthweight less than 2500 g:

To do this we first calculate the Standard Normal deviate (□ Converting to the Standard Normal distribution, p. 223):

$$\frac{2500-3397}{445} = \frac{-897}{445} = -2.02$$

The probability of a value less than −2.02 is 0.0217 and so we estimate that approximately 2.2% of term births are below 2500 g.

2. Calculate the central range:

90% of a Normal distribution lies within the range, mean ± 1.64 standard deviations (SD), 95% within mean ± 1.96 SD and 99% within mean ± 2.58 SD.

For the birthweight data we get the following ranges:

90%	2667 to 4127
95%	2525 to 4269
99%	2249 to 4545

Thus we can use the Normal distribution to estimate centiles of the distribution of birthweight among this population of term births.

Central limit theorem

What is the central limit theorem?

The central limit theorem is a very important mathematical theorem that **links the Normal distribution with other distributions** in a unique and surprising way and is therefore very useful in statistics.

- The sum of a large number of independent random variables will follow an approximately Normal distribution irrespective of their underlying distributions
- This means that any random variable which can be regarded as the sum of a large number of small, independent contributions is likely to follow the Normal distribution

Consequences of the central limit theorem

Binomial distribution:

- The Normal distribution can be used as an approximation to the Binomial distribution **when n is large**
- **In practice** this works if np **and** $n(1-p)$ **are both greater than 5** (where np and $n(1-p)$ are number of successes and number of failures)

Poisson distribution:

- The Normal distribution can be used as an approximation to the Poisson distribution **as the mean of the Poisson distribution increases**
- **In practice** this works when the **mean is greater than 10**

Advantages of using the Normal distribution

The main advantage in using the Normal rather than the Binomial or the Poisson distribution is that it makes it easier to calculate probabilities and confidence intervals (📖 Chapter 8, p. 237).

Central limit theorem (continued)

Illustrations: Binomial distribution

We can see from the histograms of the Binomial distribution with p=0.5 (Fig. 7.9) that as *n* increases from 1 to 2 to 4, that the Binomial distribution becomes more symmetrical and more closely resembles the Normal distribution.

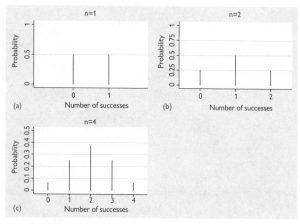

Fig. 7.9a–c Binomial distribution with p=0.5 and increasing values of *n*.

Illustrations: Poisson distribution

In a similar way, the histograms in Figure 7.10 show that as the Poisson mean increases from 1 to 5 and then to 25, the distribution becomes more symmetrical and looks more like the Normal distribution.

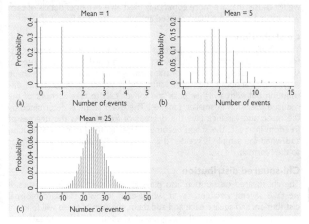

Fig. 7.10a–c Poisson distribution with increasing values of the mean.

Other distributions: t, chi-squared, F, etc.

There are many other probability distributions used in statistics. Below we list those that are more commonly used. We give brief details of each with examples of how they are used and what they look like.

t distribution

The t distribution plays an important role in statistics as the sampling distribution of the sample mean divided by its standard error and is used in significance testing (📖 Tests of statistical significance, p. 246). The shape is symmetrical about the mean value, and is similar to the Normal distribution but with a higher peak and longer tails to take account of the reduced precision in smaller samples. The exact shape is determined by the mean and variance plus the degrees of freedom. As the degrees of freedom increase, the shape becomes closer to the Normal distribution and when the sample is greater than 30, the t distribution is very similar to the Normal.

Chi-squared distribution

The chi-squared distribution also plays an important role in statistics. If we take several variables, say n, which each follow a standard Normal distribution, and square each and add them, the sum of these will follow a chi-squared distribution with n degrees of freedom. This theoretical result is very useful and widely used in statistical testing, particularly the chi-squared test (📖 Chi-squared test, p. 262). The chi-squared distribution is always positive and its shape is uniquely determined by the degrees of freedom. The distribution becomes more symmetrical as the degrees of freedom increases.

F distribution

This is the distribution of the ratio of two chi-squared distributions and is used in hypothesis testing when we want to compare variances, such as in doing analysis of variance (📖 One-way analysis of variance, p. 280). It is always positive, but the exact shape depends on the degrees of freedom for the two chi-squared distributions that determine it.

Uniform distribution

The uniform distribution has a rectangular shape so that each possible value occurs with equal probability within a given range. It can be useful in Bayesian analysis as the prior distribution of an unknown parameter where all values within a given range are thought to be equally likely (📖 Prior distributions, p. 482).

Lognormal distribution

Sometimes data may follow a positively skewed distribution which becomes a Normal distribution when each data point is log-transformed (using logarithms to base e). In this case the original data can be said to follow a lognormal distribution. The transformation of such data from lognormal to Normal is very useful in allowing skewed data to be analysed using methods based on the Normal distribution since these are usually more powerful than alternative methods (📖 Transforming data, p. 330).

Other distributions

Other distribution used by statisticians and which may be referred to in research articles are listed below. The full details of these distributions are beyond the scope of this book. Some are forms of other distributions that we have already discussed:

- Half-Normal distribution – Normal distribution with mean 0, cut at zero
- Bivariate Normal distribution – distribution followed jointly by two Normal variables
- Negative binomial distribution
- Beta distribution
- Gamma distribution

Summary: general features of probability distributions

Probability distributions
- Underpin many of the methods and tests used in medical statistics
- Are used to calculate probabilities
- Have a shape which is uniquely defined by specific parameters such as the mean, variance, sample size and degrees of freedom

Further reading

Further details of probability and probability distributions can be found in Bland, Chapter 6,[1] and Armitage, Chapter 2.[2]

References

1 Bland M. *An introduction to medical statistics.* 3rd ed. Oxford: Oxford University Press, 2000.
2 Armitage P, Berry G, Matthews JNS. *Statistical methods in medical research.* 4th ed. Oxford: Blackwell Science, 2002.

Bayes' theorem

Conditional probability

A conditional probability is a probability of one event happening given that another event has also happened. For example, we may wish to know the probability that a patient has a particular disease given that they have a positive result on a diagnostic test. This conditional probability can be calculated using Bayes' theorem.

Note that it is not the same as the underlying probability of having the disease and neither is it the same as the probability of a patient getting a positive test result if they have the disease. We give some examples here.

Bayes' theorem

Bayes' theorem enables us to reverse conditional probabilities and underpins the Bayesian statistical methods described in 📖 Chapter 14, p. 477).

Notation:

- We have two events A and B
- $Pr(A|B)$ means 'the probability of A happening given that B has already happened'. This is often shortened to 'the probability of A given B'

Bayes' theorem formula

$$Pr(A \mid B) = \frac{Pr(B \mid A) \times Pr(A)}{Pr(B)}$$

---

❶ The probability of A given B, Pr(A|B), is NOT the same as the probability of B given A, Pr(B|A), unless Pr(A)=Pr(B).

Example: conditional probabilities and court cases

Conditional probabilities are sometimes used in court cases but not always correctly. People tend to assume that just because those found guilty of a particular crime in the past tend to have a particular characteristic, then anyone subsequently arrested and who has that characteristic, must therefore be guilty.

The incorrect logic is shown in this hypothetical scenario:
House burglars are often small and agile, but if a suspect is small and agile, then he is not necessarily guilty on that basis alone. Many people are small and agile, but only a small proportion of small agile people are house burglars.

Example: conditional probabilities and diagnostic testing

Bayes' theorem can be used to calculate the conditional probability that a patient with a positive result on a diagnostic test really has the disease. (For more details of diagnostic tests, sensitivity and specificity, positive and negative predictive value, see 📖 Chapter 9 p. 339).

A study investigated a new D-dimer test for the diagnosis of venous thromboembolism (VTE):[1]
The **sensitivity** was found to be 0.79
The **prevalence** of VTE among those studied (VTE+) was 0.14
The **probability** of getting a positive test (D+) was 0.32

Therefore the probability of VTE given a positive test is:

$$Pr(VTE+ \mid D+) = \frac{Pr(D+ \mid VTE+)\, Pr(VTE+)}{Pr(D+)}$$

$$= \frac{sensitivity \times prevalence}{probability\ of\ positive\ test} = \frac{0.79 \times 0.14}{0.32} = 0.346 = 34.6\%$$

This probability is the **positive predictive value** of the test.

Reference

1 Kovacs MJ, Mackinnon KM, Anderson D, O'Rourke K, Keeney M, Kearon C et al. A comparison of three rapid D-dimer methods for the diagnosis of venous thromboembolism. *Br J Haematol* 2001; **115**(1):140–4.

Statistical tests

Introduction

Statistical tests are widely used to evaluate numerical evidence. In this chapter we discuss the rationale behind statistical tests and explain how estimates, P values, and confidence intervals are used to make inferences about a population using sample data in a variety of situations. All statistical tests and methods are described in terms of when to use them, what assumptions are involved, and how the results can be presented and interpreted. Formulae are given for the most common simple tests to allow the reader to do the tests themselves and to understand the mathematics behind them should they wish. More complex statistical methods and tests are included largely without formulae. The emphasis is on the correct use of statistics and the interpretation of statistical results. All methods are illustrated with examples and references are given for further details.

Samples and populations

Introduction

In research studies it is common to wish to draw general conclusions from a relatively small amount of data. We often have only a subset or sample (Fig. 8.1) of the whole population that we are really interested in. This is usually because it is impractical or impossible to study the whole population. If we are answering specific questions or hypotheses then the answers will tell us something about the whole population but, because we only have a sample, the answer will be imprecise in some sense. In other words data collected from the sample will never be able to provide full information about the whole population.

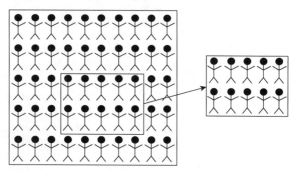

Fig. 8.1 Drawing a sample from a larger population.

Dealing with uncertainty

There will always be an element of uncertainty when we do not have 'all' of the data. Statistical methods based on probability theory are therefore used to quantify this uncertainty:

- If we are estimating some quantity from our data, for example, the proportion of patients who have a particular attribute, then we can quantify the imprecision in the estimate using a **confidence interval**
- If we are testing a hypothesis, for example, comparing blood pressure in two groups, then we can do a **statistical significance test** which helps us to weigh the evidence that the sample difference we have observed is in fact a real difference

Sampling distributions

The concept of a distribution for individual values can be extended to the hypothetical situation where there are different samples all taken from the same population. If we select one sample from a population and calculate the mean value, then the sample mean will provide some information about the overall mean in the population.

Sampling distribution of the mean

In general, different samples from the same population will give different means and so when we only choose one sample, as we usually do, we get only one of a range of possible means. Hence in a theoretical way we can imagine that if we looked at all possible samples and calculated their sample means, then we could look at the distribution of these sample means. This distribution is called the **sampling distribution of the mean**.

These sampling distributions are interpreted in a similar way to data distributions: values of sample means close to the overall population mean are more likely (more common) than extreme values.

Summary points

- Sample data are used to draw conclusions about populations
- Sample data are imprecise – estimates vary from sample to sample
- Statistical tests and confidence intervals allow us to take the imprecision into account
- Note that statistical analysis, however, sophisticated, cannot correct poor study design

---

Confidence interval for a mean

Standard error of the mean

Suppose we selected many samples, then the sample means would follow a distribution known as the **sampling distribution of the mean**. We could calculate the mean of these sample means, and the standard deviation. The standard deviation of the sample means is known as the **standard error of the mean** and provides an estimate of the precision of the sample mean.

Standard error of the sample mean SE (mean)

$$\frac{SD}{\sqrt{n}}$$

where SD is the standard deviation for the data and n is the sample size

Note as n increases, SE decreases and so precision is greater for larger samples

---

The standard error of the mean is sometimes denoted by 'se' or 'SE', or 'SEM'. The derivation of this can be found in Bland, Chapter 8.[1] If the samples are large then the sample means will follow a Normal distribution because of the **central limit theorem** (📖 Central limit theorem, p. 228). Therefore we can use the Normal distribution to calculate a range of possible values for the true population mean. The 95% confidence interval is calculated using the formula below. The derivation of this formula can be found in Bland, Chapter 8.[1]

95% confidence interval for a mean from a large sample

   mean − 1.96 SE (mean)   to   *mean + 1.96 SE (mean)*

Choice of percentage for confidence intervals (CI)

- 95% is the most commonly used percentage for CIs and the multiplier is **1.96 for large samples** (📖 What is a large sample, p. 244)
- Other percentages can be used such as 90% or 99%
- 90% CI has a probability of 90% of containing the true value and uses the multiplier **1.64** rather than 1.96
- 99% CI has a probability of 99% of containing the true value and uses the multiplier **2.58**

How to interpret the 95% confidence interval (95% CI)

- A 95% CI is a range of values which has a 95% probability of containing the true population value in the sense that if an infinite number of samples were drawn to estimate the value of interest, 95% of their 95% CIs would contain the true population value
- In other words, we have 95% confidence that the true value in the population from which the sample was taken lies within the 95% CI
- Hence a 95% CI is a margin of error around the estimate that indicates how precise the estimate is.

Example

Suppose we have a sample of 1513 babies and we calculate their mean birthweight:

Mean = 3325g
SD   = 528g

95% CI given by:

$$mean - 1.96\ SE\ (mean) \quad to \quad mean + 1.96\ SE(mean)$$

$$3325 - 1.96 \times \frac{528}{\sqrt{1513}} \quad to \quad 3325 + 1.96 \times \frac{528}{\sqrt{1513}}$$

$$3298 \quad to \quad 3352$$

Hence from these data we can be 95% confident that the population mean birthweight lies between 3298 g and 3352 g

Reference

1 Bland M. *An introduction to medical statistics.* 3rd ed. Oxford: Oxford University Press, 2000.

95% confidence interval for a proportion

Standard error of a proportion

As the sample size increases, the sampling distribution of any estimated quantity is Normal. This property is used to calculate confidence intervals for means and other estimates. Using this we can calculate the standard error of a proportion and then estimate the 95% confidence interval for a sample proportion. Suppose a certain proportion in the population has a condition. If we have n individuals altogether and r with the condition then we estimate the population proportion by $p = r/n$. The standard error of the proportion is given by:

Standard error of a proportion $SE(p)$

$$\sqrt{p(1-p)/n}$$

The 95% confidence interval for a proportion uses the Normal distribution assuming that the sample is large. The derivation of these formulae can be found in Bland, Chapter 8.[1]

95% confidence interval for a proportion from a large sample

$p - 1.96\ SE(p)$ to $p + 1.96\ SE(p)$

How to interpret 95% confidence interval for a proportion

- A 95% confidence interval for a proportion is a range of values which has 95% probability of containing the true population proportion
- In other words, we have 95% confidence that the true value of the proportion in the population from which the sample was taken lies within the interval

---

What is a large sample?

- **Means**: for a sample mean, a sample size of 100 is considered large and will lead to the sample mean following an approximately Normal distribution irrespective of the underlying distribution of the data. In this case the multiplier 1.96 can be used to calculate confidence intervals. If the sample is smaller than this, the data needs to follow a Normal distribution and the t distribution is used to calculate the confidence interval (see Bland, Chapter 10[1]).
- **Proportions:** for a sample proportion, the sample size can be considered large if r and $n - r$ are both greater than 5. If this does not hold, an exact Binomial confidence interval can be calculated[2].

Example

An Australian study compared the prevalence of asthma and allergy in schoolchildren over a 20-year period.[3] The researchers reported the prevalence of diagnosed asthma in 2002 as 31% (249/804). What is the 95% confidence interval for this estimate?

$r/n = 249/804 = 0.310$

95% CI given by:-

$$0.310 - 1.96\sqrt{0.310(1-0.310)/804} \quad \text{to}$$

$$0.310 + 1.96\sqrt{0.310(1-0.310)/804}$$

$0.310 - 1.96 \times 0.016 \quad \text{to} \quad 0.310 + 1.96 \times 0.016$

$0.28 \quad \text{to} \quad 0.34$

or 28% to 34%

Therefore the prevalence of diagnosed asthma is 31% (95% CI: 28% to 34%).

References

1 Bland M. *An introduction to medical statistics.* 3rd ed. Oxford: Oxford University Press, 2000.

2 Altman DG, Machin D, Bryant TN, Gardner MJ. *Statistics with confidence: confidence intervals and statistical guide.* London: BMJ Publishing Group, 2000.

3 Toelle BG, Ng K, Belousova E, Salome CM, Peat JK, Marks GB. Prevalence of asthma and allergy in schoolchildren in Belmont, Australia: three cross sectional surveys over 20 years. *BMJ* 2004; **328**(7436):386–7.

Tests of statistical significance

Rationale

A significance test uses data from a sample to show the likelihood that a hypothesis about a population is true. There are always two mutually exclusive hypotheses since, if the hypothesis being tested is not true, then the opposite hypothesis must be true. A measure of the evidence for or against the hypothesis is provided by a **P value**.

Null hypothesis and alternate hypothesis

The **null hypothesis** is the baseline hypothesis which is usually of the form 'there is no difference' or 'there is no association'. The corresponding **alternative hypothesis** is 'there is a difference' or 'there is an association'.

Examples

- Does a new treatment reduce blood pressure more than an existing treatment?
  The null hypothesis is that mean blood pressure is the same in the two treatment groups
  The alternative hypothesis is that mean blood pressure is different in the two treatment groups
- Is there an association between blood pressure and risk of cardiovascular disease?
  The null hypothesis is that there is no association between blood pressure and risk of cardiovascular disease
  The alternative hypothesis is that blood pressure is associated with a change in risk of cardiovascular disease

Two-sided tests (two-tailed tests)

In the examples above, the alternative hypothesis is general and allows the difference to be in either direction. In the first example, patients given the new treatment could have lower mean blood pressure or they could have higher mean blood pressure. This is known as a **two-sided or two-tailed test.**

One-sided tests (one-tailed tests)

In the first example, **a one-sided or one-tailed test** could have the alternative hypothesis that mean blood pressure is lower in patients taking the new treatment than patients taking the existing treatment.

This means that the **null hypothesis is now composite** and that either the two groups have the same mean blood pressure or that patients taking the existing treatment have lower blood pressure. In other words, a one-sided test does not distinguish between 'no difference' and a 'harmful effect' of the new treatment. In virtually all situations this would be unacceptable, since it is important to know if a new treatment is harmful.

Two-sided tests should always be used unless there is clear justification at the outset to use a one-sided test.

Steps in doing a significance test (adapted from Bland, Chapter 9[1])

1. Specify the hypothesis of interest as a null and alternative hypothesis
2. Decide what statistical test is appropriate
3. Use the test to calculate the P value
4. Weigh the evidence from the P value in favour of the null or alternative hypothesis

Errors in significance testing

- Since a significance test uses sample data to make inferences about populations, **using the results from a sample may lead to wrong conclusion.**
- **Type 1 error**: this is getting a significant result in a sample when the null hypothesis is in fact true in the underlying population ('false significant' result).
- We usually set a limit of 0.05 (5%) for the probability of a type 1 error, which is equivalent to a 0.05 cut-off for statistical significance.
- **Type 2 error**: this is getting a non-significant result in a sample when the null hypothesis is in fact false in the underlying population ('false non-significant' result).
  It is widely accepted that the probability of a type 2 error should be no more than 0.20 (20%).

Reference

1 Bland M. *An introduction to medical statistics.* 3rd ed. Oxford: Oxford University Press, 2000.

P values

What is a P value?

- A P value is a probability, and therefore lies between 0 and 1
- It comes from a statistical test that is testing a particular null hypothesis
- It expresses the weight of evidence in favour of or against the stated null hypothesis
- **Precise definition**: P value is the probability, given that the null hypothesis is true, of obtaining data as extreme or more extreme than that observed
- 0.05 or 5% is commonly used as a cut-off, such that if the observed P is less than this (P<0.05) we consider that there is good evidence that the null hypothesis is not true. This is directly related to the type 1 error rate.
- If 0.05 is the cut-off then P<0.05 is commonly described as **statistically significant** and P≥0.05 is described as **not statistically significant**

Interpreting significant results (P<0.05)

The calculation of a statistical significance test assumes that the null hypothesis is true. Hence the P value expresses the probability of getting the given data if that hypothesis were in fact true. In this way, a very small P value indicates that the observed data are not consistent with the null hypothesis – they are unlikely to have occurred if the null hypothesis were really true. It is in this sense that the P value provides evidence for or against the null hypothesis.

❶ A P value is not the probability that the null hypothesis is true.

Interpreting non-significant results (P≥0.05)

If P is greater than or equal to 0.05 then we usually say the finding is not significant. We cannot take this to mean that the null hypothesis is in fact true. We can only conclude that there is insufficient evidence to show a difference. This distinction is important because small samples often show non-significant differences simply because there are too few data (type 2 error). It may be misleading and wrong to conclude that in such cases, 'not significant' means 'there is no real difference'. Such incorrect interpretation of non-significance may lead to real differences being missed.

If a study is large and adequately powered, and the calculated confidence interval excludes any clinically important difference, then only in this case is it reasonable to conclude that there is no meaningful difference (📖 Statistical significance and clinical significance, p. 250).

Reporting P values

It is best always to report the exact P value from a test rather than report findings as P<0.05 or P≥0.05 or worse 'P=NS' (meaning non-significant). If the exact P value is given, then the readers have all of the available evidence and can interpret the findings themselves. The evidence provided by P=0.045, which would be regarded as statistically significant, is hardly different from the evidence provided by P=0.055, which would be regarded as non-significant. If the exact value is always provided this allows a full interpretation of the evidence.

In addition, estimates and confidence intervals should be given wherever possible.

Summary points
- A P value is the probability of observing data as extreme or more extreme than that observed, if the null hypothesis is true
- P<0.05 is usually regarded as statistically significant and P≥0.05 regarded as non-significant
- Not significant does not mean 'there is no difference' or 'there is no effect'. It means there is insufficient evidence for a difference or effect
- Exact P values should be given with estimates and confidence intervals wherever possible

---

Statistical significance and clinical significance

Statistical significance

Much caution is needed in interpreting statistical significance because the size of the P value is driven by the following factors:

- The size of the real effect in the population sampled
- The sample size
- The variability of the measure involved

Large samples are more likely to show a significant difference. In such cases it is possible for data to show a statistically significant result when the size of the effect is too small to be clinically important. Therefore it is important to look at the size of effect and confidence interval as well as the P values when interpreting a test result.

Clinical significance

This indicates that the difference observed is large enough to be clinically meaningful. It is not necessarily related to statistical significance as it is a clinical judgement and not a mathematical quantity.

A set of data may not show a statistically significant effect but the effect size may suggest that a meaningful difference is plausible. While a conclusive interpretation cannot be made in such circumstances, it may be a useful pointer to the need for further data.

Inspect the data

▶ It is important to look at the data and the summary statistics as well as the statistical test results. Interpretation of statistical significance alone as implying clinical importance may lead to incorrect interpretation of data.

Summary points

- Statistical significance does not necessarily imply the differences observed are clinically meaningful
- Non-significant results may be suggestive of clinically important effects
- Inspect summary statistics – effect sizes and confidence intervals – as well as P values

t test for two independent means

Details of the test
- It compares means from two independent samples
- It is based on the sampling distribution of the difference of two sample means (Normal)
- It allows the calculation of a difference and confidence interval for the difference
- The formula is given below, although the test can be done using a computer program
- For derivation and more details of test, see Bland, Chapter 10[1]

Null hypothesis
- Two samples come from populations with the same mean

Assumptions of test
- Continuous data, Normally distributed. The data can be checked visually for symmetry using a dot plot, histogram, or Normal plot
- Variances (standard deviations) are the same. This can be checked by inspecting the standard deviations. If they are different, the Satterthwaite approximation, available in some statistical programs, may be used
- Note, there are significance tests available to check for Normality and for similarity of variance (standard deviation). However, these are not very helpful guides as they are often non-significant for small samples even when there appears to be non-Normality or differences in variance, and they tend to be significant for large samples even if the skewness or differences in variance appear to be minor.

If assumptions do not hold
- **The statistical test is dubious and the P value may be wrong**
- Try **transformation of data** (📖 Transforming data, p. 330)
- Note that the t test is quite robust to slight skewness if two samples are the same size but is less robust if variances are clearly different
- Skewness and non-similar standard deviation often go together and correcting one by transforming the data may correct the other as well

The t distribution
- Has one parameter, the **degrees of freedom**
- 'Degrees of freedom' is related to the sample size = n_1+n_2-2 here
- There is no single t distribution. Each n_1+n_2-2 gives a different shape
- For large n_1+n_2-2 (>100), the t distribution is close to the Normal distribution

Note that the test is also known as two-sample t test.

Doing a t test for means

$$t = \frac{\text{difference in means}}{SE\ (\text{difference})} = \frac{\overline{X}_1 - \overline{X}_2}{\sqrt{\dfrac{SD_p^2}{n_1} + \dfrac{SD_p^2}{n_2}}}$$

Where $\overline{X}_1$, $\overline{X}_2$ are the means, SD_p is the pooled standard deviation calculated from the group SDs, SD_1 and SD_2 (see below) and n_1, n_2 are the totals in the two groups.

$$SD_p = \sqrt{\frac{(n_1 - 1)SD_1^2 + (n_2 - 1)SD_2^2}{n_1 + n_2 - 2}}$$

t follows a Student's t distribution with $n_1 + n_2 - 2$ degrees of freedom. P values are obtained from tabulated values of the t distribution or a computer program.

Calculating a 95% confidence interval for the difference:

$$\text{difference in means} \pm t_{(n_1 + n_2 - 2)}\ SE(\text{difference in means})$$

$$= (\overline{X}_1 - \overline{X}_2) \pm t_{(n_1 + n_2 - 2)} \sqrt{\frac{SD_p^2}{n_1} + \frac{SD_p^2}{n_2}}$$

Where the value of $t_{(n_1 + n_2 - 2)}$ is the two-tailed 5% point of the t distribution with $n_1 + n_2 - 2$ degrees of freedom.

Reference
1 Bland M. *An introduction to medical statistics*. 3rd ed. Oxford: Oxford University Press, 2000.

t test for two independent means: example

The following data come from a small study of risk factors for bronchopulmonary dysplasia (BPD) in preterm babies and compares a measure of lung function, forced residual capacity (FRC), in infants with and without BPD. The FRC data have been log-transformed ([📖] Transforming data, p. 330) as they were skewed. The data were:

Group 1 No BPD: n, mean (SD): 38, 3.028 (0.276)
Group 2 BPD: n, mean (SD): 27, 2.744 (0.240)

$$SD_p = \sqrt{\frac{(n_1 - 1)SD_1^2 + (n_2 - 1)SD_2^2}{n_1 + n_2 - 2}}$$

$$= \sqrt{\frac{(38 - 1) \times 0.276^2 + (27 - 1) \times 0.240^2}{38 + 27 - 2}} = 0.2617$$

$$t = \frac{\overline{X}_1 - \overline{X}_2}{\sqrt{\frac{SD_p^2}{n_1} + \frac{SD_p^2}{n_2}}} = \frac{3.028 - 2.744}{\sqrt{\frac{0.2617^2}{38} + \frac{0.2617^2}{27}}} = 4.31$$

t follows a t distribution with 38+27−2=63 degrees of freedom. The P value associated with this is 0.0001 (from computer program).

95% confidence interval for the difference:

$$3.028 - 2.744 \pm 1.998 \times \sqrt{\frac{0.2617^2}{38} + \frac{0.2617^2}{27}} = 0.284 \pm 0.132$$

$$= 0.152 \text{ to } 0.416$$

Thus there is a significant difference of 0.284 in mean FRC (log scale). between infants without and with BPD with 95% CI 0.152 to 0.416.

Checking the assumptions

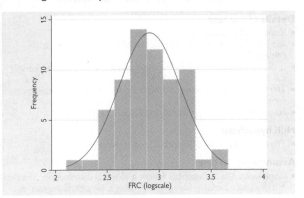

Fig. 8.2 Histogram of FRC (log scale) with the equivalent Normal distribution curve.

- Figure 8.2 shows that the data are close to symmetry and the assumption of a Normal distribution is reasonable
- The two standard deviations, 0.240 and 0.276 are similar
- Therefore the t test assumptions hold for these data
- The data were transformed for analysis but have not been back-transformed here. See 📖 Transforming data, p. 330 for how to back-transform these data

---

t test for large sample sizes

Note that with a large sample size (>50 per group), the assumptions of the two-sample t test are less critical to the validity of the test but a transformation is still worth doing with skewed data to achieve maximum statistical power and to improve the coverage of the 95% confidence interval.

Extension of t method

The t test for two independent means compares means in two groups. The method can be extended to compare more than two groups using a technique called one-way analysis of variance (📖 One-way analysis of variance, p. 280).

t test for paired (matched) data

Details of the test
- It analyses mean difference in a paired sample
- It is based on the sampling distribution of the mean difference (Normal)
- It allows the calculation of a mean difference and confidence interval for the difference
- The formula is given below, although the test can be done using a computer program
- For derivation and more details see Bland, Chapter 10[1]

Null hypothesis
- The mean change or difference is zero in the population

Assumptions of test
- Continuous data, **differences follow a Normal distribution**. The data can be checked visually for symmetry using a dot plot, histogram, or Normal plot
- Variances (standard deviations) are constant – check by plot of difference against mean, i.e. plot $(x_1 - x_2)$ against $(x_1 + x_2)/2$. This should show an even spread for $(x_1 - x_2)$ across the range of values of $(x_1 + x_2)/2$

If assumptions do not hold
- **The statistical test is dubious and the P value may be wrong**
- Try **transformation of data** ([📖] Transforming data, p. 330) – **transform the raw data not the differences**
- Note that paired t test only requires the differences to be Normal. Sometimes the original data can be skewed but when a difference or change is calculated, the difference may be Normally distributed

Note that the test is also known as one-sample t test.

Doing a paired t test

$$t = \frac{\text{mean difference}}{SE(\text{mean difference})} = \frac{\bar{d}}{\sqrt{\dfrac{SD^2}{n}}}$$

Where if $x_{i1} - x_{i2} = d_i$, then the mean of the difference d_i is $\bar{d}$, SD^2 is the standard deviation of the differences, n is the sample size.

t follows a t distribution with $n-1$ degrees of freedom

95% Confidence interval for the mean difference

mean difference $\pm t_{n-1}$ SE (mean difference)

$$= \bar{d} - t_{n-1}\sqrt{\frac{SD^2}{n}} \ to \ \bar{d} + t_{n-1}\sqrt{\frac{SD^2}{n}}$$

Where t_{n-1} is the two-tailed 5% point of the t distribution with $n-1$ degrees of freedom, which is obtained from tables or a statistical program.

References

1 Bland M. *An introduction to medical statistics.* 3rd ed. Oxford: Oxford University Press, 2000.
2 Altman DG, Machin D, Bryant TN, Gardner MJ. *Statistics with confidence: confidence intervals and statistical guidelines.* London: BMJ Publishing Group, 2000.

t test for paired data: example

Calculations

The following data are plasma cotinine levels (log scale) in 181 women measured at two points in pregnancy. The t test is used to investigate whether their cotinine levels change over pregnancy, calculating the change from early to late pregnancy. Cotinine is reported here on a logarithmic scale (log ng/ml).

Mean difference (early-late) = 0.151
SD of difference = 0.456

$$t = \frac{0.151}{\sqrt{\dfrac{0.456^2}{181}}} = 4.46$$

This has 180 degrees of freedom (i.e. 181 − 1) and a P value <0.0001

The 95% confidence interval is given by:

$$0.151 \pm 1.96\sqrt{\frac{0.456^2}{181}}$$

0.085 to 0.217

So there is good evidence that women's cotinine level decreases from early to late pregnancy by an average of 0.15 log ng/ml (95% CI: 0.09 to 0.22).

Checking the assumptions
- Fig. 8.3a shows that the data closely fit the Normal distribution
- Fig. 8.3b shows that the variability is reasonably similar across the range of values of the mean difference
- The paired t test assumptions hold for these data

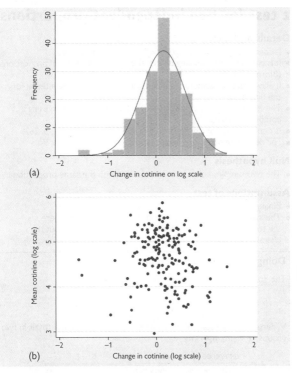

Fig. 8.3 (a) Histogram of change in plasma cotinine (log scale) with the equivalent Normal distribution curve; (b) scatter plot of change in cotinine against the mean.

Paired t test for large sample sizes

Note that with a large sample size (>100 paired observations) the assumptions of the paired t test are less critical to the validity of the test but a transformation is still worth doing with skewed data to achieve maximum statistical power and to improve the coverage of the 95% confidence interval.

---

z test for two independent proportions

Details of the test
- It compares proportions from two independent samples
- It is based on the sampling distribution of the difference of proportions (Normal)
- It allows the calculation of a difference and a confidence interval for the difference
- The formula is given below, although the test can be done using a computer program
- Is equivalent to the chi-squared test (📖 Chi-squared test, p. 262)
- For derivation and more details of test see Bland, Chapter 9[1]

Null hypothesis
- The two samples come from populations with the same proportion

Assumptions of test
- Binary data
- The sample is large: r, $n-r$ are both >5 for each group where r is the total with the characteristic and $n-r$ is the total without the characteristic (see below)

Doing a z test for proportions

The common proportion is given by:

$$p = \frac{r_1 + r_2}{n_1 + n_2}$$

Where r_1, r_2 are totals with characteristic, n_1, n_2 are overall totals in two groups; $p_1 = r_1/n_1$, $p_2 = r_2/n_2$

$$z = \frac{difference\ of\ proportions}{SE(difference\ of\ proportions)} = \frac{p_1 - p_2}{\sqrt{p(1-p)\left(\frac{1}{n_1} + \frac{1}{n_2}\right)}}$$

z follows a Normal distribution with mean 0 and standard deviation 1 when the null hypothesis is true. The P value is the probability of a value less than $-z$ and greater than $+z$ for a two-sided test. This can be obtained from tables or a computer program.

A 95% confidence interval for the difference can be calculated:

$$(p_1 - p_2) - 1.96\sqrt{\left(\frac{p_1(1-p_1)}{n_1} + \frac{p_2(1-p_2)}{n_2}\right)}$$

to

$$(p_1 - p_2) + 1.96\sqrt{\left(\frac{p_1(1-p_1)}{n_1} + \frac{p_2(1-p_2)}{n_2}\right)}$$

Example

A clinical trial for pain relief during venepuncture compared EMLA cream applied 5 minutes before injection with a placebo cream. The outcome analysed here is the proportion reporting with no pain.

Group 1 EMLA: $p_1 = 25/30 = 0.83$
Group 2 Placebo: $p_2 = 20/30 = 0.67$

$$p = \frac{25 + 20}{30 + 30} = 0.75$$

$$p_1 - p_2 = 5/30 = 0.1667$$

$$z = \frac{0.1667}{\sqrt{0.75(1 - 0.75)\left(\frac{1}{30} + \frac{1}{30}\right)}}$$

$$= 1.49$$

The P value associated with z=1.49 is 0.136 and so this difference is not significant. We therefore conclude that there is insufficient evidence from these data that EMLA for 5 minutes is effective. The 95% CI is:

$$0.1667 \pm 1.96\sqrt{\left(\frac{0.83(1 - 0.83)}{30} + \frac{0.67(1 - 0.67)}{30}\right)} = -0.048 \text{ to } 0.382$$

Note the 95% CI is quite wide because the samples are relatively small.

Reference

1 Bland M. *An introduction to medical statistics.* 3rd ed. Oxford: Oxford University Press, 2000.

Chi-squared test

Details of the test
- In general it tests for an association between two categorical variables
- Where each variable has only two categories this is equivalent to the z test for two proportions
- The test is based on the **chi-squared distribution with n degrees of freedom** where n is given by (no. of rows − 1) × (no. of columns − 1)
- It gives a P value but no direct estimate or confidence interval for the estimates unlike the z test, which gives both (📖 z test for two independent proportions, p. 260)
- For more details of test see Bland, Chapter 13[1]

Null hypothesis
- There is no association between the two variables in the population from which the samples come

Rationale of test
- It calculates the frequencies that would be expected if there were no association (i.e. null hypothesis is true)
- It compares the observed frequencies with these expected values
- If the observed frequencies are very different to the expected values this provides evidence that there is an association
- The test uses a formula based on the chi-squared distribution to give a P value

Assumptions of test
- Large sample test
- Rule of thumb for test to be valid:
  at least 80% of expected frequencies must be greater than 5
- **For a 2x2 test this means all expected values must be >5**
- If assumptions don't hold, consider collapsing the table if multi-category, use chi-squared with continuity correction (see 📖 Yates' correction, p. 263) or Fisher's exact test (📖 Fisher's exact test, p. 266)

Doing a chi-squared test
- ❶ **Always use with frequencies, never use percentages for calculations**
- The formula used works for a chi-squared test for all size tables
- The test is usually done with a computer program – the calculations are done to show how the test works

Yates' correction

The chi-squared test is based on frequencies which are discrete whilst the chi-squared distribution is continuous. The fit is good enough for large samples but breaks down when this is not so. Yates' correction is a modification of the chi-squared formula which makes the test statistic fit the continuous chi-squared distribution better.

Yates' correction is sometimes is given as an option for chi-squared tests in statistical programs and is worth using unless the sample is very large when it will make no difference to the P value. Some programs give both a Yates' corrected and the ordinary chi-squared P value. In such cases the corrected test may give a slightly bigger P value than the ordinary chi-squared test and this larger P value should be reported.

Note that using Yates' correction does not remove the need for the assumptions regarding the expected values.

Reference

1 Bland M. *An introduction to medical statistics.* 3rd ed. Oxford: Oxford University Press, 2000.

Chi-squared test: calculations

Doing a chi-squared test

These data in Table 8.1 come from a large US study of delayed time to defibrillation after in-hospital cardiac arrest.[1]

Table 8.1 Delayed time to defibrillation after in-hospital cardiac arrest[1]

		Event occurred after hours	
		Yes	No
Time to	>2 min	2094 (44%)	836 (41%)
defibrillation	≤2 min	2650 (56%)	1209 (59%)
Total		4744	2045

- Overall proportion with time >2 min:
  = (2094+836)/(4744+2045) = 2930/6789 = 0.431580
- Overall proportion with time ≤2 min:
  = (2650+1209)/(4744+2045) = 3859/6789 = 0.568420
- Expected values are given by multiplying these by each column total:
  4744×0.431 580=2047.4155, 2045×0.431 580=882.5811
  4744×0.568 420=2696.5845, 2045×0.568 420=1162.4189
- The chi-squared test statistic is given by the following formula where O and E are the observed and expected frequencies for all cells of table:

$$\sum_{all\ cells} \frac{(O-E)^2}{E}$$

$$= \frac{(2094-2047.4155)^2}{2047.4155} + \frac{(836-882.5811)^2}{882.5811}$$

$$+ \frac{(2650-2696.5845)^2}{2696.5845} + \frac{(1209-1162.4189)^2}{1162.4189}$$

$$= 6.19$$

With degrees of freedom: $(2-1)\times(2-1)=1$

This has a P value of 0.013 which is statistically significant. Hence we have good evidence of a relationship between out of hours occurrence of cardiac events and delayed time to defibrillation.

Reference

1 Chan PS, Krumholz HM, Nichol G, Nallamothu BK. Delayed time to defibrillation after in-hospital cardiac arrest. *N Engl J Med* 2008; **358**(1):9–17.

Fisher's exact test

Details of the test
- It is useful for small samples where chi-squared test is invalid
- In general it tests for an association between two categorical variables
- It is normally only used for 2×2 tables but some statistical programs allow bigger tables to be analysed
- For 2×2 tables, the method involves evaluating the probabilities associated with all possible tables which have the same row totals and the same column totals as the observed data, assuming the null hypothesis is true
- Since the test is **based on exact probabilities**, it is computationally intensive and may be slow or fail to compute for large sample sizes
- The test gives P value but no direct estimate or a confidence interval for estimates
- For more details of test including a worked example, see Bland, Chapter 13[1]

Null hypothesis
- There is no association between the two variables in the population from which the samples come
- This tests same null hypothesis as the chi-squared test

Assumptions of test
- None

Using Fisher's exact test
- ❶ **Always use with frequencies, never use percentages for calculations**
- There is **no simple formula** and so the test is normally calculated using a statistical program
- The test is one-sided and there is no unique way to get the two-sided P value. Different statistical programs therefore can give slightly different two-sided P values, although the one-sided P value should be the same. In practice this should not make any appreciable difference
- Unless there is a good reason, **use the two-sided P value**
- Fisher's exact test will give a P value which is at least as big as the chi-squared test. For large samples the two P values will be very similar but **for small samples the P value from the chi-squared test is too small**
- **If in doubt about whether the sample size is large enough for the chi-squared test to be valid, use Fisher's exact test**

Example

The example in Table 8.2 comes from a follow-up of extremely preterm infants and shows the proportions of infants still on home oxygen at age 2 according to mode of ventilation at birth, high frequency oscillation (HFOV) or conventional(CV).[2]

Table 8.2 Proportions of infants still on home oxygen at age 2 according to mode of ventilation at birth

		Ventilation at birth	
		HFOV	**CV**
On home	Yes	2 (1.2%)	4 (2.1%)
oxygen	No	171 (98.8%)	190 (97.9%)
Total		173	194

- Expected values are 2.8, 3.2, 170.2, 190.8, respectively. Hence, the chi-squared test which gives P=0.50 is not valid
- Fisher's exact test gives two sided **P = 0.69**
- Note that Fisher's P value is larger than chi-squared. Here it doesn't affect the conclusions but if P was closer to 0.05 it might do

Hence we conclude that there is no evidence that mode of ventilation is associated with the use of home oxygen at age 2.

Note that when presenting these data in a report there is no need to report both rows of the table. It would be sufficient to report 2/173 (1.2%) versus 4/194 (2.1%).

References

1 Bland M. *An introduction to medical statistics.* 3rd ed. Oxford: Oxford University Press, 2000.
2 Marlow N, Greenough A, Peacock JL, Marston L, Limb ES, Johnson AH et al. Randomised trial of high frequency oscillatory ventilation or conventional ventilation in babies of gestational age 28 weeks or less: respiratory and neurological outcomes at 2 years. *Arch Dis Child Fetal Neonatal Ed* 2006; **91**(5):F320–6.

Estimates for tests of proportions

Reporting estimates

The chi-squared test and Fisher's exact test are tests of statistical significance and only give a P value. They do not provide an estimate of the size of effect that is observed since neither the chi-squared test value nor the P value measure the effect size or strength of relationship. An estimate is therefore needed to summarize the size of effect observed.

Choosing which estimate to use for a 2x2 table

The choice of estimate may be driven by the type of data or study design, or may simply be a matter of preference. The following suggestions come from Peacock and Kerry, Chapter 7.[1] Table 8.3 gives an example.

Risk difference: $p_1 - p_2$

- Use if actual size of difference is of interest
- Most straightforward estimate and useful for surveys

Relative risk: p_1 / p_2

- **Use if the relative difference is of interest**
- Useful when comparing the size of effect for several factors particularly if they are ordered
- Easier to interpret than the odds ratio
- Do not use for case–control studies

Odds ratio: $\dfrac{p_1}{(1-p_1)} \bigg/ \dfrac{p_2}{(1-p_2)}$

(or $\dfrac{ad}{bc}$ where a, b, c, d are 2x2 table frequencies)

- **Use for case–control studies**
- Approximately equal to relative risk when the outcome is rare
- Can be misinterpreted when the outcome is common
- Can adjust for other factors using logistic regression

Example

Table 8.3 Timing of cardiac event and time to defibrillation (📖 see Table 8.1, p. 264)

		Event occurred after hours	
		Yes	No
Time to	>2 min	2094	836
defibrillation	≤2 min	2650	1209
Total		4744	2045

To quantify the relationship between time of the cardiac event and the rate of delayed defibrillation we could use any one of three estimates:

1. Risk difference (difference of proportions)
$p_1 = 2094/4744 = 0.4414$, $p_2 = 836/2045 = 0.4088$
$p_1 - p_2 = 0.4414 - 0.4088 = 0.0326$ or 3.2%

2. Relative risk (ratio of proportions, rate ratio)
$p_1/p_2 = 0.4414/0.4088 = 1.08$

3. Odds ratio (ratio of odds)

$$\frac{p_1}{(1-p_1)} \Big/ \frac{p_2}{(1-p_2)} = \frac{0.4414}{(1-0.4414)} \Big/ \frac{0.4088}{(1-0.4088)} = 1.14$$

❶ Note of caution: relative risk does not equal odds ratio

- The relative risk and odds ratio are different measures of association and will only give similar values if the event is rare
- This is demonstrated in the example where the relative risk is 1.08 which implies an 8% increase in risk and the odds ratio is 1.14 which implies a 14% increase in odds. The event, delayed defibrillation, is not rare as the average rate is 0.43 or 43%
- Odds ratios should therefore **only** be interpreted as if they were relative risks **if the event was rare**

Reference

1 Peacock J, Kerry SM. *Presenting medical statistics from proposal to publication.* Oxford: Oxford University Press, 2006.

Confidence intervals for tests of proportions

It is important to calculate a 95% confidence interval for an estimated proportion to show how precise the estimate is.

All formulae assume that the samples are large as defined in the section 📖 95% confidence interval for a proportion, p. 244. If this is not true then other methods are needed. These are often available in statistical programs. Altman[1] has worked examples.

Below are worked examples of the calculations using the defibrillation data shown in 📖 Table 8.3, p. 269). These calculations can usually be done using a statistical program but having an understanding of where they come from is helpful when interpreting the computer output and reports where results may be presented on logarithmic scales.

95% confidence interval for risk difference

(See 📖 z test for two independent proportions, p. 260, for the formula; p_1 and p_2 are the proportions in groups 1 and 2, n_1 and n_2 are the totals in groups 1 and 2).

$$(p_1 - p_2) \pm 1.96 \sqrt{\frac{p_1(1-p_1)}{n_1} + \frac{p_2(1-p_2)}{n_2}}$$

$$= 0.0326 \pm 1.96 \sqrt{\frac{0.4414(1-0.4414)}{4744} + \frac{0.4088(1-0.4088)}{2045}}$$

$$= 0.0326 \pm 0.0256 = 0.007 \text{ to } 0.058$$

95% confidence interval for a relative risk

Assuming sample is large (📖 What is a large sample?, p. 244); if sample is small use an exact method[1])

This calculation has to be done on the logarithmic scale using logs to base e. If the relative risk is $RR = p_1/p_2$, and the sample sizes are n_1, n_2, the standard error (*SE*) of the logarithm is given by:

$$SE(\log_e RR) = \sqrt{\frac{(1-p_1)}{p_1 n_1} + \frac{(1-p_2)}{p_2 n_2}}$$

If the sample is large, the $\log_e RR$ follows a Normal distribution and the 95% confidence interval is given by:

$\log_e RR - 1.96\ SE(\log_e RR)$ to $\log_e RR + 1.96\ SE(\log_e RR)$

The *CI* for *RR* by obtained by taking the exponential of these limits:. The *RR* is 1.08 and its logarithm is 0.0770. The standard error of this is:

$$SE(\log_e RR) = \sqrt{\frac{(1-0.4414)}{0.4414 \times 4744} + \frac{(1-0.4088)}{0.4088 \times 2045}} = 0.0312$$

The 95% CI for the $\log_e RR$ is then:

$0.077 \pm 1.96 \times 0.0312$

$= 0.0158$ to 0.1382

The 95% CI for the *RR* is found by taking the exponential:

1.02 to 1.15

Reference

1 Altman DG, Machin D, Bryant TN, Gardner MJ. *Statistics with confidence: confidence intervals and statistical guidelines.* London: BMJ Publishing Group, 2000.

Confidence intervals for tests of proportions (continued)

> ## 95% confidence interval for an odds ratio
>
> **Assuming sample is large ([📖] What is a large sample?, p. 244; if sample is small use an exact method[1]):**
>
> This is calculated in a similar way to the CI for the RR using the logarithmic scale. We calculate the log odds ratio and SE of log odds ratio (OR):
>
> $$SE(log_e\,OR) = \sqrt{\frac{1}{n_1 p_1 (1-p_1)} + \frac{1}{n_2 p_2 (1-p_2)}}$$
>
> If the sample is large, the $log_e OR$ follows a Normal distribution and the 95% confidence interval is given by:
>
> $log_e OR - 1.96\,SE(log_e OR)$ to $log_e OR + 1.96\,SE(log_e OR)$
>
> OR=1.143, its logarithm is 0.1334. The standard error of this is:
>
> $$SE(log_e\,OR) = \sqrt{\frac{1}{4744 \times 0.4414(1-0.4144)} + \frac{1}{2045 \times 0.4088(1-0.4088)}}$$
>
> $$= 0.0536$$
>
> The 95% CI for the $log_e OR$ is:
>
> $0.1334 \pm 1.96 \times 0.0536 = 0.0283$ to 0.2384
>
> The 95% CI for the OR is found by taking the exponential:
>
> 1.03 to 1.27

Interpreting the confidence intervals

A 95% confidence interval for an estimate may be used to deduce statistical significance by checking if the interval contains the null hypothesis value. If a 95% CI excludes the appropriate null value, then the estimate is **statistically significant at the 5% level**. The null values are given below:

- For differences in proportions: null value = 0
- For relative risk: null value = 1.0
- For odds ratio: null value = 1.0
- If a 95% CI excludes the null value, then P<0.05

Footnote

When testing the difference of two proportions the calculated standard error is slightly different for the test to the confidence interval. In practice this will make little difference.

Reference

1 Altman DG, Machin D, Bryant TN, Gardner MJ. *Statistics with confidence: confidence intervals and statistical guidelines.* London: BMJ Publishing Group, 2000.

Chi-squared test for trend

Rationale

When we wish to compare proportions among groups which have an ordering, it is important to use the ordering to increase the power of the statistical analysis. The 'ordinary' chi-squared test takes no account of ordering – if the columns were re-arranged in any order in a $2 \times k$ table then the chi-squared test result would be exactly the same. This is because the chi-squared test looks for deviations from the null hypothesis that there is no association at all and does not test for any trend. The chi-squared test for trend is a specific test that investigates the linear trend in a set of proportions.

Details of the test

- It fits a linear trend through the ordered proportions
- It effectively partitions variability in data into two components:
  - Variability due to the trend
  - Remaining variability not due to trend
- If there is a real trend then the variability due to the trend will be much greater than the remaining variability
- The test statistic follows a chi-squared distribution with 1 degree of freedom

Null hypothesis

- There is no linear trend in a set of ordered proportions

Example

Table 8.4 Death rates by gestational age in extremely preterm babies[1]

	Gestational age (weeks)					
	23	24	25	26	27	28
Deaths n (%)	32 (84)	41 (40)	46 (32)	38 (25)	32 (16)	16 (10)
Total	38	102	144	155	201	157

Chi-squared test for trend (details omitted – see Bland[2] chapter 13)
- Overall chi-squared without taking ordering into account gives:
  $\chi^2 = 112.2$, degrees of freedom $= 5$, $P < 0.0001$
- Test for trend gives:
  $\chi^2 = 91.8$, degrees of freedom $= 1$, $P < 0.0001$

Hence there is good evidence for overall variability in survival by gestational age among extremely preterm babies and also good evidence that the trend is linear.

(Note that the trend does not explain all of the variability, the remaining component has $\chi^2 = 20.4$, degrees of freedom $= 4$, $P = 0.0004$).

Calculating and presenting estimates

In the example (Table 8.4) we have shown the actual proportions that died in each gestational age category. We could use a relative measure such as the relative risk or odds ratio (📖 Estimates for tests of proportions, p. 268) instead. To do this we have to define one category as the **reference category** and relate all others to that category. If we do this using relative risks (RR) with 28 weeks as the reference category we get the relative risks shown in Table 8.5.

Table 8.5 Relative risk of death by gestational age in extremely preterm babies[1]

	Gestational age (weeks)					
	23	24	25	26	27	28
RR	8.3	3.9	3.1	2.4	1.6	1.0

This shows the trend in a relative way rather than an absolute way as with proportions. The choice of summary measure is a judgement.

Large tables with ordered categories

Suppose we have a large table with >2 rows and >2 columns:
- Both variables ordered, use rank correlation (📖 Rank correlation, p. 312)
- Only one variable ordered, use Kruskal–Wallis test (see Conover[3])

References

1 Johnson AH, Peacock JL, Greenough A, Marlow N, Limb ES, Marston L et al. High-frequency oscillatory ventilation for the prevention of chronic lung disease of prematurity. *N Engl J Med* 2002; **347**(9):633–42.

2 Bland M. *An introduction to medical statistics*. 3rd ed. Oxford: Oxford University Press, 2000.

3 Conover WJ. *Practical nonparametric statistics*. 3rd ed. New York: Wiley, 1999.

McNemar's test for paired proportions

Details of the test
- It tests for an association between two paired proportions
- It can be used with matched case–control study data or a 'before and after' study
- The test is based on the **chi-squared distribution with 1 degree of freedom**
- It gives a P value, estimates and a confidence interval
- For more details of the test, see Bland, Chapter 13[1]

Null hypothesis
- The population prevalence is the same under the two conditions

Rationale of test
- It is based on the discordant pairs where exposure is different (yes/no, no/yes). Concordant pairs (yes/yes, no/no) are ignored as they contribute no information about differences within pairs
- Expected frequencies are calculated assuming there is no association (null hypothesis true), i.e. the frequencies are the same in both discordant pairs (yes/no, no/yes)
- Observed frequencies are compared with expected values. If the observed frequencies are very different from the expected values, this provides evidence for a real association
- The test uses a formula based on chi-squared distribution to give a P value

Assumptions of test
- Large sample test
- Rule of thumb for test to be valid: each expected frequency is greater than 5

If assumptions don't hold
- P value will be too small leading to potentially false significant results
- If numbers are small but the rule of thumb holds, use the version of the test with a continuity correction (see Bland, Chapter 13)[1]

Doing McNemar's test
- ❶ **Always use with frequencies, never use percentages for calculations**
- The test is usually done with a computer program – the calculations following Table 8.6 have been done to show how the test works

Example

This study investigated risk factors for death in patients admitted to hospital with an acute asthma attack. Each patient who was admitted and died was matched to a similar patient who was admitted but survived. The data below show the analysis of the effect of short-acting β_2 agonist for the 532 patient pairs.

Table 8.6a,b Data from a matched case-control study of asthma death and use of short-acting β_2 agonist[2] presented in two ways

(a)

	Died (case)	Survived (control)	No. of pairs	Notation
Used	Yes	Yes	411	a
short	Yes	No	69	b
acting	No	Yes	45	c
β_2 agonist	No	No	7	d
	Total		532	N

(b) Results arranged as a 2×2 table

		Died (case)		
	Used β_2 agonist	Yes	No	Total
Survived	Yes	411	45	456
(control)	No	69	7	76
	Total	480	52	532

- Expected frequency = $(b+c)/2 = (69+45)/2 = 57$
- Test statistic is:

$$\sum_{discordant\ cells} \frac{(O-E)^2}{E}$$

$$= \frac{(69-57)^2}{57} + \frac{(45-57)^2}{57} = 5.05$$

This follows a chi-squared distribution with 1 degree of freedom and has $P=0.031$ showing that there was a relationship between use of short-acting β_2 agonist and death from asthma.

References

1 Bland M. *An introduction to medical statistics*. 3rd ed. Oxford: Oxford University Press, 2000.
2 Anderson HR, Ayres JG, Sturdy PM, Bland JM, Butland BK, Peckitt C *et al.* Bronchodilator treatment and deaths from asthma: case-control study. *BMJ* 2005; **330**(7483):117.

Estimates and 95% confidence intervals for paired proportions

Estimates for paired proportions

As with independent proportions, there are three estimates for paired proportions (📖 Estimates for tests of proportions, p. 268):
- Difference between proportions
- Relative risk
- Odds ratio

In the example shown in 📖 McNemar's test for paired proportions, p. 276, the data are from a case–control study and so the relative risk cannot be calculated. The calculations for the estimated difference in proportions and matched odds ratio are shown below.

Calculating the difference in proportions of cases and controls using short-acting β_2 agonist[1]

Proportion of cases who used short-acting β_2 agonist
  = (411+69)/532 = 480/532

Proportion of controls who used short-acting β_2 agonist
  = (411+45)/532 =456/532

Difference = 24/532 = 0.0451

$$\text{SE (difference)} = \sqrt{\left(\frac{(b+c)}{n^2} - \frac{(b-c)^2}{n^3} \right)} \quad \textit{(proof omitted)}$$

$$= \sqrt{\left(\frac{(69+45)}{532^2} - \frac{(69-45)^2}{532^3} \right)} = 0.01997$$

Hence 95% CI: 0.0451 ± 1.96 x 0.01997
0.006 to 0.084

Calculating the odds ratio for cases and controls using short-acting β_2 agonist[1]

Odds ratio for use of short-acting β_2 agonist is given by the ratio of the odds of the $b+c$ discordant pairs:

$$\frac{b/(b+c)}{c/(b+c)} = b/c$$

Hence OR = 69/45=1.53

There is no simple formula for the 95% CI for this but it can be calculated using Confidence Interval Analysis (CIA) software[2] which gives 95% CI: 1.038 to 2.284

Further examples

For more details on paired proportions and an example of paired cohort data, see Peacock and Kerry,[3] Chapter 8.

References

1 Anderson HR, Ayres JG, Sturdy PM, Bland JM, Butland BK, Peckitt C et al. Bronchodilator treatment and deaths from asthma: case-control study. *BMJ* 2005; **330**(7483):117.
2 Altman DG, Machin D, Bryant TN, Gardner MJ. *Statistics with confidence: confidence intervals and statistical guidelines*. London BMJ Publishing Group, 2000.
3 Peacock J, Kerry SM. *Presenting medical statistics from proposal to publication*. Oxford: Oxford University Press, 2006.

One-way analysis of variance

Details of the method

- This is an extension of the t test and compares means from three or more independent samples
- It gives one overall P value comparing all groups based on a test statistic which follows an **F distribution**

Null hypothesis

- The samples for each group come from populations with the same mean values

❶ Wrong approach

- It is wrong to do t tests for all possible combinations of groups because the more groups we have, the more likely it is that two groups will be far enough apart by chance to be significantly different. Thus some comparisons will be significant *by chance alone* ('type 1 error' 📖 Errors in significance testing, p. 247).

Rationale of one-way analysis of variance

- One-way analysis of variance is based on the variability ('variance') between the group means: if group means are far enough apart, this suggests that the groups are from different populations
- It works by partitioning the overall variability into two components of variability:
  (i) The variability between the group means: '**between group variance**'
  (ii) The remaining variability not due to differences between the groups: '**residual variance**'
- If the groups are truly different, the between-group variance will be much greater than the residual variance
- This is tested using the **ratio of the two variances: the F ratio**
- If the variability between groups is no more than we would expect due to randomness alone then the two estimates will be similar and the F ratio will be close to 1.0
- If the F ratio is much greater than 1.0, the two estimates must be very different, providing evidence that the group means are different

Assumptions of method

- Continuous data, Normally distributed within each group: plot *observation-group mean* (📖 One-way analysis of variance: example, p. 282)
- Equal variance (standard deviation) in each group
- Checking the assumptions: see t test (📖 t test for two independent means: example p. 254)

If assumptions do not hold

- **The P value may be wrong**
- Try **transforming the data** (📖 Transforming data, p. 330)

- Note that when the data are positively skewed, the standard deviation (SD) in each group increases as the group means increase. In this situation a logarithmic transformation may correct the skewness and stabilize the standard deviation

The F distribution

- The F ratio follows an F distribution if null hypothesis is true, i.e. if there is no difference between the means
- The F distribution is determined by its two parameters, the degrees of freedom of the two variance estimates:
  (i) number of groups − 1
  (ii) total observations − number of groups
- The F ratio has a corresponding P value. $P < 0.05$ is interpreted as indicating that the group means are different from each other overall

The calculations

- These are usually done using a computer package but can be done by hand – see Bland, Chapter 10[1] for a worked example
- The results are given as an **analysis of variance table** (📖 Analysis of variance table, p. 284) and/or as **group means** with confidence intervals

❶ Further tests

- If the analysis shows that there is variability between the means overall, then pairs of means may be tested (📖 Multiple comparisons, p. 286)
- It is **poor research practice to compare the smallest and largest means unless this was a prior hypothesis** since an analysis of groups selected because the difference was big is likely to be statistically significant

Reference

1 Bland M. *An introduction to medical statistics.* 3rd ed. Oxford: Oxford University Press, 2000.

One-way analysis of variance: example

The data

The data in Table 8.7 come from a double-blind experiment of the effect of caffeine on the speed of finger tapping as a measure of performance.[1] Thirty subjects were given one of three doses of caffeine, 0 mg, 100 mg, or 200 mg. The number of taps per minute was recorded. The data were analysed using a statistical package and summary results are given in Table 8.8.

Table 8.7 Number of taps per minute in 30 subjects by caffeine dose

Dose (mg)	Number of taps per minute in each subject									
0	242	245	244	248	247	248	242	244	246	242
100	248	246	245	247	248	250	247	246	243	244
200	246	248	250	252	248	250	246	248	245	250

Summary statistics

Table 8.8 Summary statistics by caffeine group

Dose (mg)	Number	Mean (SD)	95% CI for mean
0	10	244.8 (2.39)	243.1 to 246.5
100	10	246.4 (2.07)	244.9 to 247.9
200	10	248.3 (2.21)	246.7 to 249.9

Testing assumptions

Since the sample is small, a Normal plot has been used to check that the data are reasonably close to a Normal distribution. The Normal plot is a plot of the cumulative frequency distribution for the data against the cumulative frequency distribution for the corresponding Normal distribution – an 'observed versus expected' plot. If the points lie close to the line of equality then there is good reason to assume that the data are Normally distributed. For more details on Normal plots, see Bland, Chapter 7.[2]

Figure 8.4 shows that the data points are scattered around the line of equality but since they stay reasonably close to the line, the data are close enough to a Normal distribution. Further, Table 8.8 shows that the standard deviations are similar in the three groups and so the analysis is valid.

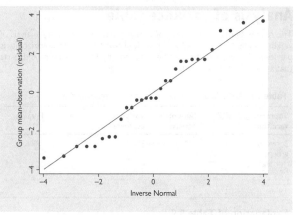

Fig. 8.4 Normal plot for one-way analysis of variance.

Note

The Normal plot was drawn using each observation minus its group mean: the **within-group residual.** The assumption of one-way analysis of variance is that the data are Normally distributed within each group and by examining the within-group residuals it is possible to examine all the data together. This is useful when the dataset is too small to examine the distribution within the groups separately.

References

1 Hand DJ. *A handbook of small data sets.* London: Chapman & Hall, 1994.
2 Bland M. *An introduction to medical statistics.* 3rd ed. Oxford: Oxford University Press, 2000.

Analysis of variance table

The results of one-way analysis of variance may be given in an analysis of variance table (see Table 8.9). This table shows how the total variability is partitioned into parts that can be explained by known factors and parts that are random (unknown).

Table 8.9 Analysis of variance table for caffeine experiment

Source of variation	DF	Sum of squares	Variance estimate	F ratio	P value
Between groups	2	61.4	30.7	6.18	0.006
Residual	27	134.1	4.97		
Total	29	195.5			

Explanation of Table 8.9

- Row 2 gives the statistics for the 'between-groups' variability
- Row 3 gives the statistics for the 'residual' variability
- Row 4 gives the overall totals
- **DF** is degrees of freedom; it is *number of groups – 1* = 2, for row 2, *total number observations – 1* = 29, for row 4 and the difference between these, 29–2=27, for row 3
- **Total sum of squares** is calculated in a similar way to a sum of squares for a standard deviation (📖 Summarizing quantitative data, p. 182):
  $(242–246.5)^2 + (245–246.5)^2 + (244–246.5)^2 +…+ (250–246.5)^2 = 195.5$
- **Between groups sum of squares** is based on the sum of the squared differences between each group mean and the overall mean:
  $10 \times [(244.8–246.5)^2 + (246.4–246.5)^2 + (248.3–246.5)^2] = 61.4$
- **Residual sum of squares** is obtained by subtraction:
  195.5–61.4=134.1
- **Variance estimate** is the sum of squares/DF:
  Between-groups variance = 61.4/2 = 30.7
  Residual variance = 134.1/27 = 4.97
- **F ratio** is ratio of 2 variances:
  30.7/4.97 = 6.18
- **P value** is probability associated with an F value of 6.18 if the null hypothesis of no difference between the groups, were true. As it is very small, we conclude that the group means are different from each other.
- Hence there is good evidence that caffeine affects performance.

Multiple comparisons

Introduction

After doing a one-way analysis of variance, it may be desirable to compare particular pairs of means. Care needs to be taken in how this is done to prevent the spurious significant results which will arise when many comparisons are done, despite there being no real differences in the underlying populations.

Approaches to multiple testing

- ❶ t tests should not be used to test all combinations of the group means since this will lead to an excess of false significant results
- t tests can be used as a guide for a small number of comparisons **if the overall variation between groups is significant**
- Better methods are available which take multiple testing into account by preserving the type 1 error rate at 5%, such as **Bonferroni** (see 'Bonferroni correction'), Scheffé, Newman–Keuls, studentized range tests, Duncan, Gabriel's test etc. The choice depends on the data and the statistical program available
- The disadvantage of these methods is that they **tend to be conservative**, i.e. they err on the side of non-significance
- If there is an ordering in the groups then use a **test for a trend** across them using linear contrasts: for the caffeine data this gives P(trend)=0.006 (details omitted)

Bonferroni correction

The Bonferroni correction is a simple method to correct the cut-off for statistical significance for multiple testing. It is based on the fact that if the null hypothesis of no differences between groups is true and a test is performed with P<0.05 taken as significant, then the probability of a non-significant result is 0.95. From this it follows that if 10 independent tests are done, then the probability of none being significant is $0.95^{10} = 0.60$, by the multiplicative rule for probabilities (📖 Probability: properties, p. 208).

If α is the cut-off for significance, then to preserve the significance level at 0.05 we need $(1-\alpha)^{10} = 0.95$. Because α is small, it can be shown that $(1-\alpha)^{10}$ is approximately equal to $1-10\alpha$ (details omitted). For this to be equal to 0.95 we must have $\alpha = 0.05/10$. Hence, in general if n tests are performed, the cut-off for significance is $0.05/n$. Bonferroni's method tends to be very conservative but does avoid spurious significant results.

Extensions to the use of multiple comparisons procedures

Sometimes, a multiple comparisons procedure is used in settings other than analysis of variance, when a number of separate tests are performed and it is desirable to guard against the possibility that some may be significant purely by chance alone. In such a situation, we are **no longer testing individual hypotheses but a composite hypothesis**. For example a study in ex-preterm babies explored risk factors for later respiratory morbidity and several different respiratory outcomes were analysed. A multiple comparisons procedure was used and the authors noted that: 'the use of a multiple testing approach means that the individual hypotheses are no longer tested, but instead a composite hypothesis, *respiratory morbidity** [emphasis added] (cough, frequent cough, cough without infection, wheeze, frequent wheeze, wheeze without infection and use of chest medicine), is tested. A variable that is associated with any of the outcomes after modification of the P value is thus significantly associated with the composite outcome'.[1]

Further details and extensions

- For further reading on multiple comparisons, see Bland[2]
- For further details and examples on one-way analysis of variance, see Bland, Chapter 10,[3] Armitage, Chapter 8,[4] Altman, Chapter 9[5]
- For examples of one-way analysis of variance in SPSS and Stata, see Peacock and Kerry, Chapter 10[6]
- The method of one-way analysis of variance can be extended to include one or more covariates (□ Multiple regression and analysis of variance, p. 412)

References

1 Greenough A, Limb E, Marston L, Marlow N, Calvert S, Peacock J. Risk factors for respiratory morbidity in infancy after very premature birth. *Arch Dis Child Fetal Neonatal Ed* 2005; **90**(4):F320–3.

2 Bland JM, Altman DG. Multiple significance tests: the Bonferroni method. *BMJ* 1995; **310**(6973):170.

3 Bland M. *An introduction to medical statistics*. 3rd ed. Oxford: Oxford University Press, 2000.

4 Armitage P, Berry G, Matthews JNS. *Statistical methods in medical research*. 4th ed. Oxford: Blackwell Science, 2002.

5 Altman DG. *Practical statistics for medical research*. London: Chapman & Hall, 1991.

6 Peacock J, Kerry SM. *Presenting medical statistics from proposal to publication*. Oxford: Oxford University Press, 2006.

Correlation and regression

Introduction

Correlation and regression (simple linear regression) are used to investigate the relationship between two continuous variables. There are several forms of correlation. Pearson's correlation is based on the Normal distribution while some other methods are based on the ranks of the data (📖 Rank correlation, p. 312). In this section we consider Pearson's correlation. The choice of whether to use correlation or regression depends on the question being answered.

Examples for correlation and regression

Correlation

Fig. 8.5a shows the relationship between two scores summarizing development in infants: one score came from a paediatrician assessment (MDI) and the other from a parental questionnaire.[1] The aim was to determine how closely these two scores were related and so the correlation coefficient was calculated ($r=0.68$, 95% CI: 0.52 to 0.79, $P<0.0001$).

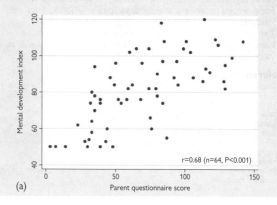

(a)

Regression

Fig. 8.5b shows the relationship between forced vital capacity (FVC) and age in a sample of school-age girls. The aim was to see how FVC increased with age and so regression analysis was used to give the equation of the line ($y = 0.305 + 0.193 \times$ age).

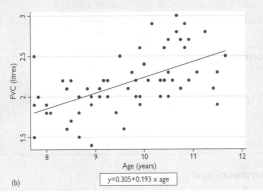

(b)

$y = 0.305 + 0.193 \times$ age

Fig. 8.5 Graphs illustrating the use of: (a) correlation and (b) regression.

Correlation or regression?

Pearson's correlation

- It investigates the **strength of a linear relationship** between two continuous variables, such as crown–heel length and head circumference in newborn babies
- It is used when neither variable can be assumed to predict the other
- It gives an estimate, the correlation coefficient, and a P value
- A confidence interval can also be calculated

Simple linear regression

- It investigates the **nature of the linear relationship** between two continuous variables, such as amount of exercise and weight in adults
- It is used when investigating how one variable (the predictor variable) affects the other (the outcome variable)
- It gives the equation of the best fitting straight line through the data in the form of the intercept and slope of the line, with confidence intervals
- It allows the estimated slope to be tested against a null value of 0
- It enables predictions to be made with confidence intervals

Reference

1 Johnson S, Marlow N, Wolke D, Davidson L, Marston L, O'Hare A et al. Validation of a parent report measure of cognitive development in very preterm infants. *Dev Med Child Neurol* 2004; **46**(6):389–97.

Pearson's correlation

Details of the method
- It is used to estimate the **strength of linear relationship** between two continuous variables
- It gives a correlation coefficient – often denoted by 'r'

The calculations are based on the differences between the observations x_i, y_i and their means $\bar{x}$ and $\bar{y}$ as shown in the formula below:

Formula

$$r = \frac{\sum_{i=1}^{n}(x_i - \bar{x})(y_i - \bar{y})}{\sqrt{\sum_{i=1}^{n}(x_i - \bar{x})^2 \sum_{i=1}^{n}(y_i - \bar{y})^2}}$$

Where x_i, y_i are values of the n pairs of two variables

Interpretation of r
- r tells us how close is the linear relationship between the two variables
- r lies between -1 and $+1$
- Negative values indicate a **negative linear relationship**, i.e. as one variable increases, the other decreases
- Positive values indicate a **positive linear relationship**, i.e. as one variable increases, so does the other
- $r=0$ indicates **no linear relationship**, i.e. the values of each variable are independent of each other
- Values closer to -1 and $+1$ indicate stronger relationships, with -1 showing a perfect negative linear relationship and $+1$ showing a perfect positive linear relationship

Tests and estimates
- A significance test can be done to test the **null hypothesis that $r=0$** using a statistical program or using tables of cut-off points for significance such as those given in Bland, Chapter 11.[1] An abridged version is shown in Table 8.10.
- A confidence interval can also be calculated by hand but has a complicated formula – see Bland, Chapter 11[1] or use a statistical program. A 95% confidence interval is rarely seen but provides useful additional information, particularly with small samples with a strong correlation but with a wide confidence interval.

Statistical significance and sample size
As with other estimates, statistical significance of r is directly related to the sample size and so for small samples the correlation needs to be bigger to be significant (see Table 8.10). But this also means that for large samples, small values of r may be statistically significant even though the relationship is weak (see Fig. 8.6).

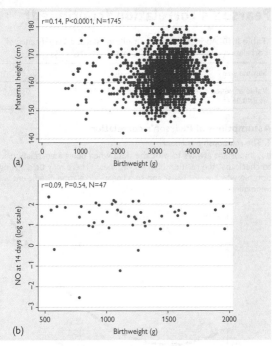

Fig. 8.6 (a) The sample size is large (*n* = 1745) and so, although the correlation is very weak, *r* = 0.14, it is highly significant. (b) The sample size is small (*n* = 64) and the correlation is very weak, *r* = 0.09, and is not significant.

Reference

1 Bland M. *An introduction to medical statistics.* 3rd ed. Oxford: Oxford University Press, 2000.

Pearson's correlation (continued)

Table 8.10 Abridged table of cut-offs for statistical significance of correlation coefficient *r* at P<0.05 by sample size

Sample size	10	20	50	100	500	1000
Value at which *r* becomes significant at P<0.05	0.63	0.44	0.28	0.20	0.09	0.06

Assumptions of Pearson's correlation

1. The relationship is linear

It is important **always** to **plot the data** when doing a correlation analysis to check that the relationship really is linear. There may be a strong relationship which is not linear and so a linear correlation coefficient will give misleading results – see below.

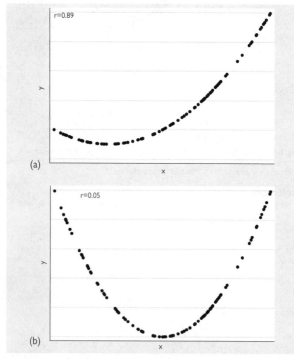

Fig. 8.7 Scatterplots illustrating non-linear relationships.

Figure 8.7 shows simulated data with perfect relationships:

Figure 8.7a has $r=0.89$, suggesting a strong linear correlation, but the scatterplot clearly shows that the relationship is not linear

Figure 8.7b has $r=0.05$, suggesting no linear relationship. The scatterplot shows a strong relationship that is not linear, but quadratic.

2. Normal distribution

For the significance test to be valid **at least one of the two variables must follow a Normal distribution** and for the confidence interval to be valid, **both variables must follow a Normal distribution.** To check these assumptions, plot histograms/Normal plots. If the assumptions are not met, a transformation of the data may be used to correct for non-Normality (📖 Transforming data, p. 330) or a rank correlation used (📖 Rank correlation, p. 312).

❶ Note that if the data are transformed, the correlation coefficient is not back-transformed.

3. Random sample

The sample of points x_i, y_i are assumed to be **a random sample** within the range of values of interest. This is important since the range of values affects r. If the range is artificially restricted, r will be too small. Conversely if two samples with different ranges are joined, r will be artificially inflated – Figure 8.8 illustrates this.

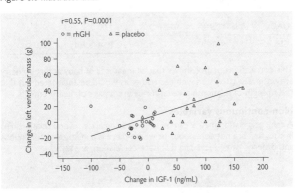

Fig. 8.8 Scatterplot of change in insulin growth factor (IGF)-1 and change in left ventricular mass in two treatment groups.

Figure 8.8 shows the relationship between change in insulin growth factor (IGF)-1 and change in left ventricular mass in two treatment groups. The overall r value was 0.55 but the authors reported values of 0.28 in the treatment group (rhGH) and 0.36 in the placebo group. The graph shows that the two samples hardly overlap and so by putting them together the range has been stretched and the correlation has been artificially inflated (Bland and Peacock, p. 126[1]).

Reference

1 Bland M, Peacock J. *Statistical questions in evidence-based medicine.* Oxford: Oxford University Press, 2000.

Correlation matrix

Exploring inter-relationships between variables

The correlation coefficient can be used to summarize how strong the relationship is between several pairs of continuous variables. This is particularly useful before doing multifactorial analyses as it shows how different variables are inter-related. This can be used to guide the analyses and help with the interpretation of results. An example of this is given in Table 8.11.

Example

Table 8.11 Correlation matrix showing the inter-relationships between baby anthropometry. BW, birthweight; HC, head circumference; UAC, upper arm circumference; CHL, crown–heel length

Correlations (P values) between four measures of anthropometry in 198 newborn infants

	BW	HC	UAC	CHL
BW	1.00			
HC	0.78 (<0.01)	1.00		
UAC	0.83 (<0.01)	0.63 (<0.01)	1.00	
CHL	0.79 (<0.01)	0.65 (<0.01)	0.59 (<0.01)	1.00

This correlations matrix shows that all measures of baby anthropometry are positively associated with each other as would be anticipated but that the strength of relationship varies for different pairs of measurements.

Non-continuous variables

A rank correlation matrix can be used to summarize several relationships in data that are not continuous or where there is a mixture of continuous and ordered categorical data (☐ Rank correlation, p. 312).

Simple linear regression

Details of the method

- Simple linear regression is used to estimate the **nature of the linear relationship** between two continuous variables where one is regarded as the **outcome** and the other **predicts** the outcome. It gives the equation of the best straight line through the observed data:

  $y = a + bx$

  where y is the outcome, a is the intercept, b is the slope of the line, and x is the predictor variable

- The calculations are based on formulae derived from minimizing the differences between the observed values and the mean values predicted by the line – '**least squares method**'. Details of the derivation are given in Bland, Chapter 11.[1] For each observed value, the difference between it and the value predicted by the model is known as the **residual**. The method of least squares is so called because it minimizes the sum of the squares of these residuals to give the line through the points that is closest to the data overall (Fig. 8.9)

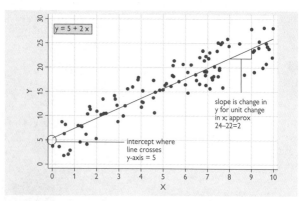

Fig. 8.9 A regression line showing the slope and intercept.

Terminology

There is some variation in terminology for regression:

- The **outcome variable** is sometimes called the **dependent** or **response variable**
- The **predictor variable** is sometimes called the **explanatory** or **independent variable**
- The **slope** or **gradient** of the line is often called a **regression coefficient** This leads to general terminology for estimates in models with more than one predictor, as in multifactorial analysis (□ Chapter 12, p. 393)

Calculations for simple linear regression

Simple linear regression can be done in all good statistical programs, but the calculations are reasonably straightforward and can be done by hand in small datasets using the following formulae:

Slope or regression coefficient is given by:

$$b = \frac{\sum_{i=1}^{n}(x_i - \bar{x})(y_i - \bar{y})}{\sum_{i=1}^{n}(x_i - \bar{x})^2}$$

The line goes through the mean point: $(\bar{x}, \bar{y})$

Therefore the intercept is given by: $a = \bar{y} - b\bar{x}$

Interpretation of the equation

- The **regression coefficient** gives the **change in the outcome (y) for a unit change in the predictor variable (x)**
- The intercept gives the value of y when x is 0
- The line gives the **mean or expected value of y for each value of x**

Reference

1 Bland M. *An introduction to medical statistics.* 3rd ed. Oxford: Oxford University Press, 2000.

Simple linear regression (continued)

Tests and estimates

- If there is no relationship between x and y then the true regression coefficient b will be 0 (null value)
- This can be tested using a form of t test
- The regression coefficient b can be a useful summary of the relationship if interested simply in how the two variables are related
- 95% confidence intervals can also be calculated for b
- The equation of the line can be used for predictions (see below)

Assumptions of the regression method

1. The relationship is linear

As with correlation, it is important to plot the data before doing a regression analysis to check that the relationship is linear. If the relationship is steadily increasing (monotonic) but not linear, it may be possible to transform the data to linearize the relationship (📖 Transforming data, p. 330).

Some non-monotonic relationships cannot be linearized and in this case it may be necessary to calculate a function of the data to make a good fit, for example if the relationship is quadratic, this will need a function which includes x and x^2. Such analyses need to be done using multiple regression (📖 Multiple regression, p. 406).

2. The distribution of the residuals is Normal

The statistical test for the regression coefficient and the calculation of the confidence intervals are based on the t distribution and only hold if the residuals follow a Normal distribution. To test this, plot a histogram or do a Normal plot of the residuals.

3. The variance (standard deviation) of the outcome y is constant over x

The statistical test for the regression coefficient also makes the assumption of constant variance. This can be checked from the scatterplot. Alternatively plot the residuals against the predictor variable to see if the spread of the residuals varies across the range of the predictor (non-constant variance).

Notes on assumptions

Sometimes **non-linearity**, **non-Normality**, and **non-constant variance occur together** and a transformation of the data may correct all three problems at the same time. If data are transformed, such as by applying a logarithmic transformation, the interpretation of the regression coefficient changes. See Peacock and Kerry, Chapter 9,[2] for worked examples of this.

❶ If we do the regression calculations the other way around (i.e. we **swap x and y), we get a different equation** and so it is important to use the right variables as the outcome and predictor variables.

Predictions

The regression equation can be used to estimate the mean value of the outcome for a given value of the predictor. These can apply in two situations: **within** and **outside the sample**.

Within-sample predictions provide the mean or expected value for the observed data using the estimated line. A 95% confidence interval can be calculated for the prediction (details are given in Bland, Chapter 11,[1] and can be calculated using a statistical program).

Predictions outside the sample can also be made. These give the expected value for a new individual with a given value of the predictor. The prediction value is the same as for the within-sample prediction but the 95% confidence interval is wider to reflect the uncertainty about predictions in a new sample. Again details can be found in Bland.[1]

Two things are particularly important to note when using a regression equation to make predictions outside the sample:

❶ Use the correct confidence interval (see Fig. 8.11) otherwise the prediction will appear to be more precise than it should be

❶ Don't make predictions outside the range of the original data since the the form of the relationship may not be the same (see 📖 Simple linear regression: example p. 300)

References

1 Bland M. *An introduction to medical statistics*. 3rd ed. Oxford: Oxford University Press, 2000.
2 Peacock J, Kerry SM. *Presenting medical statistics from proposal to publication*. Oxford: Oxford University Press, 2006.

Simple linear regression: example

This example uses data from a sample of school-age girls and investigates the relationship between their age in years and their forced vital capacity (FVC, in litres). A statistical program was used to do the calculations:

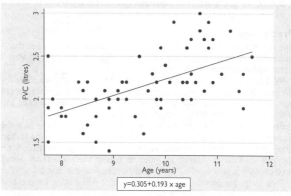

Fig. 8.10 Scatterplot of lung function against age in school-age girls.

The regression equation is **y = 0.305 + 0.193x age**
- As age increases by 1 year, FVC increases by 0.193 litres
- The significance test for the coefficient for age gave t=5.34, P<0.001 showing that there is strong evidence for a linear relationship
- 95% CI for the coefficient is 0. 121 to 0.266
- The residuals were a good fit to a Normal distribution (Fig. 8.11a)
- There is no evidence that the relationship is not linear – see scatter plot above and plot of age x residuals (Fig. 8.11b)

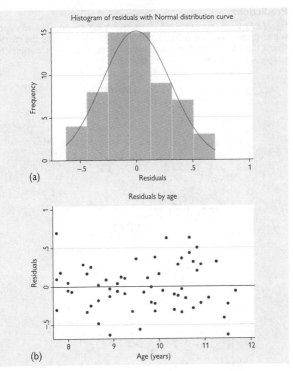

Fig. 8.11 (a) Histogram of residuals. (b) Scatterplot of residuals by age.

Predictions

Figure 8.12 shows the predicted values, with a 95% confidence interval for within-sample predictions (Fig. 8.12a) and predictions outside the sample (Fig. 8.12b). It is clear that the precision of the predictions outside the sample is much greater.

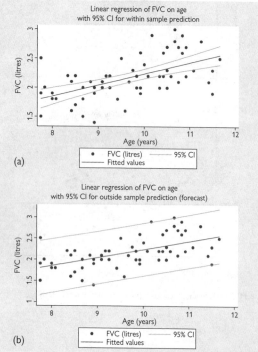

❶ Note the dangers of extrapolating outside the range of the data such as predicting mean FVC at age 50 from these data. It gives mean FVC=9.96 litres. This is clearly nonsensical and arises because FVC would not cont nue to increase once the girls reach adulthood. This extreme example illustrates the dangers of extrapolating outside the range of the data.

Fig. 8.12 Scatterplot with 95% confidence interval for (a) within-sample predictions and (b) predictions outside the sample.

Wilcoxon two-sample signed rank test (Mann Whitney U test)

Introduction to rank tests

The tests described previously, such as the two forms of the t test (for two independent means; for paired data) and regression and correlation, make fairly strong assumptions about the distribution of the data. In some circumstances these assumptions are not met either because the data have a non-standard distribution which cannot be transformed or because the data are inherently discrete rather than continuous. In these situations, tests based on the ranks of the data can be used.

All rank tests are based on the ranks or ordering of the data rather than on the actual data values themselves. This obviously leads to data being discarded and so, in general, rank tests are less powerful than tests which use all of the data, such as the t test when its assumptions are upheld.

Rank tests are sometimes called **non-parametric tests** because in general they make no assumptions about the distribution of the data. In fact the paired rank test does require the differences to follow a symmetrical distribution, and so some distributional assumptions are made although they are much less restrictive than the assumptions for the tests described previously in this chapter. For more details of rank tests see Conover.[1]

Details of the test

- **It is the analogue of the t test** for two independent means
- It compares ordinal data from two independent groups
- **It is based on the ranks** of the data in each group
- **It gives a P value but no estimate** of the difference between the groups
- Given a table of cut-offs, the test is easy to do by hand for small samples, but harder for larger samples as the data have to be ordered by hand
- Note that it is often thought of as a test for small samples but this is not so. In fact if the sample is very small (both smaller than four observations) then statistical significance is impossible
- **The Wilcoxon signed rank test is mathematically equivalent to the Mann Whitney U test** and gives exactly the same P value. However, the calculations are different and the tables are different. The Wilcoxon calculations are slightly easier to do by hand and so these are shown here.

Null hypothesis

- Observations from one group do not tend to have a higher or lower ranking than observations from the other group
- Note that this test **does not test the medians** of the data as is commonly thought, it tests the whole distribution

Assumptions of test

- The data are in two groups and can be ranked

Reference

1 Conover WJ. *Practical nonparametric statistics*. 3rd ed. New York: Wiley, 1999.

Wilcoxon two-sample signed rank test: calculations

How the Wilcoxon signed rank test works

- The test is based on the probability distribution for the arrangement of ranks, given a null hypothesis of no difference
- Cut-off points are tabulated (see Table 8.12) or the test can be done using a statistical program

To perform the test

Assume the two samples have sizes n_1, n_2:

1. Rank the data ignoring the groups
2. Give tied values the mean of their ranks
3. Add the ranks in each group separately to give T_1 and T_2
4. Compare the smallest of T_1 and T_2 with the tabulated values (Table 8.12[1]) to determine statistical significance. The test is statistically significant if the observed value, T, is *less than* the tabulated value

Table 8.12 Two-sided 5% cut-offs for the Wilcoxon two-sample test

n_1 \ n_2	4	5	6	7	8	9	10	11	12
4	10	11	12	13	14	14	15	16	17
5		17	18	20	21	22	23	24	26
6			26	27	29	31	32	34	35
7				36	38	40	42	44	46
8					49	51	53	55	58
9						62	65	68	71
10							78	81	84
11								96	99
12									115

Note: n_1 is the smaller sample size, i.e. $n_1 < n_2$. The test is statistically significant if T is *less than* the tabulated value.

Summary statistics

The median or mean, or another percentile can be used as a summary measure. The choice is guided by the shape of the distribution – if it is symmetrical, then a mean may be best, otherwise the median or a more extreme percentile may be most useful. A 95% confidence interval can be calculated for the difference in means or medians if the distributions are similar in shape (see Altman[2] for details).

Reference

1 Armitage P, Berry G, Matthews JNS. *Statistical methods in medical research*. 4th ed. Oxford: Blackwell Science, 2002.

2 Altman DG, Machin D, Bryant TN, Gardner MJ. *Statistics with confidence: confidence intervals and statistical guidelines*. London BMJ Publishing Group, 2000.

Wilcoxon two-sample signed rank test: example

The data shows urinary β-thromoglobulin excretion in 12 healthy and 12 diabetic patients[1]

Healthy patients	Diabetic patients
4.1	11.5
6.3	12.1
7.8	16.1
8.5	17.8
8.9	24
10.4	28.8
11.5	33.9
12.0	40.7
13.8	51.3
17.6	56.2
24.3	61.7
37.2	69.2

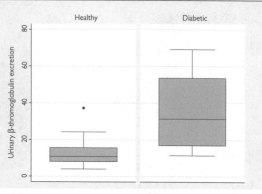

Fig. 8.13 Box plots comparing distributions in two groups.

The box plots show that the values in the two groups have different shaped distributions. The differences between the two groups can be tested using a rank test.

Table 8.13 shows the data ranked ignoring the group and with the name of the group given alongside.

Table 8.13 Urinary β-thromoglobulin excretion values and ranks in diabetic patients and in healthy patients

β-thromoglobulin	Rank	Group
4.1	1	Healthy
6.3	2	Healthy
7.8	3	Healthy
8.5	4	Healthy
8.9	5	Healthy
10.4	6	Healthy
11.5	7.5	Healthy
11.5	7.5	Diabetic
12	9	Healthy
12.1	10	Diabetic
13.8	11	Healthy
16.1	12	Diabetic
17.6	13	Healthy
17.8	14	Diabetic
24	15	Diabetic
24.3	16	Healthy
28.8	17	Diabetic
33.9	18	Diabetic
37.2	19	Healthy
40.7	20	Diabetic
51.3	21	Diabetic
56.2	22	Diabetic
61.7	23	Diabetic
69.2	24	Diabetic

- The sum of ranks in the healthy patients is:
  1+2+3+4+5+6+7.5+9+11+13+16+19=96.5
- The sum of ranks in the diabetic patients is:
  7.5+10+12+14+15+17+18+20+21+22+23+24=203.5
- From the table of cut-offs, the smaller total, 96.5, is less than the cut-off (115) for n_1=12, n_2=12 and so P<0.05

Hence there is good evidence that urinary β-thromboglobulin excretion is greater in diabetic patients than in healthy patients.

Reference

1 Hand DJ. *A handbook of small data sets.* London: Chapman & Hall,1994.

Wilcoxon matched pairs test

Details of the test

- This is the analogue of the t test for paired (matched) data
- It compares ordinal data from paired samples
- It is based on the signs of the differences in the pairs and the relative sizes of differences rather than the actual values
- **It gives a P value but no estimate of the difference between the groups**
- Given a table of cut-offs, the test is easy to do by hand for small samples, but harder for larger samples as it requires the data to be manually ordered
- It is often thought of as a test for small samples but this is not so. In fact if the **sample is smaller than 6, then statistical significance is impossible**

Null hypothesis

- The distribution of differences is symmetrical about zero

Assumptions of test

- The data are one-to-one matched and differences can be calculated and ranked, i.e. data must be interval (📖 Types of data, p. 178)
- The sample differences come from a population with a symmetrical distribution
- If the differences are skewed, a transformation may correct this (📖 Transforming data, p. 330)
- Note that the test cannot be used if many differences are zero, as zero differences are omitted (see opposite)

How the Wilcoxon matched pairs test works

- The test is based on the probability distribution for the arrangements of the ranks of the differences, given the null hypothesis of symmetry about 0
- Cut-off points are tabulated for small sample sizes (Table 8.14) or the test can be done using a statistical program

To perform the test

1. Rank the differences ignoring the sign and omitting any zero differences
2. Give tied values the mean of their ranks
3. Add the ranks of the positive and negative differences, T_+, T_-
4. If the distribution of differences is symmetrical about zero, then T_+, T_- will be similar
5. The smaller of T_+, T_- is compared with tabulated values (see Table 8.14) to determine statistical significance

Table 8.14 Two-sided 5% cut-off points for Wilcoxon matched pairs test (Bland[1])

Sample size	Cut-off
6	1
7	2
8	4
9	6
10	8
11	11
12	14
13	17
14	21
15	25
16	30
17	35
18	40
19	46
20	52
21	59
22	66
23	73
24	81
25	90

Note: the smaller of T_+, T_- is used. The test is statistically significant if the observed value, T, is *less than* the tabulated value.

Reference

1 Bland M. *An introduction to medical statistics*. 3rd ed. Oxford: Oxford University Press, 2000.

Wilcoxon matched pairs test: example

Table 8.15a,b Thickness of the cornea (microns) in patients with one eye affected by glaucoma; the other eye is unaffected[1]

(a)

Patient no.	Affected eye	Unaffected eye	Difference	Summary statistics for differences:
1	488	484	+4	Mean: −4
2	478	478	0	Median: −3
3	480	492	−12	Range: −16 to +12
4	426	444	−18	
5	440	436	+4	Differences are reasonably symmetrical so test can be used
6	410	398	+12	
7	458	464	−6	
8	460	476	−16	

(b) The test:

Patient no.	Affected eye	Unaffected eye	Difference	Rank (ignoring sign)
1	488	484	+4	1.5
2	478	478	0	
3	480	492	−12	4.5
4	426	444	−18	7
5	440	436	+4	1.5
6	410	398	+12	4.5
7	458	464	−6	3
8	460	476	−16	6

$T_+ = 1.5 + 1.5 + 4.5 = 7.5$
$T_- = 4.5 + 7 + 3 + 6 = 20.5$

From the table, when n=8, the cut-off for significance is 4.
7.5 is greater than this so the differences are not significant, P>0.05 (the exact P value is 0.32 from a statistical program).

Therefore we conclude that there is no evidence for any difference in corneal thickness in affected and unaffected eyes.

Sign test for matched pairs

The sign test can also be used for matched data. It is simpler than the Wilcoxon test and is based on the number of positive and negative differences only. It does not take account of the size of the differences at all. If the distribution of the differences were truly symmetrical about zero (null hypothesis) then the number of positive and negative differences would be similar. The test is based on the exact Binomial distribution to calculate the probability of the observed number of positive and negative differences to see if this is implausibly small (i.e. <0.05).

Since the sign test ignores the sizes of the differences it is less powerful than the Wilcoxon matched pairs test. This can be seen if we use the sign test with the corneal thickness data in Table 8.15.

Sign test using the corneal thickness data

- This can be done using a statistical program and we get P=1.00
- The calculations below are given to show how it works and to give another demonstration of the Binomial distribution (🕮 Binomial distribution: formula, p. 212)
- For the corneal thickness data there are four negative and three positive differences
- If the null hypothesis were true then Prob(positive difference) = Prob(negative difference) = 0.5
- Therefore the probability of the observed data or data more extreme is given by:

[Prob(4 negative + 3 positive) + Prob(5 negative + 2 positive) + Prob(6 negative + 1 positive) + Prob(7 negative)] × 2

(it is multiplied by 2 to give the two-sided test)

- Each of these probabilities can be calculated using the Binomial distribution formula (🕮 Binomial distribution: formula, p. 212)
- The overall probability can be shown to be:
  $(35 \times 0.5^7 + 21 \times 0.5^7 + 7 \times 0.5^7 + 0.5^7) \times 2 = 1.0$ as given by the statistical program

Note that the sign test is clearly non-significant. It gives a greater P value than the P value from the Wilcoxon matched pairs test, reflecting the lower statistical power.

Reference

1 Hand DJ. *A handbook of small data sets*. London: Chapman & Hall, 1994.

Rank correlation

Introduction

Pearson's correlation requires that at least one of the two variables follows a Normal distribution and that the relationship is linear. If these assumptions do not hold and the data cannot be transformed, then rank correlation may be used. There are two forms of the rank correlation coefficient: **Spearman's rho** and **Kendall's tau**. Both test the same null hypothesis and have the same assumptions but they work in different ways and for some situations, one may be preferred to the other (see boxes on this page).

Null hypothesis for rank correlation

- There is no tendency for one variable either to increase or to decrease as the other increases

Assumptions

- The variables can be ranked
- The relationship between the variables either increases or decreases (i.e. it is monotonic)

Spearman's rho (ρ)

- This is calculated using same formula as for Pearson's correlation but **uses the ranks of the data** rather than the data values themselves
- It gives a value between −1 and +1 but there is no straightforward interpretation of ρ regarding the strength of association
- P values can be obtained from a statistical program
- For sample sizes greater than 10, the coefficient ρ follows an approximate Normal distribution and P values can be obtained from Normal distribution tables by calculating:

  $\rho\sqrt{n-1}$, which follows a Standard Normal distribution with mean 0 and standard deviation 1
- ❶ **If there are ties use Kendall's tau-b**

Kendall's tau

- This is more complicated to calculate than Spearman's ρ and is based on the probability distribution of the orderings of the pairs of variables – whether they are concordant, discordant or tied
- Kendall's tau is the proportion of concordant pairs minus the proportion of discordant pairs. For a worked example, see Bland, Chapter 12[1]
- It gives a value between −1 and +1 where +1 indicates all pairs are ordered in the same way and −1 indicates they are all ordered in the opposite way. This is therefore a **meaningful measure** of strength of association
- **If there are ties use modified formula: tau-b**
- tau-a and tau-c give alternative ways of dealing with ties
- For further reading see Conover[2]

Which rank correlation to use: Spearman's or Kendall's?

- If a significance test only is required it doesn't matter which is used
- Spearman's ρ is easier to calculate and may be preferable if the calculations need to be done by hand
- If an estimate of the strength of correlation is needed use Kendall's tau
- If there are many ties use Kendall's tau-b

References

1 Bland M. *An introduction to medical statistics.* 3rd ed. Oxford: Oxford University Press, 2000.
2 Conover WJ. *Practical nonparametric statistics.* 3rd ed. New York: Wiley, 1999.

Rank correlation: example

The data in Figure 8.14 and Table 8.16 show the relationship between percentage unemployed and suicide rate per million in 11 US cities.[1]

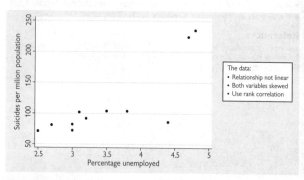

The data:
- Relationship not linear
- Both variables skewed
- Use rank correlation

Fig. 8.14 Scatterplot of unemployment against suicide rate in 11 US cities.

Table 8.16 Percentage unemployment and suicide rates in 11 US cities[1]

City	Unemployed	Suicide rate	Rank (unempl)	Rank (suicide)
Boston	2.5	71	1	1
New York	3	72	3.5	2
Washington	2.7	81	2	3
Chicago	3	82	3.5	4
Pittsburgh	4.4	86	9	5
Philadelphia	3.2	92	6	6
St Louis	3.1	102	5	7
Detroit	3.8	104	8	8.5
Cleveland	3.5	104	7	8.5
Los Angeles	4.7	224	10	10
San Francisco	4.8	235	11	11

- Since there are some ties we will use Kendall's tau-b rather than Spearman's ρ
- Looking at the data, we see that the ordering of ranks for unemployment is mostly the same as that of suicide and so we would expect that Kendall's tau-b will be positive and reasonably close to 1.0
- Using a statistical program gives tau-b = 0.76, P=0.002
- **This therefore shows that there is a moderately strong positive correlation between city-level unemployment and suicide rates and this is statistically significant.**

Footnote: There were two outlying points in the upper right hand portion of the graph (Los Angeles and San Francisco). The calculations were repeated without these as a sensitivity analysis. This gave a smaller value for tau-b, 0.63 with P=0.03, illustrating how outlying points can affect the correlation coefficient, although in this case the conclusions are broadly unchanged.

Reference

1 Hand DJ. *A handbook of small data sets*. London: Chapman & Hall, 1994.

Survival data

Introduction

Survival or time-to-event data are used when the focus of attention is a length of time between two events such as diagnosis and death, or treatment for fertility and conception. **Survival methods are used to calculate survival (time-to-event) probabilities**. For example, in studies of survival after breast cancer diagnosis, survival methods are used to calculate the probability that women will survive for 5 or 10 years. Such techniques are used to compare treatments and to provide information to patients about their likely prognosis.

Censoring

One of the problems with survival data is that at the time the data are analysed some patients will not have experienced the event of interest and so their time of survival will only be known up to that point. Also, some patients are lost to follow-up before the study ends. Both types of data without firm survival times are known as **censored data**.

Survival methods are clever in that they allow censored data to be incorporated into the calculations so that they effectively contribute information up to the point at which no further information is known. Figure 8.15 depicts data such as those described where some patients have a known event and for some the outcome is unknown.

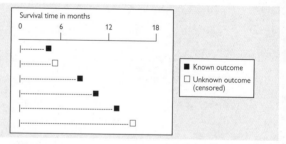

Fig. 8.15 Schematic diagram showing patient outcome in a survival study.

Calculating survival probabilities

We will illustrate the calculations using all data from a health district register of babies born with cystic fibrosis who were analysed 30 years after the register began. The data are shown in Table 8.17.

Table 8.17 Survival times for a sample of patients with cystic fibrosis

ID no.	Length of survival (years)	Outcome D/C	ID no.	Length of survival (years)	Outcome D/C
1	14	D	17	0	D
2	29	C	18	0	D
3	28	C	19	11	C
4	12	D	20	10	C
5	8	D	21	9	C
6	27	C	22	9	C
7	27	C	23	9	C
8	25	C	24	7	C
9	21	C	25	7	C
10	14	D	26	5	C
11	20	C	27	4	C
12	11	D	28	3	C
13	17	C	29	3	C
14	16	C	30	3	C
15	16	C	31	3	C
16	12	C	32	2	C

D=died; C=censored

To calculate the survival probabilities we calculate the following:
- x = age in years
- n_x = no. at that age
- c_x = no. censored at that age
- d_x = no. of deaths
- q_x = probability of death = d_x/n_x
- p_x = probability of surviving to age x = $1 - q_x$
- P_x = cumulative probability of surviving x years), i.e. probability of surviving in year x given that they survived to the start of year x)
  = $p_x \, P_{x-1}$

Survival data (continued)

Calculating survival probabilities for the cystic fibrosis data

Table 8.18 Calculations of survival probability for cystic fibrosis data

x	n_x	c_x	d_x	q_x	p_x	P_x
0	32	0	2	0.0625	0.9375	0.9375
1	30	0	0	0	1	0.9375
2	30	1	0	0	1	0.9375
3	29	4	0	0	1	0.9375
4	25	1	0	0	1	0.9375
5	24	1	0	0	1	0.9375
6	23	0	0	0	1	0.9375
7	23	2	0	0	1	0.9375
8	21	0	1	0.0476	0.9524	0.8929
9	20	3	0	0	1	0.8929
10	17	1	0	0	1	0.8929
11	16	1	1	0.0625	0.9375	0.8371
12	14	1	1	0.0714	0.9286	0.7773
13	12	0	0	0	1	0.7773
14	12	0	2	0.1667	0.8333	0.6478
15	10	0	0	0	1	0.6478
16	10	2	0	0	1	0.6478
17	8	1	0	0	1	0.6478
18	7	0	0	0	1	0.6478
19	7	0	0	0	1	0.6478
20	7	1	0	0	1	0.6478
21	6	1	0	0	1	0.6478
22	5	0	0	0	1	0.6478
23	5	0	0	0	1	0.6478
24	5	0	0	0	1	0.6478
25	5	1	0	0	1	0.6478
26	4	0	0	0	1	0.6478
27	4	2	0	0	1	0.6478
28	2	1	0	0	1	0.6478
29	1	1	0	0	1	0.6478

Explanation of calculations

- It is possible to estimate the probability of dying at each time point when there is a death
- At birth (x=0) there were 32 babies, of whom 2 died during the first year so the estimated probability of death is 2/32=0.0625, giving a probability of survival of 1−0.0625=0.9375
- No baby died during the second year (x=1) so the estimated probability of death is 0 for that time period and the probability of survival is 1. The cumulative probability of survival remains the same at 0.9375
- During the third year (x=2), 1 baby was censored but none died so the probability of death is 0 and probability of survival is 1 for that time period and the cumulative probability of survival remains the same at 0.9375
- The calculations continue in this way with the n_x reducing as subjects are removed due to death or censoring
- During the ninth year (x=8) one subject died. There were 21 alive at the beginning of the interval so the probability of death is estimated as 1/21=0.0476 and probability of survival is 1 − 0.0476=0.9524. The cumulative probability of survival changes to 0.9375 × 0.9524=0.8929
- Where there is a death and a censored patient in the same time period, it is assumed that the censored subject is still 'at risk' when the subject dies so that the censored subject is counted in the number at risk when calculating the probability of death
- The calculations continue until all deaths have been accounted for
- The calculations show the estimated probability of surviving different numbers of years. For example the probability of surviving to age 12 is 0.83 or 83% (to age 12, x=11 row)
- The calculations show that 65% of subjects with cystic fibrosis lived for 28 years (to age 29)

Kaplan–Meier curves

Graphs for survival data

Survival probabilities can be depicted graphically in a Kaplan–Meier curve (Fig. 8.16). The x-axis depicts the length of survival time and the y-axis depicts the cumulative survival probability. This only changes when there is a death and so the graph is not smooth but is stepped. The vertical dashes on the line show the points at which subjects were censored.

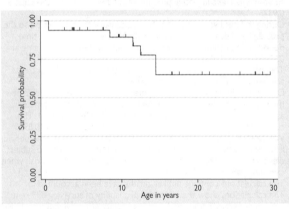

Fig. 8.16 Kaplan–Meier curve for the cystic fibrosis data.

Interpreting the curve

- We can read off the cumulative survival probabilities from the curve
- Note that at the extremes of the curve, the estimated survival probability is based on few subjects and so is not very precise. Figure 8.17 shows the 95% confidence bands around the curve. These illustrate the precision at different points on the curve. The numbers surviving are shown below the x-axis.
- Median survival which is the time for which half of the subjects survive, can be a useful summary measure and is often reported in research reports. This can be read off the Kaplan–Meier curve as long as the curve dips below the '0.50 survival' point on the y-axis, which is not the case for these data

Precision of the survival estimates

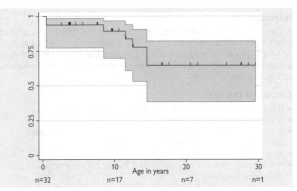

Fig. 8.17 Kaplan–Meier curve for cystic fibrosis data with 95% confidence interval bands.

- The 95% confidence interval bands show the reduced precision at the right hand end of the curve where the calculations of survival are based on fewer subjects
- The cumulative survival probability at age 29 is 65% and this has a wide 95% confidence interval from 38% to 82%

Assumptions of calculations

- The censored cases are from the same population as those who died during the study period
- If cases are censored because they were still alive when the study ended, then we are assuming that survival rates are constant over time
- This can be checked by comparing survival of early and late entrants
- When cases are censored because they cannot be traced, the censoring is self-selected. If there are many like this, the calculations may not be valid, especially if the non-contact is related to survival.

Logrank test

Introduction

If there is more than one group we can draw multiple curves on one graph. If we want to compare the survival in two groups using a statistical test then we need a method that will compare the whole curve for each group, rather than choose only certain time points for testing. The logrank test will do this.

Details of the test

- It is based on comparing the whole curve for each group
- It uses all of the survival data
- It is based on differences between observed and expected values assuming survival is the same in two groups
- It uses a form of chi-squared test
- It is a significance test only and gives a P value but no estimate of the difference in survival

Null hypothesis

- There is no tendency for survival time to be shorter in one group than in the other

Assumptions

- Subjects who are censored have the same probability of an event as those who are fully followed up, i.e. censoring is not related to prognosis
- There is no tendency for one group to have better survival at early time points and worse at later time points. If this were true the curves would diverge and then cross
- The test makes no assumptions about shape of survival curve

The calculations

To illustrate the logrank test we will use data from a study of survival in 2820 women with bilateral carcinoma of the breast,[1] and will compare survival among 51 women with synchronous tumours and 49 with metachronous tumours (Tables 8.19–8.22 and Fig. 8.18). Women still alive at the time of analysis were regarded as 'censored' (56) as were those lost to follow-up (6) and those who died of unrelated causes (4).

The calculations are usually done using a statistical program but hand calculations are given to show how the method works.

Reference

1 Graham MD, Yelland A, Peacock J, Beck N, Ford H, Gazet JC. Bilateral carcinoma of the breast. *Eur J Surg Oncol* 1993; **19**(3):259–64.

Logrank test: example

Table 8.19 Group 1: women with synchronous tumours (*n*=51)

ID	Time (months)	Outcome	ID	Time (months)	Outcome
1	0.5	Censored	27	51	Died
2	0.5	Censored	28	52	Censored
3	1	Died	29	52	Died
4	1	Died	30	55	Censored
5	2	Censored	31	59	Censored
6	3	Died	32	59	Censored
7	4	Died	33	68	Died
8	5	Died	34	73	Censored
9	6	Censored	35	75	Died
10	6	Censored	36	76	Censored
11	8	Died	37	81	Censored
12	9	Censored	38	81	Censored
13	9	Died	39	84	Died
14	14	Died	40	89	Died
15	17	Censored	41	105	Censored
16	18	Censored	42	112	Censored
17	18	Censored	43	115	Censored
18	18	Censored	44	119	Censored
19	24	Censored	45	119	Censored
20	24	Died	46	129	Censored
21	26	Censored	47	130	Died
22	26	Censored	48	131	Censored
23	31	Censored	49	146	Censored
24	39	Censored	50	163	Censored
25	48	Died	51	179	Died
26	50	Died			

Table 8.20 Group 2: women with metachronous tumours (n=49)

ID	Time (months)	Outcome	ID	Time (months)	Outcome
52	4	Died	77	110	Died
53	15	Died	78	117	Censored
54	23	Died	79	118	Censored
55	26	Censored	80	119	Died
56	30	Died	81	124	Censored
57	34	Died	82	129	Censored
58	36	Died	83	130	Censored
59	42	Died	84	133	Died
60	49	Censored	85	138	Censored
61	57	Censored	86	140	Censored
62	58	Died	87	142	Died
63	69	Censored	88	144	Censored
64	74	Censored	89	145	Censored
65	80	Censored	90	146	Censored
66	81	Censored	91	149	Censored
67	81	Censored	92	155	Censored
68	81	Censored	93	155	Censored
69	81	Censored	94	156	Censored
70	86	Censored	95	168	Censored
71	89	Died	96	182	Censored
72	89	Died	97	206	Censored
73	92	Censored	98	211	Censored
74	92	Died	99	218	Censored
75	93	Censored	100	219	Censored
76	94	Censored			

Table 8.21 Extract of table of calculations for logrank test

Time (months)	Group	Outcome	Number at risk			Number of deaths			Probability death	Expected numbers	
			synchro	metach	total	synchr	metach	total		synchro	metach
0	synchron	0	51	49	100	0	0	0	0	0	0
0	synchron	0						0		0	0
1	synchron	1	49	49	98	2	0	2	0.020408	1	1
1	synchron	1						0		0	0
2	synchron	0	47	49	96	0	0	0	0	0	0
3	synchron	1	46	49	95	1	0	1	0.010526	0.484211	0.515789
4	synchron	1	45	49	94	1	1	2	0.021277	0.957447	1.042553
4	metachro	1						0		0	0
And so on until......											
179	synchron	1	1	5	6	1	0	1	0.166667	0.166667	0.833333
182	metachro	0	0	5	5	0	0	0	0	0	0
206	metachro	0	0	4	4	0	0	0	0	0	0
211	metachro	0	0	3	3	0	0	0	0	0	0
218	metachro	0	0	2	2	0	0	0	0	0	0
219	metachro	0	0	1	1	0	0	0	0	0	0
									TOTALS	12.37882	21.62118

Table 8.22 Explanation of calculations for the logrank test

How the calculations work

The synchronous and metachronous groups are denoted by **S** and **M**, respectively

- The logrank test works by dividing survival scale into intervals according to the observed survival times. Censored survival times are ignored
- For each time period the observed data are compared with the expected values if the null hypothesis is true, i.e. there is no difference in survival between the groups
- In the first month (rows 1–2) there were 2 censored observations in **S** (denoted by '0'). These give no information about the probability of death in this interval so the estimated probability of death is 0
- In the second month (rows 3–4) the number at risk was reduced by 2 to allow for 2 subjects censored in the first month. There were 2 deaths in **S**
- 98 subjects were therefore at risk and 2 died so assuming equal risk of death in **S** and **M**, the estimated probability of death is 2/98=0.020 408
- The probability is multiplied by the number of subjects in **S** and **M** to give the expected numbers of deaths: $49 \times 0.020408 = 1$ and $49 \times 0.020408 = 1$
- Note that the expected numbers are 1 in each group because there are equal numbers in the groups at this point. This is not usually the case, as can be seen in row 6, 3 months, where there is one death giving a the probability of death, $1/95 = 0.010526$ and expected numbers in the two groups $46 \times 0.010526 = 0.484211$ and $49 \times 0.010526 = 0.515789$
- The calculations continue in this way until all events have been accounted for
- The expected numbers of deaths are then summed for both **S** and **M**
- Observed numbers are compared to those expected using a chi-squared test as for a two-way table.
- We therefore calculate:

$$\frac{(O_s - E_s)^2}{E_s} + \frac{(O_m - E_m)^2}{E_m}$$

Where O_s is the observed number of deaths in group **S** and E_s is the expected number and conversely O_m, E_m for deaths in group **M**. If the null hypothesis is true, then this expression follows a chi-squared distribution with 1 degree of freedom.

For these data this gives:

$$\frac{(19 - 12.38)^2}{12.38} + \frac{(15 - 21.62)^2}{21.62} = 5.57 \quad P = 0.018$$

Logrank test: interpreting the results

Kaplan–Meier curves for the two groups

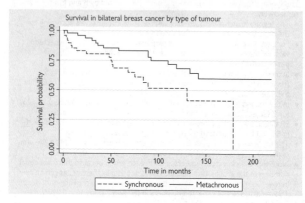

Fig. 8.18 Kaplan–Meier curves comparing two groups.

The results

- The P value is 0.018 which is clearly significant and gives good evidence that there is a difference in survival between women with synchronous and metachronous tumours, with the former group having poorer survival rates
- The method assumes that the censored women have the same probability of survival as those who were fully followed up. If many women were lost to follow-up this would cast doubt on the calculations, particularly if this was related to survival
- An estimate of the difference in survival between the two groups can be obtained using Cox regression – the **hazard ratio**, but this requires firmer assumptions about the relationships, namely that the hazards or death rates are proportional at all time points (see 📖 Cox proportional hazards regression, p. 428)
- The logrank test can be extended for comparing more than two groups

Transforming data

Introduction

Many statistical methods make assumptions about the data that, if not met, will lead to dubious test results. Transformations can be used for the following reasons:

> **Common reasons for transforming data**
> - **Normal distribution**: to make skewed data more closely fit a Normal distribution
> - **Variance:** to stabilize variance, i.e. make the variability more constant either in groups or across a range, as appropriate
> - **Linearity**: to make curved relationships linear

Logarithmic transformation

- Used for data that are quite highly skewed to the right (positive skew) or where the group standard deviations increases with the group means
- Raw data are transformed and calculations done on the log scale, then the estimates are back-transformed
- ❶ P values are **not** back-transformed

Example

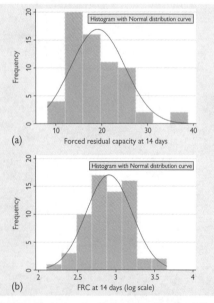

Fig. 8.19 Histograms showing forced residual capacity in 65 preterm babies at 14 days (a) before and (b) after a logarithmic transformation.

The data

Figure 8.19 shows that the raw data are positively skewed but that after log-transformation, the distribution is reasonably symmetrical.

Table 8.23 Data for the first 10 babies, as measured and log-transformed [$\log_e$(FRC)]

ID	FRC	$\log_e$(FRC)
1	11.31	2.426
2	38.90	3.661
3	23.00	3.135
4	20.60	3.025
5	26.00	3.258
6	19.30	2.960
7	22.20	3.100
8	17.20	2.845
9	12.70	2.542
10	15.90	2.766
etc to subject 65		

Calculations for all 65 babies

- Mean FRC = 19.17
- Mean log(FRC) = 2.910
- Anti-log to give: geometric mean = 18.36

Back-transforming log-transformed data for single group

- To back-transform log data use the **anti-log** or **exponential function**
- Back-transformed means given **geometric mean** (📖 Geometric mean, p. 188)
- **Standard deviation (SD) cannot be back-transformed** because the antilog of the SD on log scale will not be in the original units and so is meaningless
- To get confidence intervals, do the calculations on the log scale and back-transform the 2 limits. This gives the **confidence interval for the geometric mean**

Transforming data: comparing means

Using transformations to compare means in two groups

Example

For example, to compare FRC at 14 days in babies who developed bronchopulmonary dysplasia (BPD) and in those who did not (📖 t test for two independent means: example, p. 254). The data were positively skewed (Fig. 8.19). To allow for this, data were log-transformed and a t test done on the log scale data. This gave:

Table 8.24 Results of t test before and after transformation

Raw data (not transformed)				
BPD	No.	Mean	SD	95% CI
No	38	21.44	6.07	
Yes	27	15.97	3.82	
Log-transformed data				
No	38	3.0277	0.2761	
Yes	27	2.7436	0.2403	
Difference		0.2841		0.1524 to 0.4158

t = 4.31, degrees of freedom = 63, P = 0.0001

- Note that the SDs are quite different for the raw data but the log-transformation has corrected this (Table 8.24)
- Antilog difference (0.2841) to give **ratio of geometric means = 1.33**
- Antilog 95% CI for difference to give **95% CI for ratio of geometric means: 1.16 to 1.52**
- This is interpreted as showing that mean FRC at 14 days was 33% greater for babies with BPD than for babies without BPD, with a 95% CI 16% to 52%

Using transformations with paired means
- If differences do not follow a Normal distribution, then a transformation can be used
- **Transform the individual data** not the differences
- Back-transform the mean difference to give the **ratio of the geometric means.** If the paired data are before and after measurements then this is interpreted as the ratio of the two geometric mean measurements

Transforming data: regression and correlation

Regression and correlation

Regression and correlation make assumptions about the distribution of the data, the homogeneity of the variance for different values of x, and the linearity of the relationship. In general, where data follow a positive skewed distribution, the variance will increase as the mean increases and relationships with other variables may not be linear. In such situations, the logarithmic transformation will reduce the skewness and make the variance more homogeneous, and linearize relationships with other variables.

Figure 8.20 shows the effect of transformation on data in an ecological study of free school meals and tuberculosis (TB) rates (☐ Bland and Peacock, p. 122–3[1]).

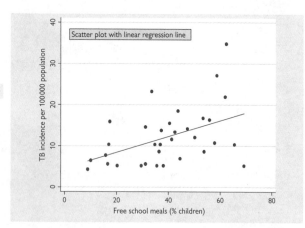

Fig. 8.20 Relationship between free school meals and tuberculosis rate.

- There are more TB values in the lower half of the graph showing that TB rate is positively skewed
- The variance is not constant but increases from left to right

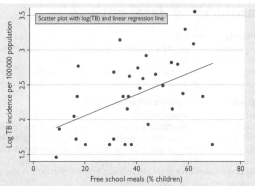

- Log TB rate is more symmetrical in Figure 8.21
- The variance (spread) is more even as we move from left to right
- The straight line is a slightly better fit than in the graph opposite

Fig. 8.21 Relationship between free school meals and log-transformed tuberculosis rate.

Comments

- In this example, transformation has corrected the skewness, non-constant variance and slight non-linearity. However, the effect is modest and the correlation coefficient only increases from 0.44 to 0.46
- In other situations the effect may be more marked, particularly with a larger dataset
- Note that in some situations the relationship between two variables may be approximately linear within a given range but not outside that range. An example of this is the age and lung function data in children (☐ Simple linear regression: example, p. 300) where a straight line relationship gave a reasonable fit between the limited ages studied but would not hold if the age range was extended towards adulthood

Reference

1 Bland M, Peacock J. *Statistical questions in evidence-based medicine*. Oxford: Oxford University Press, 2000.

Transforming data: options

Positively skewed data

- **Log transform** – good for moderate skewness such as found in many biochemical variables
- **Reciprocal** – good for high skewness such as survival data
- **Square root** – good for slight skewness such as often seen in counts

Angular transformation for proportions

- This transformation can be useful when summarizing a set of proportions. For example, in a study comparing proportions of patients referred for X-ray in all general practice surgeries in two regions where we calculate the proportion referred in each practice and then average these proportions in each of the two regions
- The proportions do not usually follow a Normal distribution and the variances are not constant

To correct this, we can use the **arcsine square root transformation** where p is the proportion, $arcsin(\sqrt{p})$ is the angle whose sine is the square root of p. Values of this can be found in tables or using a statistical program (for further details see Bland, Chapter 10[1]).

Size of sample

- If the sample is small, use experience and trial-and-error to get best fit to Normal distribution
- If the sample is large, there are mathematical methods to help decide which to use (see Healy[2])

Zeros

❶ Zeros cause difficulty with many transformations: for example log(0) does not exist, and 1/0 is undefined

- Therefore, zeros have to be dealt with differently
- One possibility is to add a very small number, such 0.1, to any zeros to allow a transformation to be made
- If there are many zeros, then a suitable transformation may not be found because of the shape of the distribution

Preference

Sometimes no transformation completely corrects the skewness in a dataset – one transformation may slightly over-correct and another may slightly under-correct. In such cases, and where the log-transformation improves the symmetry, use this transformation since its results can be back-transformed to provide estimates and confidence intervals.

Back-transforming means

After using log transform

- Means, and differences of means, on the transformed scale are back-transformed to give geometric means, and ratios of geometric means, respectively
- Confidence intervals are back-transformed to give limits for geometric mean, and ratio of geometric mean, respectively
- ❶ SDs and variances cannot be back-transformed

After using reciprocal transformation
- Single means and their confidence intervals can be back-transformed (harmonic mean)

❶ Differences of means and their confidence intervals cannot be back-transformed

❶ SDs can never be back-transformed

After using a square root transformation
- Single means and their confidence intervals can be back-transformed

❶ Differences of means and their confidence intervals cannot be back-transformed

❶ SDs can never be back-transformed

Back-transforming in regression and correlation
Regression: y-variable log-transformed
- The regression coefficients and their confidence intervals are anti-logged
- Interpretation: back-transformed coefficients are ratio of outcome divided by the outcome with one unit lower value of x

Correlation: either or both variables log-transformed
- Correlation coefficient is dimensionless and so is not back-transformed

P values
❶ These are never back-transformed

Further examples
For several worked examples where data were transformed and the results back-transformed, see Peacock and Kerry, Chapter 9[3].

References
1 Bland M. *An introduction to medical statistics.* 3rd ed. Oxford: Oxford University Press, 2000.
2 Healy MJ. The disciplining of medical data. *Br Med Bull* 1968; **24**(3):210–14.
3 Peacock J, Kerry SM. *Presenting medical statistics from proposal to publication.* Oxford: Oxford University Press, 2006.

Diagnostic studies

Introduction

In this chapter we describe how statistical methods are used in diagnostic testing to obtain different measures of a test's performance. We describe how to calculate sensitivity, specificity, and positive and negative predictive values, and show the relevance of pre- and post-test odds and likelihood ratio in evaluating a test in a clinical situation. We also describe the receiver operating characteristic curve and show how this links with logistic regression analysis. All methods are illustrated with examples.

Sensitivity and specificity

Introduction

A diagnostic test or procedure is used in clinical practice to determine whether a patient is likely to have a particular disease or condition. A diagnostic test is used in preference to a definitive '**gold standard**' test when the definitive test is invasive, and/or expensive, and/or time-consuming, and so impractical for use in routine clinical practice.

A diagnostic test may be used to classify individuals into one of two categories such as:
- **Diseased or non-diseased**, e.g. HIV test
- **Positive or negative** physiological state, e.g. pregnancy test
- **High or low risk**, e.g. cervical smear screening
- **Exposed or unexposed**, e.g. paracetamol and salicylate levels in suspected overdose

Diagnostic tests do not always give the 'correct' answer and so it is important to be able to quantify how accurate a particular test is. There is no single statistical measure that can summarize accuracy, since a test result may either fail to detect a case (false negative) or falsely identify a case (false positive). Four measures are commonly used to summarize a test's performance:
- Sensitivity
- Specificity
- Positive predictive value
- Negative predictive value

Gold standard

Sometimes it is not possible to determine the true diagnosis without invasive procedures which would be harmful to the patient and so the gold standard is the best diagnosis possible. For example Alzheimer's dementia can only be accurately confirmed at post mortem.

- **Sensitivity and specificity are characteristics of the test**
- **Sensitivity** is the proportion of those who have the disease who are correctly identified by the test as positive
- **Specificity** is the proportion of those who do not have the disease who are correctly identified by the test as negative

---

Hence sensitivity measures how good the test is at correctly identifying 'diseased' individuals and specificity measures how good the test is at correctly identifying 'non-diseased' individuals.

Ideally tests should have both sensitivity and specificity close to 1.0 (or 100% if they are presented as percentages), although it is often difficult in reality to have both high sensitivity and specificity. The consequences of a false positive or false negative depends on the setting. For example:
- A false negative test for a sexually transmitted disease could falsely reassure and lead to further transmission
- In a pregnant woman, a false positive test for Down's syndrome may result in an unnecessary abortion

- A false positive smear test for cervical cancer would be overturned on further testing, although the anxiety associated with a positive test result that turns out to be false is also an important consideration in evaluating a test's performance. Conversely, a false negative smear test may lead to delayed diagnosis of cancer, causing a worse prognosis.

Example

Table 9.1 Commonly used diagnostic tests with sensitivity and specificity

Test	Sensitivity	Specificity
(a) Conventional cervical smear[1]	72%	94%
(b) Faecal occult blood test for colorectal cancer or adenomatous polyps[2]	43%	92%
(c) Previous history of cancer to indicate cancer in patients with low back pain[3]	31%	98%
(d) Unrelieved symptoms following bed rest to indicate cancer in patients with low back pain[3]	90%	46%
(e) Quadruple test in pregnancy for Down's syndrome[4]	81%	93%

- The examples in Table 9.1 illustrate the range of values for sensitivity and specificity commonly seen in diagnostic tests (assuming that a value of 80% or more for sensitivity or specificity is 'good')
- Some tests are 'good' at correctly identifying those with the disease (d, e)
- Some are 'good' at correctly identifying those without disease (a, b, c, e)
- Only one test is 'good' at both (e)

References

1 Coste J, Cochand-Priollet B, de CP, Le GC, Cartier I, Molinie V *et al.* Cross sectional study of conventional cervical smear, monolayer cytology, and human papillomavirus DNA testing for cervical cancer screening. *BMJ* 2003; **326**(7392):733.

2 Tibble J, Sigthorsson G, Foster R, Sherwood R, Fagerhol M, Bjarnason I. Faecal calprotectin and faecal occult blood tests in the diagnosis of colorectal carcinoma and adenoma. *Gut* 2001; **49**(3):402–8.

3 Deyo RA, Rainville J, Kent DL. What can the history and physical examination tell us about low back pain? *JAMA* 1992; **268**(6):760–5.

4 Wald NJ, Huttly WJ, Hackshaw AK. Antenatal screening for Down's syndrome with the quadruple test. *Lancet* 2003; **361**(9360):835–6.

Calculations for sensitivity and specificity

Notation for calculations in a diagnostic test

Assuming that the diagnostic test can either be positive or negative, indicating the presence or absence of disease, the different test results can be represented as follows.

		Disease status (gold standard)		
		Positive	Negative	Total
Test	Positive	a	b	a+b
	Negative	c	d	c+d
	Total	a+c	b+d	n

Sensitivity = a/(a+c)
(proportion of true positives who are test positive)
Specificity = d/(b+d)
(proportion of true negatives who are test negative)

Positive and negative predictive values

Sensitivity and specificity are characteristics of the test but they do not help a clinician to interpret the results of an individual test. Positive and negative predictive values are useful in a clinical setting as they give the probabilities that an individual is truly positive given that they tested positive, or truly negative given that they tested negative. More precisely they are defined as follows.

Positive predictive value (PPV) = a/(a+b)
(proportion of test positives who are true positive)
Negative predictive value (NPV) = d/(c+d)
(proportion of test negatives who are true negative)

Note that the prevalence of disease is given by:
Prevalence of disease = (a+c)/n
(proportion of all individuals who have the disease, i.e. are positive)

Example

To illustrate the calculations we use data from a paediatric study in which clinicians derived a score from a chest x-ray (CXR) in preterm babies to predict frequent wheeze in the infants at 6 months of age.[1]

		Frequent wheeze at 6 months		
		Yes	No	Total
Chest x-ray score	3+	30	106	136
	<3	7	42	49
	Total	37	148	185

Sensitivity $= \dfrac{\text{Score } 3+ \text{ and frequent wheeze}}{\text{Total with frequent wheeze}}$ = 30/37 = 81%

Specificity $= \dfrac{\text{Score} <3 \text{ and no frequent wheeze}}{\text{Total without frequent wheeze}}$ = 42/148 = 28%

Positive predictive value (PPV) $= \dfrac{\text{Score } 3+ \text{ and frequent wheeze}}{\text{Total with score } 3+}$ = 30/136 = 22%

Negative predictive value (NPV) $= \dfrac{\text{Score} <3 \text{ and no frequent wheeze}}{\text{Total with score} <3}$ = 42/49 = 86%

Prevalence $= \dfrac{\text{Total with frequent wheeze}}{\text{Total patients}}$ = 37/185 = 20%

- The relatively high NPV of 86% means that the majority of those who have a CXR score of <3 (test negative) will not have frequent wheeze at 6 months of age (disease negative)
- The relatively low PPV of 22% means that even with a CXR score of ≥3 (test positive), there is a fairly low probability of having frequent wheeze at 6 months (disease positive)
- NPV and PPV depend on the prevalence of the disease in question (see 📖 Effect of prevalence, p. 344)

Reference

1 Thomas M, Greenough A, Johnson A, Limb E, Marlow N, Peacock JL et al. Frequent wheeze at follow up of very preterm infants: which factors are predictive? *Arch Dis Child Fetal Neonatal Ed* 2003; **88**(4):F329–32.

Effect of prevalence

Performance of a diagnostic test and PPV, NPV

PPV and NPV depend on the prevalence of the disease in the population being tested. If the sensitivity and specificity for a test are known but we wish to use the test on a different population from the one it was developed in, the PPV and NPV can be calculated using standard formulae based on Bayes' theorem (📖 Bayes' theorem, p. 234).

$$PPV = \frac{\text{sensitivity} \times \text{prevalence}}{[\text{sensitivity} \times \text{prevalence}] + [(1-\text{specificity}) \times (1-\text{prevalence})]}$$

$$NPV = \frac{\text{specificity} \times (1-\text{prevalence})}{[(1-\text{sensitivity}) \times \text{prevalence}] + [\text{specificity} \times (1-\text{prevalence})]}$$

Note that the prevalence of disease can also be interpreted as the probability of disease before the test is carried out, the **prior probability** of disease. PPV gives a revised estimate of disease given the extra information provided by the test and is known as the **posterior probability.**

Examples

The effect of prevalence on PPV and NPV can be substantial as the three scenarios below demonstrate.

1. Low prevalence: 100/1100 (9%), high sensitivity, and high specificity

		Disease status		
		+	–	Total
	+	95	50	145
Test result	–	5	950	955
	Total	100	1000	1100

Sensitivity = 95/100 = 95%   PPV = 95/145 = 66%
Specificity = 950/1000 = 95%   NPV = 950/955 = 99%

- Low prevalence and high specificity → NPV is high
- Test negatives are likely to be true negatives but a proportion of those who test positive will actually be negative (34%)

2. Moderate prevalence: 550/1100 (50%), high sensitivity, and high specificity

		Disease status		
		+	−	Total
Test result	+	523	27	550
	−	27	523	550
	Total	550	550	1100

Sensitivity = 523/550 = 95% PPV = 523/550 = 95%
Specificity = 523/550 = 95% NPV = 523/550 = 95%

- Prevalence = 50%, high sensitivity, high specificity → PPV and NPV both high
- Test results are likely to be right, both positive and negative

3. High prevalence: 1000/1100 (91%), high sensitivity, and high specificity

		Disease status		
		+	−	Total
Test result	+	950	5	955
	−	50	95	145
	Total	1000	100	1100

Sensitivity = 950/1000 = 95% PPV = 950/955 = 99%
Specificity = 95/100 = 95% NPV = 95/145 = 66%

- High prevalence, high specificity → PPV high
- Test positives are likely to be true positives, but a proportion of those who test negative will actually be positive (34%)

Likelihood ratio, pre-test odds, post-test odds

Likelihood ratio

The **likelihood ratio** (LR) gives another measure of the performance of a test and is defined as follows.

> LR = sensitivity/(1−specificity)

Therefore, for a particular test, the LR compares the probability of a positive test result in an individual with the disease of interest with the probability of a positive test result if they were healthy. An LR greater than 1.0 indicates that the test is more likely to give a positive result if the individual had the disease than if they did not, and the greater the value of the LR, the more discriminating is the test.[1]

The LR can be combined with the **odds** of having the condition, to quantify the information given by the test that an individual with a positive test result actually has the disease.

The odds of having the disease is defined as follows.

> Odds = prevalence/(1−prevalence)   (= pre-test odds)

This is often referred to as the **pre-test odds** because it relates to the underlying prevalence in all individuals in the population of interest.

Following a positive test result, the **post-test odds** is given as follows.

> Post-test odds = pre-test odds x LR

The post-test odds is another way of quantifying the information that a positive test result provides about whether an individual truly has the disease. Table 9.2 shows data from a cohort study of just under 800 000 patients, which investigated alarm symptoms in early diagnosis of cancer in primary care. Since general practitioners see relatively few new cases of cancer in the primary care setting, this study compared four common symptoms in relation to a subsequent diagnosis of cancer.

Example

Table 9.2 Observed related diagnoses of cancer in the first 6 months after first alarm symptom. Positive predicted value (PPV) and likelihood ratio for cancer after symptom[2]

	PPV (%)	Likelihood ratio
Haematuria:		
Men	5.5	111
Women	2.5	215
Haemoptysis:		
Men	5.8	117
Women	3.3	153
Dysphagia:		
Men	5.3	348
Women	2.1	266
Rectal bleeding:		
Men	1.8	75
Women	1.5	78

- **The likelihood ratios (LRs) are all high**, showing that the presence of the symptom makes it much more likely that the patient has cancer than if they did not have the symptom
  For example, the LRs for dysphagia (348 in men, 266 in women) mean that those with the symptom are approximately 300 times as likely to have cancer as patients without the symptom.
- **However, the PPVs are very low** showing that most patients with these symptoms will not have cancer:
  For example, for dysphagia, only 5% of men and 2% of women with this symptom actually have cancer.
- Note that both PPVs and LRs vary by symptom

References

1 Deeks JJ, Altman DG. Diagnostic tests 4: likelihood ratios. *BMJ* 2004; **329**(7458):168–9.
2 Jones R, Latinovic R, Charlton J, Gulliford MC. Alarm symptoms in early diagnosis of cancer in primary care: cohort study using General Practice Research Database. *BMJ* 2007; **334**(7602):1040.

Receiver operating characteristic (ROC) curves

Introduction

The discussions about sensitivity and specificity so far have assumed that the diagnostic test gives one of two results, positive or negative. In practice, a clinical assessment may have a range of possible values such as a score or a measurement. The Normal or reference range can be used to determine the cut-off for abnormality, for example troponin I for diagnosing myocardial infarction (cut-off 0.6 ng/mL: sensitivity=94%, specificity=81%; cut-off 2.0ng/mL: sensitivity=85%, specificity=91%[1]).

As an alternative we can use a graphical method, the **receiver operating characteristic (ROC) curve** to compare the sensitivity and specificity for all possible cut-offs. This allows the most appropriate cut-off to be chosen for the particular context.

Description

- ROC curves usually plot 1–specificity (x-axis) against sensitivity (y-axis). A horizontal line is shown at 45° and the 'curve' joins the points (Fig. 9.1). Each point indicates a different cut-off and therefore gives a different combination of sensitivity and specificity
- Sensitivity and specificity are inversely related – if we change the cut-off for sensitivity, to improve the performance of the test, this will automatically reduce the specificity
- If the diagnostic test performs well then the curve will be distinctly above the 45° line. If the curve rises steeply and is close to the y-axis and then flattens out, the 'best' possible cut-off will give high sensitivity and specificity
- The area under the curve is sometimes used as a summary measure of how well a variable or set of variables predict a binary outcome

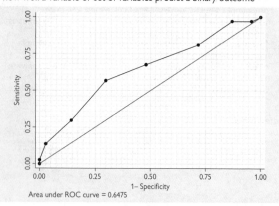

Area under ROC curve = 0.6475

Fig. 9.1 Example of a receiver operating characteristic (ROC) curve.

To illustrate the use of ROC curves to determine the best cut-off, we use the data from the paediatric study shown earlier in this chapter (Calculations for sensitivity and specificity, p. 343).[2] The chest x-ray score was discrete and ranged from 0 to 8. The ROC curve in Figure 9.1 shows that the curve is well above the 45° line but is not steep.

Table 9.3 Sensitivity and specificity for each possible cut-off of chest x-ray score

Cut-off	Sensitivity	Specificity
≥0	100%	0%
≥1	97%	4%
≥2	97%	13%
≥3	81%	28%
≥4	68%	52%
≥5	57%	70%
≥6	30%	86%
≥7	14%	97%
8	3%	100%

- No cut-off gives both high sensitivity and high specificity
- In this particular clinical setting it was desirable to have a low rate of false negatives (high sensitivity) since infants who were likely to have later respiratory disease would benefit from extra treatment in infancy
- The cut-off chosen was ≥3 giving sensitivity 81%, and specificity 28%
- The area under the curve was 0.65 (maximum = 1.0). Thus the predictive power of this test in general is moderately high
- The **accuracy of the test** (proportion of all individuals who were correctly identified by the test) is (30+42)/185 = 39%

Extensions to two cut-offs

A diagnostic test can have two cut-offs: one to rule out disease with high probability and another to rule in disease with high probability. Values in-between are inconclusive. This principle is often applied informally in clinical practice. For example, a blood pressure reading of 120/80 mmHg would generally rule out hypertension, with a reading of 160/100 usually demonstrating disease. A reading in the middle may be deemed inconclusive, with the resulting decision being to repeat at a later date. For some published examples see the work on diagnosing non-alcoholic fatty liver disease.[3–5]

References

1 Ross G, Bever FN, Uddin Z, Hockman EM. Troponin I sensitivity and specificity for the diagnosis of acute myocardial infarction. *J Am Osteopath Assoc* 2000; **100**(1):29–32.

2 Thomas M, Greenough A, Johnson A, Limb E, Marlow N, Peacock JL et al. Frequent wheeze at follow up of very preterm infants: which factors are predictive? *Arch Dis Child Fetal Neonatal Ed* 2003; **88**(4):F329–32.

3 Guha IN, Parkes J, Roderick P, Chattopadhyay D, Cross R, Harris S et al. Noninvasive markers of fibrosis in nonalcoholic fatty liver disease: Validating the European Liver Fibrosis Panel and exploring simple markers. *Hepatology* 2008; **47**(2):455–60.

4 Guha IN, Parkes J, Roderick PR, Harris S, Rosenberg WM. Non-invasive markers associated with liver fibrosis in non-alcoholic fatty liver disease. *Gut* 2006; **55**(11):1650–60.

5 Parkes J, Guha IN, Roderick P, Rosenberg W. Performance of serum marker panels for liver fibrosis in chronic hepatitis C. *J Hepatol* 2006; **44**(3):462–74.

Links to other statistics

1. Link to logistic regression

Logistic regression can be used to calculate the area under the curve for a particular combination of 'gold standard' variable and 'test' variable. This can be useful if there are several possible variables which could be used to derive a test, for example there might be several possible scores that may be useful in predicting frequent wheeze. To determine which of these is best we can compare the area under the curves, and the variable with the highest area is the best predictor of the disease of interest. Alternatively, it may be possible to combine the different scores to produce an even better measure.

2. Confidence intervals and significance tests

- Sensitivity, specificity, PPV, and NPV are all proportions and confidence intervals (CI) are useful to indicate precision
- CIs are calculated in the same way as for other proportions (📖 95% confidence intervals for a proportion, p. 244)[1]
- Sometimes these proportions, particularly sensitivity, come from a small sample and so CIs may be wide
- For example, in the paediatric data given previously (📖 Calculations for sensitivity and specificity, p. 342): sensitivity = 30/37 = 81%, 95% CI: 65% to 92%
- Sensitivity, specificity, etc. can be compared but care needs to be taken:
  (i) When two diagnostic tests have been developed using the same dataset then **paired tests need to be used**, see Hawass for worked details[2]
  (ii) When two diagnostic tests have been developed using different datasets then **unpaired tests should be used**, such as the chi-squared test (📖 Chi-squared test, p. 262)
- A significance test is available to compare two or more ROC curves. This can be useful when exploring the ability of different factors to predict an outcome as described in point 1 above (📖 Logistic regression, p. 420)
  Likelihood ratios are ratios of proportions, and so CIs can be calculated and significance tests performed in the same way as for relative risks (📖 Confidence interval for tests of proportions, p. 270)

3. Effect of prevalence on sensitivity and specificity

- Sensitivity and specificity are not affected by the prevalence of disease if the true diagnosis (gold standard) is always correct
- In practice there may be an error in the true diagnosis and in such cases the sensitivity and specificity are measuring the ability of the test to predict the *diagnosis* rather than the true disease state
- Hence, if it is known that errors are possible in the true diagnosis, then it is safer to evaluate a diagnostic test in a sample with a similar prevalence to that in which it is planned to use the test in future[3]

References

1 Altman DG, Machin D, Bryant TN, Gardner MJ. *Statistics with confidence: confidence intervals and statistical guidelines.* London: BMJ Publishing Group, 2000.
2 Hawass NE. Comparing the sensitivities and specificities of two diagnostic procedures performed on the same group of patients. *Br J Radiol* 1997; **70**(832):360–6.
3 Begg CB. Biases in the assessment of diagnostic tests. *Stat Med* 1987; **6**(4):411–23.

Other statistical methods

Introduction

In this chapter we describe several individual statistical methods that do not fit neatly in the other chapters but which are commonly used in medical research. These include methods used to assess agreement in measurement and reliability studies, the number needed to treat as a measure of efficacy in a trial, and life tables. All methods are illustrated with examples.

Kappa for inter-rater agreement

Introduction

Kappa is a statistic that measures the agreement between two raters where responses can fall into any of a number of categories. For example Table 10.1 shows data from ultrasound scans in preterm babies to determine how well different doctors agree with the grading of the scans. Each baby's scan can be classified as normal or abnormal using a published grading system.

Table 10.1 Grading of ultrasound scans into normal or abnormal by two doctors: the hospital doctor and an independent doctor

Hospital Doctor	Independent Doctor		
	Normal	Abnormal	Total
Normal	490	45	535
Abnormal	18	57	75
Total	508	102	610

❶ Percentage agreement is misleading

One approach commonly used with data such as these is to calculate the percentage agreement. Here this is (490+57)/610=0.897 or approximately 90%. This looks impressive but is misleading because it ignores agreement that could have occurred by chance.

To illustrate this suppose we had the only the hospital doctor grading and that we tossed a coin to get the second opinion. We assume that a head is 'Normal' and a tail is 'Abnormal'. We used a computer program to simulate the coin tossing and obtained the data shown in Table 10.2.

Table 10.2 Grading of ultrasound scans by hospital doctor with the second opinion obtained by tossing a coin (head='normal', tail='abnormal')

Hospital Doctor	Second opinion (toss coin)		
	Normal	Abnormal	Total
Normal	274	261	535
Abnormal	34	41	75
Total	308	302	610

Here the percentage agreement is (274+41)/610=0.516 or approximately 52%. This is clearly less impressive than the real data but shows that simply by chance alone we can get a value of over 50%. If the second opinion always chooses 'normal' then we get Table 10.3, which has a percentage agreement of (535+0)/610=0.877 or approximately 88%, which is close to the value of 90% obtained with the actual data.

Table 10.3 Grading of ultrasound scans by hospital doctor with the second opinion obtained always grading scans as 'normal'

| Hospital Doctor | Second opinion (grade all scans 'normal') | | |
	Normal	Abnormal	Total
Normal	535	0	535
Abnormal	75	0	75
Total	610	0	610

Kappa

We therefore need a method that will measure agreement over and beyond agreement that happens by chance alone. Kappa does this. It works by adjusting the observed proportion agreeing for the agreement that would happen by chance.

Calculating kappa
1. **Calculate the proportion of categories where there is agreement, Pa**
2. **Calculate the proportion agreeing by chance, Pc, as below:**
    - Expected values are calculated as in the chi-squared test (📖 Chi-squared test, p. 262) as row total × column total/grand total
    - Proportion agreeing by chance is sum of expected numbers divided by grand total
3. **Kappa = (Pa – Pc)/(1 – Pc)**

Example of calculations

From Table 10.1:
1. Proportion of categories where there is agreement = 0.897
2. Proportion agreeing by chance:
    normal/normal: 535/610 × 508/610 = 0.730
    abnormal/abnormal: 102/610 × 75/610 = 0.021
    Proportion agreeing by chance:
    0.730 + 0.021 = 0.751
3. Kappa = (0.897 – 0.751)/(1 – 0.751)
         = 0.59

Kappa (continued)

Interpreting kappa

Table 10.4 gives a qualitative interpretation of kappa devised by Landis and Koch.[1] This has been widely adopted as a useful guide.

Table 10.4 Interpretation of kappa[1]

Value of kappa	Strength of agreement
<0.00	Poor (worse than chance)
0.00–0.20	Slight
0.21–0.40	Fair
0.41–0.60	Moderate
0.61–0.80	Good
0.81–1.00	Very good

Note that kappa can be negative, and although this is unlikely in practice, negative values imply that agreement is worse than that expected by chance. For the example (Table 10.1), the kappa value, 0.59 can be described as representing moderate agreement between the two doctors.

Confidence interval for kappa

A confidence interval (CI) can be calculated for kappa provided the sample is large enough. In practice this works as long as $n \times Pc$ and $n \times (1 - Pc)$ are both greater than 5, where n is the overall total.

Calculation of CI for kappa

1. **Standard error** of kappa (SE) is given by:

$$SE = \sqrt{\frac{Pa(1-Pa)}{n(1-Pc)^2}}$$

Where n is the overall total and Pc and Pa are as before.

2. **95% CI:**
   $Kappa \pm 1.96 \times SE$

Example of calculation of 95% CI

From previous section ([Calculation of CI for kappa, p. 355):
$Pa = 0.897$
$Pc = 0.751$
$n = 610$
Kappa $= 0.586$

$$SE = \sqrt{\frac{Pa(1-Pa)}{n(1-Pc)^2}} = \sqrt{\frac{0.897(1-0.897)}{610(1-0.751)^2}}$$

$$= 0.049$$

95% CI:
$0.586 \pm 1.96 \times 0.049$
0.49 to 0.68

Significance test

A significance test for kappa can be calculated to test the null hypothesis that the population value of kappa is zero. The calculation of this involves a slightly modified standard error and is shown below.

Calculation of significance test for kappa

For the significance test use the following test statistic:

$$\frac{Kappa}{\sqrt{\frac{Pc}{n(1-Pc)}}} = \frac{0.586}{\sqrt{\frac{0.751}{610(1-0.751)}}}$$

$$= 8.33, P < 0.001$$

So we have good evidence for real agreement but it is only moderately strong.

Reference

1 Landis JR, Koch GG. The measurement of observer agreement for categorical data. *Biometrics* 1977; **33**(1):159–74.

Extensions to kappa

More than two categories

Table 10.5 shows data from a study to validate a new five-level triage instrument. The instrument was trialled in 351 patients by both a nurse and a doctor.[1] The kappa calculation can be extended to more than two categories (details omitted), and gives kappa=0.70.

Table 10.5 The agreement in triage ratings patients by a nurse and a doctor in 351 using the Emergency severity index (ESI).[1] The shaded cells indicate agreement

Doctor triage	Nurse triage					Total
	ESI-1	ESI-2	ESI-3	ESI-4	ESI-5	
ESI-1	4	0	0	0	0	4
ESI-2	2	84	12	1	0	99
ESI-3	0	13	81	12	1	107
ESI-4	0	0	5	66	22	93
ESI-5	0	0	1	10	37	48
Total	6	97	99	89	60	351

Weighted kappa

The calculation of kappa for Table 10.5 has not taken into account the ordering in the categories. This may be important if the extent of the disagreement has a useful meaning. With these data, a disagreement by one category may be less serious than a disagreement by two categories or more.

A weighted version of kappa can be calculated which takes account of how far apart any disagreements are. In the example above, for the ESI-2 row, 84 were also graded as ESI-2 by the nurse but 2 were graded ESI-1, 12 were graded ESI-3, and 1 was graded ESI-4 by the nurse. Weighted kappa takes into account the degree of disagreement.

An obvious choice for weights would be 0 for agree, 1 for a disagreement by one category, 2 for a disagreement of two categories, etc. Using this weighting system, weighted kappa is 0.80 (details of calculations omitted). This indicates a greater level of agreement than the unweighted kappa value.

A 95% confidence interval can also be calculated for the weighted kappa and is 0.76 to 0.84 here.

Choice of weights matters

The weights used above are known as **linear weights**. Other weighting systems can be used such as **quadratic weights** where the weights are the squares of the linear weights, i.e. they are 0, 1, 4, 9, 16. This gives a different kappa, 0.89.

❶ Since the choice of weights affects kappa, it is clearly important to **choose the weights in advance on theoretical grounds** and not to try different weights and use the set which give the biggest kappa value.

More than two observers

Kappa can be extended still further to allow for multiple observers. For example in a study of interobserver agreement for the assessment of handicap in stroke patients, 10 senior neurologists and 24 junior doctors interviewed 100 patients in different combinations of pairs.[2] The degree of handicap was recorded by each observer on the modified Rankin scale, which measures the degree of disability in stroke patients on a six-point scale. The authors reported a weighted kappa of 0.91, using quadratic weights (details omitted). A further extension is where multiple observers rate each subject (see Streiner and Norman[3]).

Calculations

These extensions to kappa are not easily calculated by hand and require specialized statistical software, such as Stata,[4] which will calculate all methods discussed here.

Cautions in using kappa

Using kappa is not trouble-free and potential problems in using and interpreting kappa include:

- Kappa depends on the true proportions of subjects in each category. It is greatest when the proportion is 0.5. Hence unless there is perfect agreement, when one category is much smaller than the other(s), kappa will be small irrespective of the degree of agreement
- The calculation of kappa assumes that the sample is representative of the underlying population. If for example the sample is stratified to have a larger number in a rare category, then the sample kappa will be artificially inflated and will not reflect the true agreement

Further information on kappa

See the following books and papers:

- Theory: Cohen,[5,6] Fleiss[7]
- Practical description: Altman[8] (Chapter 14), Streiner and Norman[3]

References

1 Wuerz RC, Milne LW, Eitel DR, Travers D, Gilboy N. Reliability and validity of a new five-level triage instrument. *Acad Emerg Med* 2000; **7**(3):236–42.

2 van Swieten JC, Koudstaal PJ, Visser MC, Schouten HJ, van GJ. Interobserver agreement for the assessment of handicap in stroke patients. *Stroke* 1988; **19**(5):604–7.

3 Streiner DL, Norman GR. *Health measurement scales: a practical guide to their development and use.* 3rd ed. Oxford: Oxford University Press, 2003.

4 Stata: Data analysis and statistical software. ℞ www.stats.com.

5 Cohen J. A coefficient of agreement for nominal scales. *Educational and Psychological Measurement* 1960; **20**(1):37–46.

6 Cohen J. Weighted kappa: nominal scale agreement provision for scaled disagreement or partial credit. *Psychol Bull* 1968; **70**:213–20.

7 Fleiss J.L. Measuring nominal scale agreement among many raters. *Psychol Bull* 1971; **76**:378–82.

8 Altman DG. *Practical statistics for medical research.* London: Chapman & Hall, 1991.

Bland–Altman method to measure agreement

Comparing methods of measurements

It is common in medicine to compare two different methods of measuring the same quantity. For example the data in Table 10.6 show airway resistance, a measure of lung function, measured in infants using an invasive method (Raw) and using a non-invasive method (Rint).[1]

Table 10.6 Airway resistance measured in two ways – Raw and Rint in 26 infants

Raw	Rint	Raw	Rint	Raw	Rint
2.35	3	2.64	1.8	4.12	3.5
2.08	2.1	2.44	2.5	3.31	2.1
6.92	5	3.83	2.4	3.59	2.3
6.87	3.4	2.24	3.3	3.55	2.6
3.76	3	2.54	1.8	4.4	3.1
3	1.7	2.13	2.2	2.53	3
4.66	4	2.92	3.6	1.65	2.7
3.62	2.1	3.07	3.8	3.22	2.2
4.55	3.6	3.68	3.1		

❶ Correlation is inappropriate

It is common but inappropriate to analyse data such as these by plotting them and calculating a correlation coefficient as in Figure 10.1.

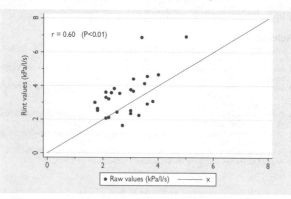

Fig. 10.1 Scatter plot of Raw and Rint in 26 infants.

Figure 10.1 shows the Raw and Rint values with the line of equality. The correlation coefficient of 0.60 is statistically significant showing that there is good evidence of a real linear relationship between Raw and Rint. However the statistically significant correlation does not indicate that the methods *agree,* as Bland explains.[2]

- Correlation r measures how strongly two variables are related to each other, not how well they agree. There would be perfect correlation and agreement if all the points were on the line of equality. However, there would be perfect correlation if the points were on any non-horizontal straight line but this would not indicate perfect agreement.
- If the scale of measurement was changed, for example by multiplying all Raw values by two, the correlation r would be exactly the same, 0.60, but there would be poor agreement between the values.
- Correlation is affected by the range of data used – a greater range gives a stronger correlation. Agreement on the other hand is not affected by the range.

Bland–Altman limits of agreement

The Bland–Altman method provides a measure of agreement by estimating how far apart the two values are on average and putting an interval around this. This is achieved by calculating the following:

- Mean difference between the methods
- Standard deviation of differences (SD)
- Range: **mean $\pm$ 2 SD** gives **limits of agreement**

Example of calculations

- Mean difference between Rint and Raw: 0.6065
- Standard deviation of differences: 1.03406
- Limits of agreement: $0.6065 \pm 2 \times 1.03406$
  Limits of agreement are: −1.46 to 2.67
- This means that for 95% of observations, the difference between Rint and Raw will lie between −1.46 and 2.67

References

1 Thomas MR, Rafferty GF, Blowes R, Peacock JL, Marlow N, Calvert S *et al.* Plethysmograph and interrupter resistance measurements in prematurely born young children. *Arch Dis Child Fetal Neonatal Ed* 2006; **91**(3):F193–6.
2 Bland JM, Altman DG. Statistical methods for assessing agreement between two methods of clinical measurement. *Lancet* 1986; **i**(8476):307–10.

Bland–Altman method (continued)

Interpretation of limits of agreement

- **Limits of agreement indicate how closely the two methods agree**
- What is regarded as **'close' is a clinical decision not a statistical one**
- If methods **agree closely they can be used interchangeably**
- If methods **do not agree closely they should not be used interchangeably**
- Check **if agreement is uniform along the range of values measured**. If not, the limits do not apply and a modified method is needed (see opposite 'extensions to Bland–Altman')

Bland–Altman plot

This is a graph that plots the mean of the two measurements against the difference to provide a visual impression of the extent of agreement. Figure 10.2 shows the plot for the Raw and Rint data. It clearly shows that Rint values tend to be higher than Raw and this does not appear to be affected by the size of the lung function measurement, except at the upper end where two high values show very poor agreement.

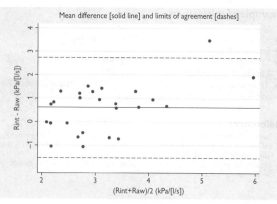

Fig. 10.2 Bland–Altman plot for Raw and Rint data[1].

For these data, the researchers concluded that there was poor agreement between Rint and Raw. This meant that Rint measurements which do not require the infant to be sedated cannot be used as a substitute for Raw measurements which do.[1]

Extensions to Bland–Altman method

- **95% confidence intervals:** these are rarely seen but can be calculated using formulae given in Bland[2] and are shown below (details omitted)
  Mean difference = 0.61 (95% CI: 0.19 to 1.02)
  Lower limit of agreement = −1.46 (95% CI: −2.18 to −0.74)
  Upper limit of agreement = 2.67 (95% CI: 1.95 to 3.39)
- **Relationship between difference and mean**: if the difference increases with the mean, try a logarithmic transformation. See Bland[2] for worked example
- **Testing repeatability**: can be done using similar methods, see Bland[2]
- **Measuring agreement with repeated measurements**: see Bland[2]
- **Multiple observations per individual:** see Bland[3]

Intraclass correlation coefficient

Whereas the correlation coefficient is not appropriate to measure agreement, the intraclass correlation coefficient (ICC) may be used. It measures the extent to which there is perfect agreement, i.e. the extent to which the points vary around a line of perfect unity. It is a dimensionless quantity and so can be useful when looking at agreement in several factors separately, i.e. to see which factors agree most closely. Unlike the limits of agreement described above, the ICC does not estimate how closely the two methods agree in absolute terms.

Further reading

- Bland and Altman have published a number of papers on their method[2–11]
- Martin Bland's website provides regular updates on this work and has helpful FAQs ✆ www.users.york.ac.uk/~mb55/

References

1 Thomas MR, Rafferty GF, Blowes R, Peacock JL, Marlow N, Calvert S et al. Plethysmograph and interrupter resistance measurements in prematurely born young children. *Arch Dis Child Fetal Neonatal Ed* 2006; **91**(3):F193–6.
2 Bland JM, Altman DG. Statistical methods for assessing agreement between two methods of clinical measurement. *Lancet* 1986; **i**(8476):307–10.
3 Bland JM, Altman DG. Agreement between methods of measurement with multiple observations per individual. *J Biopharm Stat* 2007; **17**(4):571–82.
4 Altman DG, Bland JM. Measurement in medicine: the analysis of method comparison studies. *The Statistician* 1983; **32**(307):317.
5 Altman DG, Bland JM. Comparison of methods of measuring blood pressure. *J Epidemiol Community Health* 1986; **40**(3):274–-7.
6 Bland JM, Altman DG. A note on the use of the intraclass correlation coefficient in the evaluation of agreement between two methods of measurement. *Comput Biol Med* 1990; **20**(5): 337–40.
7 Bland JM, Altman DG. Comparing two methods of clinical measurement: a personal history. *Int J Epidemiol* 1995; **24** Suppl 1:S7–14.
8 Bland JM, Altman DG. Comparing methods of measurement: why plotting difference against standard method is misleading. *Lancet* 1995; **346**(8982):1085–7.
9 Bland JM, Altman DG. Difference versus mean plots. *Ann Clin Biochem* 1997; **34**(Pt 5):570–1.
10 Bland JM, Altman DG. Measuring agreement in method comparison studies. *Stat Methods Med Res* 1999; **8**(2):135–60.
11 Bland JM, Altman DG. Applying the right statistics: analyses of measurement studies. *Ultrasound Obstet Gynecol* 2003; **22**(1):85–93.

Chi-squared goodness of fit test

Details of the test

It is used to test the null hypothesis that a frequency distribution follows a particular theoretical distribution, for example a uniform distribution, the Poisson distribution or Normal distribution.

How it works

- It works by calculating expected values (**E**) for the data and comparing them with the observed values (**O**) using a chi-squared test
- Expected numbers are calculated by multiplying the frequency in a category by the probability that an individual falls in that category
- The format of the test is the same as for contingency tables, i.e.:

$$\sum_{all\ cells} \frac{(O-E)^2}{E}$$

- The degrees of freedom are given by:
  (no. of groups − 1) − (no. of parameters estimated from the data)
- If a Normal distribution is fitted to some data then two parameters are estimated from the data – the mean and the standard deviation. For the Poisson distribution there is one parameter – the mean. In some situations as in the following example, no parameters were estimated.
- ❶ Do not use the chi-squared goodness of fit test if more than a small proportion of expected frequencies are less than 5 or if any are less than 1

Example

The cause of sudden unexpected death in epilepsy (SUDEP) is by definition unknown and there have been many studies investigating possible risk factors. It was recently suggested that winter temperatures might be a risk factor but no data were presented, and so Bell and colleagues sought to explore this hypothesis using data from the UK. They cross-classified deaths by month, season, and temperature to see if the number of deaths varied by any of the seasonal factors.[1] Numbers by month are given in Table 10.7.

Hypothesis

If there were no differences in the incidence of SUDEP by month, then the distribution of deaths would be even across all months and the numbers expected could be calculated by equally dividing the total deaths across the months. If cold temperatures did lead to more deaths in winter then the observed deaths would not be evenly distributed. To test this, a chi-squared goodness of fit test can be used to compare the observed number of deaths with the expected number.

Table 10.7 Distribution of SUDEP by month of death

Sep 99	Oct 99	Nov 99	Dec 99	Jan 00	Feb 00	Total
35	34	41	43	44	30	
Mar 00	Apr 00	May 00	Jun 00	Jul 00	Aug 00	
27	36	33	30	32	24	409

The calculations
- The expected values are calculated as:
  total × no. of days in month/366
- For example for January: *expected no.= 409 × 31/366*
- All expected numbers are shown below

Table 10.8 Expected values for the monthly data

Sep 99	Oct 99	Nov 99	Dec 99	Jan 00	Feb 00	Total
33.52	34.64	33.52	34.64	34.64	32.41	
Mar 00	Apr 00	May 00	Jun 00	Jul 00	Aug 00	
34.64	33.52	34.64	33.52	34.64	34.64	409.00

$$\sum_{all\ cells} \frac{(O-E)^2}{E}$$

$$= \frac{(35-33.52)^2}{33.52} + \frac{(34-34.64)^2}{34.64} + ... + \frac{(24-34.64)^2}{34.64}$$

$$= 12.25$$

The degrees of freedom are: no. months − 1 = 11; P=0.35

So there is *no* evidence that the number of deaths varies by month.

Reference

1 Bell GS, Peacock JL, Sander JW. Seasonality as a risk factor for sudden unexpected death in epilepsy: A study in a large cohort. *Epilepsia* 27 Oct 2009 [epub ahead of print].

Number needed to treat

Introduction

The number need to treat (NNT) is a useful way to summarize the clinical effectiveness of a treatment that has been assessed using a binary (yes/no) outcome. NNT is widely used in the reporting of clinical trials and is calculated as the reciprocal of the absolute risk reduction.

Formula

> - Assume that two treatments A and B are being compared and A is more effective than B
> - P_A is the proportion experiencing the negative outcome in group A, P_B is the proportion experiencing the negative outcome in group B
>
> → Absolute difference is $P_B - P_A$
> → **Number needed to treat is $1/(P_B - P_A)$**

Interpretation of NNT

- Number of patients who need to be treated in order that one additional patient has a positive outcome
- A lower number indicates a more effective treatment
- When there is no difference in outcome between the treatment and control groups, i.e. difference=0, the NNT is 1/0 which is infinity (∞)

Example

> A randomized controlled trial in pregnant women with gestational diabetes investigated whether a package of care including insulin therapy reduced the risk of perinatal complications.[1] The main outcome was 'any serious perinatal complications' (yes/no) and the following results were reported:
> - Proportion with complications in the treated group: 7/506 = 0.014
> - Proportion with complications in the control group: 23/524 =0.044
> - Difference in proportions: 0.044 − 0.014 = 0.03 (95% CI: 0.010 to 0.052)
>
> To calculate the NNT, invert the difference and its 95% CI:
> 1/0.03 = 33; 1/0.052 to 1/0.010 = 19 to 100
> → **NNT is 33 (95% CI: 19 to 100)**

Non-significant results

The gestational diabetes trial obtained a statistically significant difference, as shown by a 95% confidence interval for the difference which excluded the null value 0. When the difference is not statistically significant, the confidence interval for the difference includes 0. This causes some difficulty in constructing and interpreting a confidence interval for NNT because the inverse of 0 cannot be calculated and so the confidence interval is discontinuous. In addition, one of the 95% confidence limits will be negative when a number needed to treat cannot be negative. In this case it indicates a harmful effect. The harmful effect number is called the **number needed to harm (NNH)**.

Example

In the randomized controlled trial in pregnant women with gestational diabetes, the authors reported caesarean section rates in the treated and control groups[1]:

Proportion with caesarean section in the treated group: 152/506=0.300
Proportion with complications in the control group: 164/524 =0.313
Difference in proportions: 0.313 − 0.300 = 0.013 (95% CI: −0.044 to 0.069)
NNT = 1/0.013 = 77

Superficially the 95% confidence limits are: −1/0.044 = −14 and 1/0.069 = 23

❶ **But note that**:
- **The 95% CI for the NNT cannot be the simple reciprocal** of this, −23 to 14, as this does not include the actual NNT value. It is in fact all values outside this range, i.e.:
  −∞ to −14, 23 to +∞
- As suggested by Altman,[2] this 95% CI could be reported as:
  NNT(benefit) 23 to NNT(harm) 14

This shows that NNT(benefit) is unlikely to be less than 23.

Reporting 95% CIs or not?

Some researchers do not report 95% CIs for NNTs where the difference is not statistically significant. However this is unhelpful since confidence intervals are *especially* informative where a difference is not significant. The 95% CI from a non-significant randomized controlled trial indicates that the treatment is potentially associated with either a harmful effect or a beneficial effect that is entirely consistent with the non-significant difference.

References

1 Crowther CA, Hiller JE, Moss JR, McPhee AJ, Jeffries WS, Robinson JS. Effect of treatment of gestational diabetes mellitus on pregnancy outcomes. *N Engl J Med* 2005; **352**(24):2477–86.
2 Altman DG. Confidence intervals for the number needed to treat. *BMJ* 1998; **317**(7168): 1309–12.

Number needed to treat (continued)

Number needed to harm (NNH or NNT(harm))

NNH and its 95% confidence interval is reported when treatment differences are not significant. In addition, NNH is also used where the treatment is more harmful than the control, such as when side effects are more common in the intervention group than in the control group.

Example

In the randomized controlled trial in pregnant women with gestational diabetes, the authors reported rates of admission to the neonatal nursery in the treated and control groups:[1]

Proportion with admission in the treated group: 357/506 = 0.706
Proportion with admission in the control group: 321/524 = 0.613
Difference in proportions: 0.706 − 0.613 = 0.093 (95% CI: 0.035 to 0.150)
NNH = 1/0.093 = 11
95% confidence limits: 1/0.035 = 29 and 1/0.150 = 7
→ **NNH is 11 (95% CI: 7 to 29)**

NNT in meta-analyses

When doing a meta-analysis (📖 Chapter 13, p. 447) of randomized controlled trials with binary outcomes it may be desirable to present results as NNTs as well as either absolute differences in proportions or rate ratios. This can be done by **inverting the pooled absolute difference** and its 95% confidence interval. Forest plots can be drawn using NNTs as for absolute differences or relative risks. Altman gives an example[2] reproduced in Figure 10.2.

If the meta-analysis uses relative risks then the pooled estimate can be used to obtain the NNT if the control group event rate is specified.

If P_A, P_B, are the rates in the treatment and control groups respectively, P_B is known, and the relative risk is RR, then NNT is given by:

$$NNT = \frac{1}{P_B(RR-1)}$$

Example

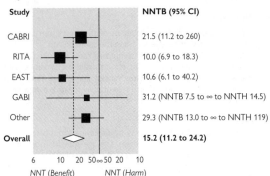

Fig. 10.3 Forest plot for meta-analysis of eight trials showing NNTB (number needed to treat for benefit) and NNTH (number needed to treat for harm).

Reproduced from *BMJ* Altman DG; 317:1309–1312 1998 with permission from BMJ Publishing Group Ltd.

❶ Problems in pooling NNTs

If the baseline event rates vary between the randomized controlled trials that have been pooled then the overall NNT obtained from the pooled estimate may be seriously misleading.[3] If baseline control rates are known to vary then the best approach is to calculate different NNTs according to the baseline rate in the target population. If the NNTs are for potential use in a range of populations, then it is useful to calculate a range of NNTs to cover the range of baseline rates that may occur. This approach was used in an effectiveness review of treatment for neuropathic pain (Fox-Rushby et al. 2010) – see extract below:

'For 50% response to pain, the placebo rate varied between studies and so the number needed to treat (NNT) has been calculated from the pooled relative risk value 2.70 using a range of placebo responses, 5%, 10%, 15%, and 20% to reflect real variation in rates among different patient groups. This gives NNT values of 12, 6, 4, and 3 respectively.'

1 Crowther CA, Hiller JE, Moss JR, McPhee AJ, Jeffries WS, Robinson JS. Effect of treatment of gestational diabetes mellitus on pregnancy outcomes. *N Engl J Med* 2005; **352**(24):2477–86.

2 Altman DG. Confidence intervals for the number needed to treat. *BMJ* 1998; **317**(7168): 1309–12.

3 Smeeth L, Haines A, Ebrahim S. Numbers needed to treat derived from meta-analyses-sometimes informative, usually misleading. *BMJ* 1999; **318**(7197):1548–51.

Life tables

Mortality rates

These are calculated from the number of deaths in a given time period divided by the number of people at risk in the same period. They are proportions although they are often presented as rates such as the number of deaths per 100 people or per 1000, etc. to make the usually small proportions easier to read. Mortality rates vary by age and so separate rates in specific age categories are often presented – these are **age-specific mortality rates**.

Life tables

Demographic life tables provide a way of displaying the mortality experience of a population. To calculate them, the age-specific mortality rates in a population are applied to a theoretical cohort of 100 000 people as shown in Table 10.9.

Table 10.9 Extract from English life table 16 for males and females combined 2000–2002[1]

Age (years)	Death rate observed per 10,000	Hypothetical number alive	Hypothetical number of deaths	Proportion of deaths
0	54.20	100000	542	0.00542000
1	3.720	99458	37	0.00037202
2	2.414	99421	24	0.00024140
3	1.7103	99397	17	0.00017103
4	1.3081	99380	13	0.00013081
5	1.3083	99367	13	0.00013083
etc				
60	84.5294	90856	768	0.00845294
61	93.0202	90088	838	0.00930202
62	102.4090	89250	914	0.01024090
63	112.1853	88336	991	0.01121853
etc				
109	5000	4	2	0.5
110	5000	2	1	0.5
111	10,000	1	1	1.0

The calculations

- The observed death rate is that seen in the population of interest, here males and females in England between 2000 and 2002
- The hypothetical number of deaths is found by multiplying the hypothetical total by the observed death rate
- The proportion of deaths is the death rate expressed as a proportion
- The number alive at a given age is the number alive at the previous age category, minus the number of deaths at the given age. For example, the number alive at age 1 is 100 000 − 542 = 99 458, the number of survivors

Expected (average) years of life

This is the average length of life after a particular age and is calculated from a full life table. For example to calculate the expected years of life from age 60, add all the numbers alive from age 60 and divide by the number alive at age 60. A half is usually added as people rarely die on their birthdays. The full life table is not given in Table 10.9 but can be found on the ONS website.[1]

Calculating expected years of life

N_x is no. surviving to age x
Expected years of life from age x is:

$$\frac{\sum_{i=x+1}^{\infty} n_i}{n_x} + 0.5$$

Expected years of life after age 60
= (90 088+89 250+88 336+...+4+2+1)/90 856+0.5
= 21.5
This means that on average people who reach age 60 will live for another 21.5 years

Life expectancy at birth

This can be calculated in the same way but starting at age 0, and therefore provides a estimate of the average length of life.

Further information

Bland, Chapter 16,[2] has further details of life tables with more examples.

References

1 Office for National Statistics. Decennial Life Tables – English Life Tables: Series DS. 2009. www.statistics.gov.uk/STATBASE/Product.asp?vlnk=333 (accessed 7 Jan 2009).
2 Bland M. *An introduction to medical statistics.* 3rd ed. Oxford: Oxford University Press, 2000.

Direct standardization

Why standardize?

It is often useful to compare overall mortality rates in different populations but the comparison will be confounded by age if the two populations have different age structures. Standardization provides a way to adjust for this. There are two ways to standardize – **direct standardization** and **indirect standardization**.

Details of direct standardization

- One population is regarded as the **standard population** and the other as the **comparison population**
- The age-specific death rates of the comparison population are applied to the age structure of the standard population
- The standardized mortality rate in the comparison population is compared with that observed

Example taken from Bland, Chapter 16[1]

In this example, mortality rates were compared in England and Wales for 1901 and 1981. The overall rates in the 2 years were: 1901: 15.7 per 1000; and 1981: 15.6. This is not a fair comparison though because the age structure of England and Wales changed over the 80-year time period. Hence direct standardization was used.

Table 10.10 Direct standardization of mortality rates in England and Wales in 1901 and 1981

Age group	Proportion in 1901 population	Death rate in 1981	Expected death rate in 1981 assuming age structure of 1901 column 2 x column 3
15–19	0.1536	0.8	0.1229
20–24	0.1407	0.8	0.1126
25–34	0.2376	0.9	0.2138
35–44	0.1846	1.8	0.3323
45–54	0.1334	6.1	0.8137
55–64	0.0868	17.7	1.5364
65–74	0.0457	45.6	2.0839
75–84	0.0158	105.2	1.6622
85+	0.0017	226.2	0.3845
TOTAL			**7.2623**

From Bland 2000 © Reproduced with kind permission from Oxford University Press.

Interpretation

The crude mortality rates are similar in the two populations but after standardization the 1981 rate, 7.26 per 1000, is much lower than the 1901 rate, 15.7 per 1000. This illustrates that:

- Comparison of crude mortality rates in populations may be misleading
- Adjusting for age structure can reveal large differences in mortality that are not seen in when comparing crude rates only

Confidence intervals

These can be calculated using a computer package such as CIA, available with *Statistics with confidence*[2] (details omitted).

❶ Note

The example here demonstrates clearly that comparison of crude death rates can be seriously misleading when the age structure of the two populations is different. The example here has shown that standardization may reveal large differences in death rates that were not apparent when simply looking at crude rates.

References

1 Bland M. *An introduction to medical statistics.* 3rd ed. Oxford: Oxford University Press, 2000.
2 Altman DG, Machin D, Bryant TN, Gardner MJ. *Statistics with confidence: confidence intervals and statistical guidelines.* London: BMJ Publishing Group, 2000.

Indirect standardization

Details of indirect standardization

- It is used when the comparison population is small and so age-specific death rates are poorly estimated, for example when studying mortality due to certain conditions or when considering an occupational group
- The age-specific death rates in the standard population are applied to the age distribution in the comparison population to get the number of deaths expected. The expected number is compared with the observed number of deaths.

Example from Bland, Chapter 16[1]

In this example, death rates were compared for cirrhosis of the liver in all men and in male doctors. The crude rates were 1423/152 479 80= 93 per million in all men and 14/435 70= 321 per million in male doctors. There are too few deaths among the doctors to calculate age-specific rates and yet it seems likely that the age structure of the two groups would differ. Therefore indirect standardization was used.

Table 10.11 Mortality rates for cirrhosis of the liver in all men and male doctors standardized using the indirect method

Age group	Death rate in standard population	Numbers of doctors in comparison population	Expected number of deaths in doctors assuming standard population death rates
15–24	0.000005859	1080	0.006 328
25–34	0.000013050	12 860	0.167 823
35–44	0.000046937	11 510	0.540 245
45–54	0.000161503	10 330	1.668 326
55–64	0.000271358	7790	2.113 879
TOTAL			4.4966

From Bland 2000 © reproduced with kind permission from Oxford University Press.

Standardized mortality ratio (SMR)

- This is 14/4.4966 = 3.11
- SMR usually multiplied by 100 to give 311
- Here this is not very different to the ratio of the crude rate, 321/93=3.44

Interpretation

The observed number (14) is more than there times the number expected (4.5) and so it is clear that mortality from cirrhosis of the liver among doctors in the UK is much greater than in the general population after standardizing for age.

Confidence interval for SMR

Assuming that the observed number of deaths follow a Poisson distribution and the observed number of deaths is more than 10, an approximate 95% CI is given as shown in the box.

$$100 \times \frac{O}{E} - 1.96 \times 100 \times \frac{\sqrt{O}}{E} \quad to \quad 100 \times \frac{O}{E} + 1.96 \times 100 \times \frac{\sqrt{O}}{E}$$

For the cirrhosis data this is:

$$100 \times \frac{14}{4.4966} - 1.96 \times 100 \times \frac{\sqrt{14}}{4.4966} \quad to \quad 100 \times \frac{14}{4.4966} + 1.96 \times 100 \times \frac{\sqrt{14}}{4.4966}$$

$$= 311 - 163 \ to \ 311 + 163$$

$$= 348 \ to \ 474$$

Since the confidence interval excludes the null value, 100, the SMR is statistically significant, i.e. the excess of deaths in doctors is likely to be a real effect.

Further points

- SMRs are sometimes used to compare mortality in a large number of populations. This is useful but care is needed in interpreting the individual SMRs, particularly any very extreme SMRs which may have occurred simply due to the multiplicity of analyses performed.
- Julious and others[2] suggest caution in using SMRs to compare several small geographical areas where the denominators vary and tend to be small.
- Other statistical methods may be used to adjust for age, such as fitting regression models. This may be a better approach if it is necessary to adjust for further variables in addition to age.

Further reading

Standardization is described in both statistics and in epidemiology books such as Bland[1] (Chapter 16), Armitage[3] Chapter 19), Kirkwood[4] (Chapter 25), and Gordis[5] (Chapter 4).

References

1 Bland M. *An introduction to medical statistics*. 3rd ed. Oxford: Oxford University Press, 2000.
2 Julious SA, Nicholl J, George S. Why do we continue to use standardized mortality ratios for small area comparisons? *J Public Health Med* 2001; **23**(1):40–6.
3 Armitage P, Berry G, Matthews JNS. *Statistical methods in medical research*. 4th ed. Oxford: Blackwell Science, 2002.
4 Kirkwood BR, Sterne JAC. *Essential medical statistics*. 2nd ed. Malden, MA: Blackwell Science, 2003.
5 Gordis L. *Epidemiology*. 3rd ed. Philadelphia, PA: Elsevier Saunders, 2004.

Analysing multiple observations per subject

Introduction

In this chapter we describe the statistical issues involved in analysing studies with more than one data point or observation per subject, such as when a series of measurements are made on each individual over time or when a group of subjects are analysed together, forming a cluster. For each of these situations, the statistical analysis needs to take account of the design of the study, and for most situations there are several possible approaches which may be used. We describe the most common approaches in terms of when the methods are appropriate, how they work, and how the results are interpreted.

Serial (longitudinal) data

Introduction

It is very common in medicine to make a series of measurements on a patient either as part of clinical care or as part of a research study. For example:

- Blood pressure measured automatically at 30-minute intervals over a 24-hour period in a patient with possible hypertension
- Lung function measured daily in patients with chronic obstructive pulmonary disease (COPD) (Fig. 11.1)
- Temperature measured every 30 seconds for 4 hours after febrile subjects are given one of two possible antipyretic drugs

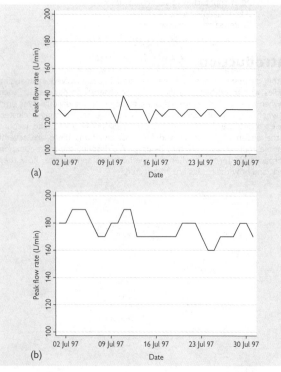

Fig. 11.1a,b Example of serial data: peak flow rate for 30 days in two patients with COPD.

Sometimes these serial measures are simply plotted and visually examined, as in the blood pressure example. There are many forms that the longitudinal relationships can take but commonly seen patterns are:

- **A flat relationship** where levels stay broadly the same, as in the first graph in Figure 11.1
- **A sloping relationship** where values either increase or decrease with time, such as in the second graph in Figure 11.1 where lung function is fluctuating but overall is decreasing over time
- **A peaked relationship** where values rise and fall, for example oestrogen levels over a month in menstruating women, which vary as a result of the monthly menstrual cycle
- **Sinusoidal relationships** where values rise and fall over time in a regular seasonal pattern, such as outdoor temperature measured daily over several years

Introduction to summarizing serial data

In research settings, it is useful to summarize serial data, especially to compare subjects in different groups, but it may not be obvious how best to do this. The appropriate method must answer the question of interest and must be suitable for the data observed. Matthews[1] provides a practical description of a range of appropriate yet simple approaches that can be used in different situations. Each method works by calculating a particular summary statistic for each subject, such as an overall mean value, a slope of the line, or the maximum or minimum value as appropriate. These individual measures can then be used as the raw data to represent an individual's experience. For example, if the summary measure is a mean, then these means can be used to compute the average of the means across all subjects and a standard deviation, and range and so on.

Summary measures

Table 11.1 lists summary measures to use under a range of circumstances.

Table 11.1 Choice of summary measure for different questions

Summary measure	Aim
Overall mean (equal time intervals)	• To estimate the overall value of the outcome for each subject
Area under the curve (equal or unequal time intervals)	
Maximum	• To estimate the highest value obtained
Minimum	• To estimate the lowest value obtained
Time to a given value	• To estimate how long it takes to reach a critical value
Slope of the line	• To estimate how the measurement changes over time

Reference

1 Matthews JN, Altman DG, Campbell MJ, Royston P. Analysis of serial measurements in medical research. *BMJ* 1990; **300**(6719):230–5.

Summarizing serial data

Comparing serial data in two groups

If the subjects come from two groups it may be informative to compare the groups. This can be done using the summary statistics for each subject and by averaging them within each group, and then comparing the group means using a statistical test such as a t test if the usual assumptions hold.

❶ Note that it is incorrect to compare two groups of subjects with serial data by calculating means at each time point and doing t tests on each pair of means, for the following reasons:

- **Non-independence of tests**
  The series of data points for each individual are not independent of each other in the sense that in a particular subject values which are close in time will be more similar than values further away in time. This means that tests performed at different time points are not independent of each other – if a test at a particular time point is statistically significant, then the tests done at the adjacent time points are likely to be significant too simply because the values in individuals are correlated.

- **Shape of the trend in means**
  The trend in means at each time point may not provide a meaningful summary of the overall trend since it might not represent a typical individual. If different individuals peak at different times then this type of averaging will produce an overall curve that has been '**over smoothed**' and does not represent any individual at all.

Procedure for summarizing serial data

- Plot the relationship for all individuals separately to determine the nature of the relationship
- Choose the appropriate summary statistic that suits the data and answers the question of interest (see Table 11.1)
- Calculate the summary for each subject and then, if helpful, summarize these as if you would if these were the raw data for the individuals
- If the individuals are in two groups, these groups can be compared using tests based on the single summary calculated for each individual such as a t test or Mann Whitney U test (📖 Chapter 8, p. 237)

Example: summarizing serial measures

These data are from a randomized controlled trial that compared multilayer bandaging followed by hosiery versus hosiery alone in cancer patients with lymphoedema of one limb.[1] The main outcome was the severity of swelling in the affected limb measured at a maximum of five time points. It was calculated as the difference in limb volume between the affected and normal limb as a percentage of the normal limb volume. This outcome was measured on day 1, day 19, week 7, week 12, and week 24 in the treatment and control group.

The aim was to see if the treated group had a greater reduction in limb volume than the control group. Since the time intervals were unequal, the area under the curve was used as the summary measure for each patient. Figure 11.2 shows individual plots in one group.

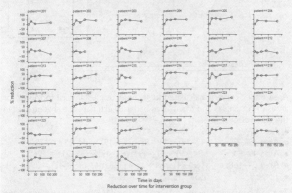

Results

- The reduction in limb volume to week 24, calculated as the area under the curve (see ◰ Calculating area under the curve, p. 382) followed a Normal distribution and so the mean reduction in the intervention and control groups was compared using a two-sample t test
- Intervention group (n=32): mean reduction = 31.0%
- Control group (n=46): mean reduction = 15.8%
- Difference (95% CI): 15.2 (6.2 to 24.2); P=0.001

Hence there was good evidence for a greater reduction in swelling in the intervention group showing that bandaging was effective.

Fig. 11.2 Individual plots for patients in one arm of the trial[1].

Reference

1 Badger CM, Peacock JL, Mortimer PS. A randomized, controlled, parallel-group clinical trial comparing multilayer bandaging followed by hosiery versus hosiery alone in the treatment of patients with lymphedema of the limb. *Cancer* 2000; **88**(12):2832–7.

Calculating area under the curve

Example

The graph below shows the serial data for one patient in the randomized controlled trial of multilayer bandaging plus hosiery versus hosiery alone in patients with lymphoedema[1] with the data listed alongside.

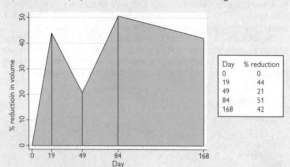

Day	% reduction
0	0
19	44
49	21
84	51
168	42

Area under curve is calculated in sections using standard formulae for areas of rectangles and triangles in order to estimate the shaded area in the graph above:

- Area 0–19:   ½ × 19 × 44 = 418
- Area 19–49:   (49–19) × 44 – ½ × (49–19) × (44–21) = 975
- Area 49–84:   (84–49) × 51 – ½ × (84–49) × (51–21) = 1260
- Area 84–168:   (168–84) × 51 – ½ × (168–84) × (51–42) = 3906
- Total: 6559

This can be divided by the total no. of days (168) to give a standardized value: 6559/168 = 39.0%

Note that here this is close to the mean value obtained by adding all values and dividing by 4 (44+21+51+42)/4 = 39.5 but in general the area under the curve is a better representation of the overall effect when time intervals are unequal.

Fig. 11.3 Serial data for one patient to illustrate the calculation of the area under the curve.

Trapezium rule

In general the area under the curve is given by the sum of the individual areas. This is called the **trapezium rule**. In symbols this is:

$$\frac{1}{2} \sum_{i=0}^{n-1} (t_{i+1} - t_i)(y_{i+1} + y_i)$$

Where t_i is the time and y_i is the value of the outcome variable.

Reference

1 Badger CM, Peacock JL, Mortimer PS. A randomized, controlled, parallel-group clinical trial comparing multilayer bandaging followed by hosiery versus hosiery alone in the treatment of patients with lymphedema of the limb. *Cancer* 2000; **88**(12):2832–7.

Other summary measures for serial data

The following examples illustrate the use of other summary measures in research studies.

Example: summarizing by the proportion of time below a given value

The PITCH randomized controlled trial compared paracetamol plus ibuprofen for treatment of fever in children with paracetamol or ibuprofen alone.[1] The primary outcome was the time without fever in the first 4 hours after the first dose was given, calculated from a series of temperature measurements recorded automatically every 30 seconds.

- The **series of data in each child was summarized by the proportion of time that child had temperature below 37.2 °C**
- This value was averaged across all children in each group and compared
- The combined treatment showed a greater length of time without fever compared with each drug alone (see paper for full details)

Example: summarizing using the slope of the line

A UK air pollution study investigated the relationship between peak flow rate in children and outdoor air pollution, over 9 weeks.[2] For each child, the relationship was analysed between pollution level and peak flow rate, giving a slope of the line (regression coefficient) for each child.

- The **series of data in each child was summarized by the slope of the line**
- This value was averaged over all children to quantify the evidence that overall there was a negative relationship between air pollution and peak flow rate
- The combined slope showed that there was no strong evidence that air pollution affected peak flow rate in healthy children (see paper for full details of analysis and results)

References

1 Hay AD, Costelloe C, Redmond NM, Montgomery AA, Fletcher M, Hollinghurst S et al. Paracetamol plus ibuprofen for the treatment of fever in children (PITCH): randomised controlled trial. *BMJ* 2008; **337**:a1302.

2 Peacock JL, Symonds P, Jackson P, Bremner SA, Scarlett JF, Strachan DP et al. Acute effects of winter air pollution on respiratory function in schoolchildren in southern England. *Occup Environ Med* 2003; **60**(2):82–9.

Summary measures approach: key points

Advantages of the summary measures approach
- They are conceptually simple and relatively easy to use
- The method and results are straightforward to understand
- They can be used when the time intervals are unequal
- They can usually still be used when there are missing data at some time points
- They can be adapted to answer a range of questions
- They are statistically valid

Disadvantages of summary measures approach
- It may be difficult to identify the best summary measure until the data are collected

Other points
- It may be appropriate to calculate more than one summary variable for a set of serial data. For example, with a series of lung function measurements both the mean value and minimum value may be informative.
- Missing observations can be accommodated:
  For example, in the multilayer bandaging trial[1] there were some missing data since a few patients did not have readings at all time points. To allow for this, three analyses were done: (i) with all data available and patients averaged over their own period of observation, (ii) with all patients with complete data up to 84 days, and (iii) with all patients with data up to 168 days. The three analyses were compared as a test of sensitivity. This showed virtually identical results under each scenario. If different results had been obtained this would suggest that there was some systematic differences in subjects with missing data.
- Multiple regression analysis may be used to adjust the analyses for other individual-level confounding variables. The summary measure is used as the outcome in the regression model and other individual-level factors are included as predictors (🕮 Multiple regression, p. 406).
- Serial discrete data such as pain scores may also be analysed using summary measures
- The method of summary measures is a two-stage method because summary statistics are calculated for each subject and then these are analysed in a separate analysis
- If the summary measure is a trend such as a slope then strictly speaking it may be necessary to take the correlation between observations in each individual into account when calculating the overall summary slope.

Further reading on summary measures
- Matthews (1990)[2] provides a full account
- Matthews (1993)[3] discusses the calculation of weighted averages of summary measures
- Armitage (2002)[4] discusses problems with summary measures and alternative approaches
- Altman (1991)[5] discusses summary measures and gives examples

References

1 Badger CM, Peacock JL, Mortimer PS. A randomized, controlled, parallel-group clinical trial comparing multilayer bandaging followed by hosiery versus hosiery alone in the treatment of patients with lymphedema of the limb. *Cancer* 2000; **88**(12):2832–7.
2 Matthews JN, Altman DG, Campbell MJ, Royston P. Analysis of serial measurements in medical research. *BMJ* 1990; **300**(6719):230–5.
3 Matthews JN. A refinement to the analysis of serial data using summary measures. *Stat Med* 1993; **12**(1):27–37.
4 Armitage P, Berry G, Matthews JNS. *Statistical methods in medical research.* 4th ed. Oxford: Blackwell Science. 2002.
5 Altman DG. *Practical statistics for medical research.* London: Chapman & Hall, 1991.

Other approaches to serial data

Levels of data

Serial data can be thought of as having a **two-level structure** in that we start with subjects, and within each subject there are multiple observations. It is often described in the following way:

- **At level 1** we have the different subjects, and so level 1 represents the **variability between the subjects**
- **At level 2** we have the serial observations within each of the subjects, and so level 2 represents the **variability within each subject**
- The correlation between observations within an individual is nearly always much greater than the correlation between individuals at similar time points

Other approaches

Rather than using the two-stage summary measures approach, other more complex approaches can be used to analyse serial data in a single, **one-stage approach**. These are listed here with some general points about their use.

Repeated measures analysis of variance

- This is an extension of one-way analysis of variance (📖 One-way analysis of variance, p. 280)
- The method **tests for general differences across time categories**, i.e. it tests whether there are any differences between mean levels of the outcome at different times
- Specific relationships such as a linear trend or rise-and-fall are not tested
- It assumes the 'time' effect is the same for all subjects
- The results need to be interpreted in the light of the actual relationship observed by plotting and summarizing the raw data, since a significant result may not necessarily imply that there is a specific relationship
- Post-hoc tests can be done to test for a specific relationship or for differences between chosen time points
- ❶ **Missing data are problematic** since an individual is omitted from analysis if they have a value missing at any time point and so the method is inefficient. It is also potentially biased if many individuals are left out and/or those left out are atypical in some way. For these reasons statisticians generally prefer to use multilevel models (also known as mixed or random effects models, see next section) since these allow individuals to be included in the analysis even if they have missing data at some time points.

Multilevel model (also known as mixed model or random effects model)

- This method accounts for the two-level structure in a single model by specifying the two sources of variation – between subjects and within subjects
- It is used to test a specific mathematical trend such as a linear or exponential rise or a quadratic rise-and-fall
- The trend to be tested must be known in advance and incorporated into the model

- Individuals with data missing at some time points can still be included as long as data are missing at random (📖 Missing data, p. 402)
- For further details and examples see 📖 Multilevel models (p. 436)

Generalized estimating equations (GEEs)

- This method accounts for the two-level structure by specifying the correlation between the serial data points in each subject
- It is used to test a specific mathematical trend such as a linear or exponential rise or a quadratic rise-and-fall
- The trend to be tested must be known in advance and incorporated into the model
- For further details and examples see 📖 Generalized estimating equations p. 438

Choice of method

This is a matter of judgement, but the following points may be helpful:
- Summary measures are relatively simple to use and interpret, and are statistically sound and robust
- The appropriate summary measure may be hard to define and so a more general one-stage model such as a multilevel model or GEE may be needed
- It is important to **plot the data for the individuals** before doing any analysis to see what the relationships look like and how much they vary between individuals
- When reading reported analyses on serial data look for information on the individual trends either as graphs or as meaningful summary statistics to guide the interpretation of the results
- If there are missing data or unequal numbers of data points in the individuals, it is important to decide how to deal with this statistically and consider the reasons they are missing, i.e. if it may lead to bias

Note

Where the outcome is a continuous variable and the dataset is reasonably large, multilevel modelling and GEEs give very similar results. The sections on multilevel models and GEEs give more details on their use and on how to decide which multifactorial method to use.

Cluster samples: units of analysis

Independent observations

Standard statistical methods make the assumption that **observations are independent** of each other. For example if the data are a set of single blood pressure measurements on 10 patients, then these values will be independent of each other, so that knowing one patient's blood pressure will not allow us to predict another's.

If we took three blood pressure measurements on each patient to give 30 readings in all, these readings would not all be independent because repeated measures in the same patient will be correlated with each other. In this example the patient is the **unit of analysis** and so the analysis should be based on the patient. One way to do this is to use a summary statistic for each patient such as the mean of the three values to give 10 independent values.

Consequences of ignoring non-independence

If non-independent data are analysed as if they were independent, the calculated overall variability is reduced and is too small. This leads to confidence intervals which are too narrow and P values that are too small, potentially leading to spurious significant results. Altman cites an example where 3944 observations from 58 patients were analysed as if they were independent and gave a spuriously tiny P value.[1] The example below illustrates how the P value changes when repeated measures are analysed as if they were independent observations.

Example

In a study in 71 preterm babies, repeated measures of lung function were made up on six occasions. Table 11.2 shows two t tests to compare mean lung function in babies who were diagnosed with moderate (15) or severe (6) bronchopulmonary dysplasia (BPD), (i) treating all observations as if they were independent (n=85 readings) and (ii) by analysing the mean measure for each baby (n=21 babies). The lung function measure shown here is resistance index analysed on a log scale.

The correct analysis gives a non-significant result (P=0.278) but the wrong analysis which treats all the data as independent obtains a smaller P value and is statistically significant (P=0.044).

Table 11.2 t test in clustered data ignoring the clustering (i) and allowing for clustering (ii)

	Group	n	Mean	P value
(i)	Moderate BPD	70	4.84	0.044
	Severe BPD	15	5.04	
	Difference	85	0.20	
(ii)	Moderate BPD	15	4.84	0.278
	Severe BPD	6	5.00	
	Difference	21	0.16	

(i) The data are **analysed incorrectly**, by treating the sets of repeated measures as if they were all from different subjects, giving $n=85$ observations.

(ii) The data are **analysed correctly** using the average of all readings for each baby, giving $n=21$ observations.

Clinical trials

In many clinical trials, individual patients are randomly allocated to a particular treatment and then the outcomes are summed and compared in each treatment group using individual patient data. In other words the **randomization is at the patient level** and so the analysis should also be conducted at the patient level. The **unit of analysis is the patient**.

By contrast, in **cluster randomized trials** whole groups are allocated to particular interventions and so the **randomization is at the group level**. In general, individuals within a group will be more alike than individuals in different groups and so their values will not be independent of each other.[2]

Therefore, in cluster randomized trials the **unit of analysis is the group**. If the analysis is done on individual patients as if they were independent observations, the statistical methods will give P values and confidence intervals which are too small and so there may be spurious positive findings.[3] In addition when planning a cluster randomized trial the **sample size calculations must be based on the groups**, otherwise the total variability will be underestimated and the calculations will give too few patients. This means that the power of the study will be less than expected and so the study may be inconclusive.[4,5]

Summary points
- Identify the correct unit of analysis and consider this in planning and analysing the study
- The assumption of independence matters – if untrue, it affects the results of statistical analyses

---

References
1 Altman DG, Bland JM. Statistics notes: units of analysis. *BMJ* 1997; **314**(7098):1874.
2 Bland JM, Kerry SM. Statistics notes. Trials randomised in clusters. *BMJ* 1997; **315**(7108):600.
3 Kerry SM, Bland JM. Analysis of a trial randomised in clusters. *BMJ* 1998; **316**(7124):54.
4 Kerry SM, Bland JM. Sample size in cluster randomisation. *BMJ* 1998; **316**(7130):549.
5 Kerry SM, Bland JM. The intracluster correlation coefficient in cluster randomisation. *BMJ* 1998; **316**(7142):1455.

Cluster samples: analysis

Appropriate analysis for cluster samples

It is important to use the right unit of analysis for cluster samples. The following methods can be used to do this:

- Summary statistics two-stage approach
- Regression with adjusted standard errors
- Multilevel modelling
- Generalized estimating equations (GEEs)

Summary statistics two-stage approach

- This is based on calculating an appropriate summary statistic for each cluster
- Treat the cluster summary statistic as an ordinary observation (as an item of raw data) and summarize these in each group that is to be compared, or across the whole sample if there is only one group
- The number of observations is the total number of clusters, not the total number of subjects
- This is a similar approach to that described for longitudinal data (📖 Serial (longitudinal) data, p. 378)

Calculating summary statistics (two-stage method) with different outcomes in a cluster trial

Continuous outcome, e.g. height of each subject

1. Calculate the mean height separately in each cluster by averaging the heights of the subjects in the cluster → cluster mean
2. Calculate the average of these cluster means for each group
3. Compare groups in the usual way with a two-sample t test (assuming the cluster means are Normally distributed)

Binary outcome, e.g. improved yes/no

1. Calculate the proportion improved in each cluster
2. Calculate the average of these cluster proportions for each group
3. Compare groups in the usual way with a two-sample t test as above

Counts, e.g. number of infections in a period of time

1. Calculate the mean number of infections in each cluster
2. Calculate the average of these cluster means for each group
3. Compare groups in the usual way with a two-sample t test as above

Notes

- Cluster means and cluster proportions may be Normally distributed even for non-Normal outcome data as a consequence of the central limit theorem (📖 Central limit theorem, p. 228)
- A further refinement is to 'weight' the analysis where there are different total numbers of individuals in the clusters (details omitted)
- These methods assume there are similar numbers of individuals in each cluster

Example: analysis of a cluster randomized trial (1)

A cluster randomized trial examined whether students use or avoid newly shaded areas at 51 secondary schools in Australia.[1] Areas with full sun were identified in each school and shades installed in these areas in the intervention schools. The primary outcome was the change in the mean number of students using these areas at time points before and after the intervention was installed.

Analysis and results
- The clusters are the schools (26 control, 25 interventions schools)
- A two-stage summary measures analysis was used
- The mean number of students using the designated areas pre- and post-intervention was calculated in each school
- The pre-and post-intervention values were subtracted to give the mean change for each school and then averaged in the two randomization groups
- These mean changes were analysed in a two-sample t test
- The mean change in control schools was −0.03 compared with +2.67 in the intervention schools (P=0.011) showing that students do use rather than avoid newly shaded areas

Regression with adjusted standard errors one-stage approach

It is possible to analyse clustered data in some statistical packages by using the individual observations but choosing an option which adjusts the standard error for the clustering. This provides confidence intervals and P values which are corrected for non-independence. The regression coefficients themselves are not changed. The advantage of this method is that it is relatively easy to carry out and to interpret but it has the disadvantage that it does not use the full data structure in the analysis.

Multilevel modelling and GEEs one-stage approach

These methods take the two-level structure into account in one single model. They have the advantage that the estimates and standard errors are mutually adjusted for clustering and it is possible to add other variables into the model that affect the outcome at either the individual or cluster level. The disadvantage is that the methods are not easy to implement and interpret, and are not available in all statistical packages (see 📖 Multilevel models, p. 436, 📖 Generalized estimating equations, p. 438).

Example: analysis of a cluster randomized trial (2)

A cluster randomized trial in 61 general practices, with 558 children compared the use of an interactive booklet on respiratory tract infections in reducing unnecessary general practitioner (GP) consultations and antibiotic use.[2]

Analysis and results
- The clusters are the general practices
- A 1-stage multilevel approach was used to account for clustering
- There was no significant difference in reconsulting with odds ratio 0.75 (95% CI: 0.41 to 1.38) but there was a reduction in antibiotic prescribing, odds ratio 0.29 (95% CI: 0.14 to 0.60)

References

1 Dobbinson SJ, White V, Wakefield MA, Jamsen KM, White V, Livingston PM *et al.* Adolescents' use of purpose built shade in secondary schools: cluster randomised controlled trial. *BMJ* 2009; **338**(feb17_1):b95.

2 Francis NA, Butler CC, Hood K, Simpson S, Wood F, Nuttall J. Effect of using an interactive booklet about childhood respiratory tract infections in primary care consultations on reconsulting and antibiotic prescribing: a cluster randomised controlled trial. *BMJ* 2009; **339**(jul29_2):b2885.

Analysing multiple variables per subject

Introduction

In this chapter we describe the statistical issues involved in analysing studies with more than one variable for each subject such as when adjusting for confounding or nuisance variables or wishing to disentangle the effect of multiple variables on a single outcome. There is a wide range of modelling techniques that can be used and so we describe the approaches commonly used when analysing different outcome variables and/or different study designs. We describe the approaches in terms of when the methods are appropriate, how they work, and how the results are interpreted.

Multiple variables per subject

Introduction

It is common in medical research to have several variables for each subject, for example:

- When collating death rates by age and sex where each subject is categorized according to their age and sex
- When exploring the effects of several factors predicting an outcome, such as baby's birthweight or risk of heart attack in adults where several factors are potentially important
- When many variables have been obtained for each individual but it is desirable to reduce these to a smaller combination of key factors. For example when deriving a simple symptom score from a wide range of symptoms
- When seeking to determine groups of variables that characterize particular groups, such as when looking for clusters of individuals who respond particularly well to an intervention

Standardization

In the first example with death rates, it may be important to adjust the death rates for age and sex in order to make meaningful comparisons between populations since these factors have strong effects. The first step is usually to produce age/sex-specific rates. If different populations are being compared then the differences in age/sex structure can be adjusted for using **direct or indirect standardization** to produce standardized death rates as described in Chapter 10 (📖 Direct standardization, p. 372, Indirect standardization, p. 374).

Multifactorial (multivariable) modelling

In the second example with an outcome such as baby's birthweight and several factors that may predict birthweight, **multifactorial** regression may be used simultaneously to analyse and disentangle the predictive factors. There are a range of modelling methods that can be used depending on the nature of the outcome and the design of the study. The commonly used ones are listed in Table 12.1 and described in detail later in this chapter.

Multivariate modelling

In the third example, **principal components analysis** can be used to reduce a large dataset to a smaller one that captures nearly all of the information. In the fourth example, **factor analysis** or **cluster analysis** may be used to identify groups of similar individuals.

Table 12.1 Multifactorial and multivariate modelling methods described in this chapter

Design or aim of study	Type of outcome variable	Modelling method
One observation per subject	Continuous	Multiple regression
One observation per subject	Binary	Logistic regression
One observation per subject	Time to an event	Proportional hazards (Cox) regression
One observation per subject	Counts	Poisson regression
More than one observation per subject: serial data or repeated measures or a cluster design	Continuous	Multilevel model (also called mixed model or random effects model)
	Binary	
	Time to an event	or generalized estimating equations (GEEs)
	Counts	
Many variables: aim is to reduce to a smaller number	Any of continuous, discrete, binary, categorical[*]	Principal components analysis
Many variables: aim to identify groups of individuals who are similar	Any of continuous, discrete, binary, categorical[*]	Cluster analysis Factor analysis

[*]Categorical variables need to be analysed as dummy variables (see 📖 Multifactorial methods: overview, p. 396).

Multifactorial methods: overview

Introduction

In this section we outline general 'nuts and bolts' issues that arise in using multifactorial methods, such as how they work, how to use them, and what the results mean. Specific details of the individual methods are given in their own sections later in this chapter.

How the methods work

- A mathematical model is fitted to a common set of variables for each subject simultaneously
- The modelling process identifies which variables are related to the outcome after adjusting for each of the others in the model
- The results are given in the form of regression coefficients, which are the estimated effect of each variable on the outcome after adjusting for all the other variables included in the model
- The calculations are complex so computer packages are used

Types of data that can be used

Outcome variables

Modelling methods are available for the following types of data:

- Continuous
- Binary
- Discrete (counts)
- Time to an event

Predictor variables

All modelling methods allow **any combination** of these types of data:

- Continuous
- Binary
- Categorical

Assumptions of methods

All modelling methods make assumptions about the data that must hold true else the results may be invalid. Examples are:

- The observations are independent of each other
- The relationship is linear
- There is similar variability in each of the groups
- The data follow a specific distribution

Meaning of coefficients

This is different for different modelling methods and depends on the nature of the outcome variable:

- Continuous data: slope of the line
- Binary data: odds ratio
- Time to an event data: hazard ratios
- Count data: rate ratios

Dummy variables

When non-ordered categorical variables are used in regression models it is necessary to set up **dummy variables**. Some statistical packages set up dummy variables automatically, but it is important to understand the meaning of a dummy variable to be able to interpret results when they are used.

If the categorical variable has three categories then there will be two dummy variables representing two of the three categories and the other is the **reference category**.

In general for any categorical variable with n categories, one category will be the reference level and there will be $n-1$ dummy variables, each of which represents a comparison with the reference category.

Example

The variable 'marital status' is recorded in three categories:
(i) married, (ii) single, (iii) divorced or widowed or separated
The two dummy variables, **variable1** and **variable2** are defined as follows:
variable1 = 1 if the woman is single, = 0 otherwise
variable2 = 1 if the woman is divorced, widowed or separated,
= 0 otherwise

Hence for a married woman, variable1 and variable2 are both be zero, and this is the **reference level**.

The two regression coefficients will therefore represent the following comparison:
variable1: *single women* versus *married women*
variable2: *divorced/widowed/separated women* versus *married women*

Multifactorial methods: model selection

Choosing the best model

Sometimes we know in advance which variables to include in a multifactorial regression model. In this situation, we test the variables of interest and omit any that are not significant, if we wish. Sometimes it may be helpful to keep a non-significant variable in the model if past experience has shown that that particular variable is important. The strategy used is driven by the purpose of the analysis. If the aim is to identify important predictor variables, it makes sense to leave out non-significant ones, i.e. ones where the evidence for a relationship is weak. If the purpose is to adjust for all important prognostic factors, then it may be best to retain all known important variables.

Automatic selection methods

Statistical packages that do multifactorial regression may offer a type of automatic selection procedure, **forward or backward stepwise methods.** These work as follows:

Forward
- Put each variable in the model alone
- Discard any that are not statistically significant
- Of the remaining variables, select the one which is most strongly related to the outcome variable
- Add the remaining variables one at a time in order of their strength of relationship with the outcome, until adding an extra variable does not contribute significantly to the model

Backward
- This uses a similar process but in reverse
- All predictor variables are put into the model and the one with the weakest relationship with the outcome is removed
- The process is repeated until all the remaining variables are significantly related to the outcome

Modelling in groups of similar variables

If there are many predictor variables it is helpful to consider them in groups of similar variables. For example in a study of survival from breast cancer three groups of variables were analysed: (i) socioeconomic/demographic factors, (ii) clinical/pathological factors, and (iii) distant metastases.[1] In this study, the best fitting model in each group was presented since this made sense clinically. In other situations, after this step, it may be helpful to combine the variables in the groups together in a single model, thus building up the model conceptually.

Chronological order

If factors affect an outcome at different time points, it may be sensible to fit a sequence of models where the factors are added in chronological order. This allows the exploration of how the outcome is affected by factors over time, and may shed light on underlying mechanisms.

Common sense

- It is important, both in fitting and interpreting models with many explanatory variables, to examine each possible predictor in relation to the outcome *on its own* to understand the relationship
- It is important to look at the **sizes of effects rather than just rely on P values** alone to determine and interpret a multifactorial regression analysis
- It is unhelpful to present an analysis that includes many predictor variables simply with P values alone and no estimates

Further details

- On quantifying how well a model fits: see 📖 How well the model fits, p. 418
- On choosing and fitting models: see Kirkwood and Sterne, Chapter 29[2]

References

1 Rezaianzadeh A, Peacock J, Reidpath D, Talei A, Hoseini SV, Mehrabani D. Survival analysis of 1148 women diagnosed with breast cancer in Southern Iran. *BMC Cancer* 2009; **9**:168.
2 Kirkwood BR, Sterne JAC. *Essential medical statistics.* 2nd ed. Malden, MA: Blackwell Science, 2003.

Multifactorial methods: challenges

Introduction
Multifactorial methods are powerful statistical tools and yet present many challenges. The topics below describe some of these.

Fitting the right model
Computer packages are tantalizingly easy to use for very complex analyses but will produce garbage if garbage is fed in! For example, we need to check that relationships we are modelling are sensible, such as whether a linear relationship is reasonable, or whether the trend flattens off. Inspection of the data and discussions between clinical and statistical colleagues is often very helpful. The same considerations apply when interpreting a multifactorial analysis in a paper or report.

Close correlation between variables (colinearity)
It is common to find that some predictive factors are correlated with each other and sometimes quite strongly so. This makes modelling tricky because two very highly correlated variables will effectively cancel each other out when modelled together. For this reason it is helpful to examine the relationship between variables that are to go into the model beforehand to guide the analysis (📖 Correlation matrix, p. 294). If the variables are highly correlated, choices may need to be made. In some situations it is reasonable to choose one of a few highly correlated variables to represent them all such as when adjusting for social class where several possible proxies for social circumstances could be chosen and it may not matter which. Alternatively, if there is a group of correlated variables it may be helpful to reduce them to a smaller set by using principal components analysis (📖 Principal components analysis, p. 441).

Influential data points
On occasion a particular data point may be very influential in that it lies away from the other data points but strongly affects the slope of the line. Such values can be detected when doing preliminary plots of the data and can then be checked to determine if the potential outlying value is correct or was wrongly recorded. Alternatively there are more formal statistics that can be used to identify influential points such as Cook's distance (see Kirkwood, Chapter 12[1]). If an outlier and influential point is a valid observation, then a sensible approach is to do a sensitivity analysis with and without it, to guide interpretation.

Missing data
This is potentially a serious problem and is dealt with in a separate section (📖 Missing data, p. 402).

Presenting the appropriate statistics in a paper or report

Computer packages which perform complex multifactorial analyses in fractions of a second often produce a seemingly disproportionate quantity of results. Hence it can be difficult to know which bits are relevant and appropriate to extract and interpret and/or present in a paper or report. Peacock and Kerry[2] give guidance on this with examples.

References

1 Kirkwood BR, Sterne JAC. *Essential medical statistics*. 2nd ed. Malden, MA: Blackwell Science, 2003.

2 Peacock J, Kerry SM. *Presenting medical statistics from proposal to publication*. Oxford: Oxford University Press, 2006.

Missing data

Why data are missing

It is common to have missing data for some variables. The extent to which data are missing often varies among variables, for example, in studies about babies, birthweight is usually recorded but gestational age, crown–heel length and head circumference may be missing for a few babies, smoking status of the mother may be missing for some more, and family income for even more! This means that any multifactorial analysis that includes all of these variables can only be done using the subjects with complete data. This is potentially problematic since the sub-sample of subjects with complete data may not be representative of all subjects, especially if the tendency for certain data to be missing is linked to the main outcome. Hence analyses based on sub-samples with complete data may provide misleading results.

Types of missing data

There are several types of missing data patterns where one variable is missing:

- *'Missing completely at random'* (MCAR)
  This means that the probability that an observation is missing does not depend on any of the other observations. In other words, there are no systematic differences between the values that are present and those that are missing. For example weight may be missing in some subjects in a study because the weighing scales were broken.

- *'Missing at random'* (MAR)
  This is weaker assumption than MCAR, and means that the probability that a data value is missing, given all other data values, is independent of its true value. Hence it may depend on other values in the dataset but not on the unknown value itself. For example missing data on weight would be higher than recorded values if more men refused to be weighed than women, since men tend to weight more.

- *Missing not at random* (MNAR)
  This means that there are systematic differences between the missing data values and the observed ones, even after the data values are taken into account. For example if weight is missing for some subjects because they were too heavy for the scales.

Dealing with missing data

There are some ad hoc methods of dealing with missing data, for example:

- ❶ To replace a missing value by the overall mean of the non-missing values. This obviously assumes that the missing values are similar to the missing ones, i.e. they have the same mean value. This is often not true and so this method is not recommended

- ❶ When the final value in a series of measurements is missing, it is common to use the last observation recorded to substitute for the missing final value. This is known as the **'last observation carried forwards' (LOCF) method.** This has been shown to be **very flawed** and is not recommended

In general, **single imputation of missing values is unreliable** because it makes untested assumptions about the missing data.

Multiple imputation

This is a complex statistical approach whereby missing data are 'recovered' and analyses performed to attempt to replicate the analyses that would have occurred if no data had been missing. It is essentially a Bayesian approach (📖 Chapter 14, p. 477). Broadly it works as follows:

- The missing data are replaced by values predicted using data from other related variables that are not missing.
- This is repeated many times to take into account the uncertainty in the estimated missing values. Statistical analyses are then performed on each of the datasets in the same way as would have been done on the single original dataset had all the data been present.
- Multiple imputation is a powerful statistical technique and can be performed using some standard statistical programs such as Stata. However, since the procedure requires the analyst to model the distribution of variables with missing values, **it is critical that this modelling is done correctly** to ensure that the resulting analyses are valid.

Further reading

- For a helpful overview of methods and pitfalls, see Sterne et al.'s article[1]
- For materials and courses see the website maintained by James Carpenter and Mike Kenward (🖰 www.missingdata.org.uk)

Reference

1 Sterne JA, White IR, Carlin JB, Spratt M, Royston P, Kenward MG et al. Multiple imputation for missing data in epidemiological and clinical research: potential and pitfalls. *BMJ* 2009; **338**:b2393.

Generalized linear models

The big picture
The modelling techniques listed in row 5 of 📖 Table 12.1, (p. 395) belong to a broad class of statistical models called **generalized linear models**. This means that many of the original multifactorial methods have been cleverly extended in recent years, and generalized to more complex situations.

> **Generalized linear models which include k predictor variables all take the following form:**
>
> $$f(y) = b_0 + b_1 x_1 + b_2 x_2 + b_3 x_3 + ... + b_k x_k$$
>
> where:
> - $f(y)$ is a function or transformation of the outcome y which converts the outcome y to a linear function of the xs. It is known as the **link function**
> - $f(y)$ depends on the type of data
> - $x_1, x_2 ...$ are the predictor variables
> - $b_0, b_1, b_2 ...$ are the regression coefficients
> - b_0 is the intercept and b_1, b_2, b_3, etc. provide the effect estimates for the variables x_1, x_2, x_3, etc.

Simple linear regression
The simple equation of a straight line $y = a + bx$ is the simplest example of a generalized linear model and the interpretation of results of all such models, whether simple or complex have much in common.

Multiple regression

Details of multiple regression

- It is used for a continuous outcome variable, e.g. birthweight, height, peak flow rate
- It enables us to disentangle the effects of several predictor variables on a continuous outcome, either to test hypotheses about predictive factors or to produce a predictive model
- The predictor variables can be any mixture of continuous, binary, or categorical data
- The method works by fitting linear relationships between the outcome and the predictors
- It gives a set of regression coefficients that represent the relationship between each predictor variable and the continuous outcome adjusted for all the other variables in the model
- It fits a model of the form:

$$y = b_0 + b_1 x_1 + b_2 x_2 + b_3 x_3 + \ldots + b_k x_k$$

where:
- y is the outcome
- x_1, x_2 … are the predictor variables
- b_0, b_1, b_2… are the regression coefficients
- b_0 is the intercept and b_1, b_2, b_3, etc. are the regression coefficients (estimates) for the variables x_1, x_2, x_3, etc.

Approach to the analysis

1. Consider which predictor variables may be important in advance
2. Investigate the relationship between each of these and the outcome variable separately before doing the multiple regression, to guide both the analysis and the interpretation:
   - *Continuous predictor variable:* draw a scatter plot and do a simple linear regression
   - *Binary predictor variable:* calculate summary statistics of the outcome such as mean, standard deviation, range in the two groups
   - *Categorical predictor variable:* calculate summary statistics of the outcome such as mean, standard deviation, range in each of the categories
3. Choose the modelling approach to be used (📖 Multifactorial methods: model selection, p. 398)

Tests and estimates

If there is no relationship between y and x_i after adjusting for the other xs, then b_i will be zero (the null value). The interpretation of the coefficients depends on whether the predictor variable is continuous, binary, or categorical. The precise meanings are given as follows.

Interpreting the coefficients from multiple regression

- **Continuous predictor variable**: slope or gradient of the line, i.e. the change in the outcome for a unit change in the predictor
- **Binary predictor variable**: difference in the mean value of the outcome between the two levels of the predictor
- **Categorical predictor variable with n categories**: gives $n-1$ values where each is the difference in mean value of the outcome for a particular category versus the reference category (see Dummy variables for more details on how this works, 📖 Multifactorial methods: overview, p. 396)

Assumptions

These mirror closely the assumptions for simple linear regression (📖 Simple linear regression, p. 296):

1. The relationship is linear

The straight line relationship can be checked by plotting the relationship for each continuous predictor variable separately before carrying out the multiple regression. If the relationship is steadily increasing but not linear, it may be possible to transform the data to linearize the relationship (📖 Transforming data, p. 330).

2. The distribution of the residuals is Normal

To test this, draw a histogram or a Normal plot of the residuals.

3. The standard deviation of the outcome y is constant over all values of each continuous predictor x

This can be checked from a scatter plot of y by x for each continuous x or plot the residuals against the x, to check that the spread of the residuals is similar across the range of x.

Note

As with simple linear regression, a transformation may simultaneously correct non-linearity, non-Normal residuals and a non-constant variance. It can be tricky to interpret a log-transformed regression coefficient – see Peacock and Kerry, Chapter 9,[1] for a worked example.

Reference

1 Peacock J, Kerry SM. *Presenting medical statistics from proposal to publication.* Oxford: Oxford University Press, 2006.

Multiple regression: examples

Using multiple regression to test hypotheses

A UK study evaluated children's language ability after early detection of permanent hearing impairment. Table 12.2 shows an extract of the results with differences between children with early versus late diagnosis of hearing loss. The differences are shown before and after adjustment for severity of hearing impairment and maternal education using multiple regression. The children's scores were normalized by using z scores, which represent the number of standard deviations by which the score differs from the mean score among a sample of age-matched control children with normal hearing.

Table 12.2 Receptive language in children with hearing impairment confirmed at ≤9months (n=45) versus >9months (n=56)

Measure	Mean z score		Mean difference (95% CI)	
	≤9 m	>9 m	Unadjusted	Adjusted[*]
Test for reception of grammar	−1.46	−2.25	0.78 (0.08 to 1.48)	0.90 (0.32 to 1.47)
British picture vocabulary scale	−1.86	−2.36	0.50 (−0.11 to 1.11)	0.64 (0.13 to 1.16)
Aggregate score	−1.76	−2.38	0.61 (−0.02 to 1.24)	0.76 (0.26 to 1.27)
Aggregate score minus non-verbal	−0.82	−1.68	0.86 (0.32 to 1.40)	0.82 (0.31 to 1.33)

[*]Adjusted for severity of hearing impairment, maternal education.

Interpretation
- Each row of the table is a separate multiple regression analysis where the outcome is the measure named in the first column
- In each multiple regression the outcome has been adjusted for the same variables, severity of hearing impairment, maternal education
- The results are presented as mean differences between the two groups, unadjusted and adjusted
- The adjustment has increased the magnitude of the difference for all measures except 'aggregate score minus non-verbal' where the difference is slightly smaller
- All adjusted differences are statistically significant as shown by the 95% confidence intervals, which exclude the null value of zero

Example (continued)

Conclusions of study
- The study concluded that early detection of hearing loss was associated with higher scores for language (see paper for more details[1])

Notes
- All mean z scores were negative, showing that these children had poorer language attainment than children of the same age without hearing loss
- This is important information to aid interpretation showing the importance of presenting the means in the two groups as well as the differences

Reference

1 Kennedy CR, McCann DC, Campbell MJ, Law CM, Mullee M, Petrou S *et al.* Language ability after early detection of permanent childhood hearing impairment. *N Engl J Med* 2006; **354**(20):2131–41.

Multiple regression: examples (continued)

Using multiple regression to produce an equation

A study of factors affecting fetal growth in 1513 singleton babies used multiple regression to adjust the babies' birthweights for their mother's height, the sex of the infant, and mother's parity. The birthweight was analysed as a ratio of the observed birthweight to the expected birthweight-for-gestational age derived from UK birthweight standards. Table 12.3 shows the adjusted coefficients.

Table 12.3 Results of multiple regression to predict birthweight

Variable	Regression coefficient	95% CI
Height (cm)	0.0036	0.0026 to 0.0046
Sex (female=1, male=2)	0.0440	0.0311 to 0.0569
Parity (1st baby=0, 2nd or later=1)	0.0353	0.0224 to 0.0482
Intercept	0.3335	0.1651 to 0.5019

Interpretation
- The coefficient for height, 0.0036, estimates the difference in birthweight ratio between two women whose height differed by 1 cm
- The coefficient for sex, 0.0440, estimates the mean difference in birthweight ratio between boys and girls
- The coefficient for parity, 0.0353, estimates the mean difference in birthweight ratio between second or later babies and first babies
- The intercept is a constant that estimates the value of the birthweight ratio when maternal height is zero
- All coefficients are statistically significant, as shown by the 95% confidence intervals, which exclude the null value, zero
- The multiple regression results correspond to the following equation

$BW\ ratio = 0.3335 + (0.0036 \times height) + (0.044 \times sex) + (0.0353 \times parity)$

- The equation was used to adjust each baby's birthweight for the maternal and infant variables which were regarded as 'nuisance' variables in this context
- The resulting adjusted birthweight ratio was used as the outcome variable in further multifactorial analyses of smoking, alcohol, and other lifestyle factors on fetal growth

Notes
- In order to use the equation it is necessary to know the coding that was used for sex of infant and parity

- Differences in birthweight ratios have an easy interpretation as a percentage difference: for example the birthweight ratios 1.05 and 1.01 have a difference of 0.04 and so the difference in the two birthweights is 4%
- In this example the **equation was used to compute an adjusted outcome** (see below for further details); in other situations an **equation may be required to compute a set of predicted values** such as when computing predicted values for lung function measurements, given a subject's age, height, and sex

Additional details: how to calculate adjusted birthweight

The researchers adjusted the birthweight ratios to height=160 cm, male sex, and parity 1 on the advice of the study obstetrician. This was achieved using the following equation derived from the original multiple regression:[1]

Adjusted BW =

BW ratio − 0.0036 × (height−160) − 0.044 × (sex−2) − 0.0353 × (parity-1)

Where sex was coded 1 (female), or 2 (male); and parity was coded 0 (first baby), 1 (second or later baby)

So for a mother of height 155 cm, who had a girl who was her first baby, with a BW ratio of 1.00, the adjusted BW was given by:

1.00 − 0.0036 × (155−160) − 0.044 × (1−2) − 0.0353 × (0−1)
=1.0973

Reference

1 Brooke OG, Anderson HR, Bland JM, Peacock JL, Stewart CM. Effects on birth weight of smoking, alcohol, caffeine, socioeconomic factors, and psychosocial stress. *BMJ* 1989; **298**(6676):795–801.

Multiple regression and analysis of variance

Analysis of variance table for multiple regression

The results of a multiple regression can be shown as an analysis of variance (anova) table, (📖 Analysis of variance table, p. 284). To illustrate, Table 12.4 shows the analysis of variance table for the multiple regression of birthweight ratio and mother's height, sex of infant, and the parity.

Table 12.4 Analysis of variance table for multiple regression to predict birthweight (📖 Table 12.3, p. 410)

Factor	DF	Sum of squares	Variance estimate	F ratio	P value

Model
  height
  sex of infant
  parity
	3	1.9082	0.6360	39.15	0.0001

Residual	1509	24.5152	0.0162		
Total	1512	26.4234			

Explanation of table
- Row 2 gives the statistics for the model that was fitted, i.e. the set of variables height, sex of infant, and parity. Row 4 gives the overall totals. Row 3 gives the residual or unexplained part of the variation.
- DF is degrees of freedom; it is the *number of variables in the model (3)* for row 2, *total number observations* −1 (1512), for row 4, and the difference between these, 1512−3=1509, for row 3
- Total sum of squares is the sum of squares of the overall mean minus each observation squared. The other sums of squares cannot be easily calculated by hand
- The model and residual sums of squares add up to the total, i.e. 1.9082+24.5152=26.4234
- Variance estimate is the sum of squares/DF:
   F ratio is ratio of 2 variances:
   0.6360/0.0162 = 39.15
- P value is probability associated with an F value of 39.15 if the null hypothesis that the model variables collectively are unrelated to the outcome, BW ratio. As it is very small, we conclude that the model variables height, sex, and parity are related to birthweight.

Two-way analysis of variance

The method of one-way analysis of variance (📖 One-way analysis of variance, p. 280) can be extended to allow two factors to be analysed together. For example, Table 12.5 shows data from a clinical trial investigating the effect of different topical analgesics and different gauge needles on reported pain on injection.[1]

Table 12.5 Median visual analogue scale (VAS; 0–10) pain score after injection in 120 subjects

Treatment	Needle size (gauge)			All
	22	**20**	**18**	
EMLA 60	0.3	0.2	1.2	0.4
EMLA 5	0.4	0.5	1.1	1.0
Placebo	0.8	1.4	2.3	1.9
Nil	1.6	1.2	2.8	2.3
All	0.5	0.9	1.9	

These data were analysed using two-way analysis of variance but could equally have been analysed using multiple regression to give the same answer since analysis of variance is a special case of multiple regression.

Balanced designs

In a two-way analysis of variance, the data are said to be **balanced if there are equal numbers of subjects for each combination of factors**. Otherwise the design is unbalanced. In balanced designs the sums of squares add up and analysis of variance can be done by hand using formulae. This is of no great importance nowadays since computers are so readily available to most people, but the issue was critical when most calculations were done manually. This is why many older textbooks describe analysis of variance and multiple regression separately.

Unbalanced designs

Unbalanced data are common in medical research. This affects the way that analyses are done in modelling situations, such as when adding another variable to a particular group of variables to see if the model is improved. In such a situation it is necessary to do the following:
- Fit the model (i) without and then (ii) with the new variable
- Test the addition of the new variable using the **extra sum of squares** that the new variable adds to the model
- For an example of this see 📖 Linear and non-linear terms, p. 416.

❶ Choice of method: analysis of variance or multiple regression

Some statistical programs will do both methods but the different commands may deal with predictor variables differently. For example, in Stata the 'anova' command assumes all variables are categorical unless the user specifies otherwise, whereas its 'regression' command assumes that all variables are continuous unless otherwise specified.

Reference

1 Nott MR, Peacock JL. Relief of injection pain in adults. EMLA cream for 5 minutes before venepuncture. *Anaesthesia* 1990; **45**(9):772–4.

Main effects and interactions

Introduction

The regression analyses considered so far have only included **main effects**. In other words, it was assumed that the effect of one predictor on an outcome was constant for all values of other predictor variables in the model. For example, in the birthweight study data presented earlier in the chapter it was assumed that the effect of maternal height on birthweight was the same for both males and females and also that that the difference in mean birthweight between males and females did not vary with mother's height. These assumptions were reasonable but in other situations they may not be so.

Example

An ecological study investigated the inter-relationships between tooth decay in children, water fluoridation, and deprivation.[1] The study found a protective effect of both natural and artificial fluoridation on tooth decay and an adverse effect of deprivation. But the study also reported an interaction such that the observed benefit of fluoridation was greater in more deprived areas than in less deprived areas. Figure 12.1 depicts this.

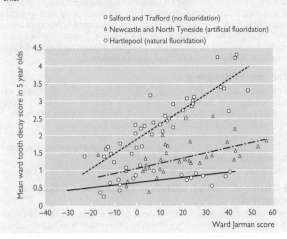

Fig. 12.1 Mean decayed, missing, or filled tooth score and Jarman underprivileged area score, by non-fluoridated, artificially fluoridated, and naturally fluoridated electoral wards.

Reproduced from *BMJ* Jones CM *et al.* **315**:514–517 1997 with permission from BMJ Publishing Group Ltd.

Example (continued)

Interpretation of graph
- Both artificial and natural fluoridation were associated with a lower ward tooth decay score than no fluoridation
- The differences in mean ward tooth decay score were small for areas with low Jarman deprivation score (left hand end of the graph) and were much greater for areas with high deprivation scores (right hand end of the graph)
- There is an interaction between fluoridation and deprivation such that the effects of fluoridation are greater in areas with high deprivation

Notes
- When there is an interaction between two factors as there is here, the regression lines are not parallel – there is a different line for each group
- If an interaction term had not been included in the model, three parallel lines would have been computed but these would not have represented the data very well
- The statistical model used here was:

  tooth decay = fluoridation + deprivation + (fluoridation × deprivation)
  - Where fluoridation is in three groups and deprivation score is continuous.
  - The multiplicative term *'fluoridation × deprivation'* is the **interaction term**

Reference
1 Jones CM, Taylor GO, Whittle JG, Evans D, Trotter DP. Water fluoridation, tooth decay in 5 year olds, and social deprivation measured by the Jarman score: analysis of data from British dental surveys. *BMJ* 1997; **315**(7107):514–17.

Linear and non-linear terms

Introduction

The basic assumption of regression is that the relationship between a predictor and outcome variable is linear. If this is not true, it may be possible to find a transformation of the variable that will give a linear relationship so that regression methods can be used. For example, if the relationship is U-shaped (quadratic), then a relationship of the following form can be used:

$$y = a + bx + cx^2$$

Example

The EMLA trial investigated whether using EMLA anaesthetic cream for just 5 minutes before injection was better than using nothing[1] (📖 Table 12.5, p. 413 has the summary data). The trial included four treatment groups: EMLA 60 applied 60 minutes before injection (known to be effective), EMLA 5 minutes before injection, placebo cream 5 minutes before injection, and nothing. Pain was assessed using a 10 cm VAS. The data were analysed firstly using two-way analysis of variance and then using a multiple regression model to adjust for the effect of the age of the patient. Age did not have a linear relationship with pain; reported pain was highest for the youngest and oldest people and lowest for those in between so the relationship was U-shaped. To model this, the factors age and age^2 were put into the multiple regression model.

Table 12.6 Analysis of variance table for multiple regression in EMLA trial

Factor	DF	Sum of squares	Variance estimate	F ratio	P value
Age + age^2	2	7.49	3.75	4.40	0.01
Needle size	2	19.39	9.70	11.39	<0.0001
Treatments	3	23.95	7.98	9.38	<0.0001
Residual	112	95.36	0.85		
Total	119	146.19			

Interpretation
1. The quadratic term 'age + age^2':
- Has 2 DF as there were two continuous factors
- It is statistically significant
- The sum of squares (SS) is the same as we get if we had included only the 'age' term in the multiple regression model, and not needle size or treatment

Example (continued)

2. The 'needles' term:
- Has 3–1=2 DF as there were three types of needle
- SS is the extra SS due to 'needles' after including 'age'
- It is statistically significant

3. The 'treatments' term:
- Has 4–1=3 DF as there were four different treatments
- SS is the extra SS due to 'treatments' after including age and needles
- It is statistically significant

Conclusion

The two-way analysis of variance had shown that EMLA applied 5 minutes before injection reduced pain slightly compared to placebo cream or nothing. The multiple regression analysis showed that the treatment effect remained statistically significant after allowing for the age of the subject and the gauge of the needle used. It was concluded that the observed treatment differences were not due to other factors.

Notes
- Since pain score was skewed and there were some zero values, the outcome was transformed for analysis by taking log(pain score + 1)
- When modelling the quadratic relationship for age, the mean age was subtracted from the age in each term to reduce the correlation between the age and age squared terms, i.e. the following was used: $(x-\bar{x})+(x-\bar{x})^2$ (see Bland, Chapter 17[2])

Tests of fit using extra sum of squares

In the example we examined the effect of treatment after allowing for needles and age. If the question of interest was to see if adding 'age' to the model improved the fit, a different approach is used:
- Fit a model with just needles and treatments
- Fit a second model adding in 'age' as a quadratic term
- Subtract the two model sums of squares, and test statistical significance of the difference using an F test

In the example above this gives model SS without age is 42.47, DF=5 and model SS with age is 50.83, DF=7. The difference is the extra SS: 50.83 – 42.47 = 8.36 with DF= 7–5=2. The F test is given by (8.36/2)/residual mean square, 4.18/0.85 = 4.92, DF = 2,112. This gives P=0.009.
- The F test for the extra SS is equivalent to a t test of the regression coefficient for a continuous predictor variable
- The above two ways of testing the effect of 'age' are very similar here. This may not always be so

References
1 Nott MR, Peacock JL. Relief of injection pain in adults. EMLA cream for 5 minutes before venepuncture. *Anaesthesia* 1990; **45**(9):772–4.
2 Bland M. *An introduction to medical statistics.* 3rd ed. Oxford: Oxford University Press, 2000.

How well the model fits

How well a multiple regression model fits the data

We can assess how well a multiple regression model fits the data by considering the proportion of the total variability, the total sum of squares, that is accounted for or 'explained' by the model that was fitted. For example in the birthweight, height, sex, and parity model, the total sum of squares was 26.423 and the model sum of squares was 1.908. Therefore, the model explained 1.908/26.423 = 0.072 or 7.2% of the variation in birthweight ratio. This means that over 90% of the total variability was not accounted for by these factors. This may be because the wrong factors had been measured or included in the model, or because there was unknown variation which cannot be quantified. (The latter is certainly true with birthweight.)

R-squared (R^2)

The proportion of variability explained is known as R-squared (R^2) and is analogous to the square of the correlation coefficient for simple linear regression. **R** is known as the **multiple correlation coefficient**.

- Note that **R^2 always increases when additional variables are added** to the model even if the additional variable is not statistically significant. Some statistical programs calculate an **adjusted R^2** which takes account of chance prediction to address this potential problem
- The basic assumptions of the multiple regression model, linearity, and Normal residuals (📖 Simple regression, p. 296) should be tested. If these are not met, then the model fit will be poorer and so estimates and tests may be unreliable

Deviance for generalized linear models

Deviance is a general measure of how well a generalized linear model fits a set of data (📖 Generalized linear models, p. 404). It is analogous to the R-squared statistic for multiple regression described above. The deviance follows an approximately chi-squared distribution with degrees of freedom equal to the difference in the number of parameters fitted by two models. Analysis of deviance is used to determine the best-fitting model, and in particular to determine if the inclusion of extra variables in a model significantly improves the fit. This is analogous to using the 'extra sum of squares' method to test the addition of new variables in multiple regression (📖 Linear and non-linear terms, p. 416). Deviance is used to test model fit in logistic regression, Cox regression, Poisson regression, and in other generalized linear models.

What is a good fit?

This depends on the purpose of the study and analysis:

- If this is to derive an equation from which predictions will be made, it is important that the model fits closely since a large residual error will lead to wide confidence intervals and poor precision
- If this is to investigate relationships and test hypotheses, high precision is less critical and so it may not matter if the proportion of variability explained is low as long as all known confounding variables are included

Sample size for multiple regression

Introduction

There is no simple way to determine the size of sample required for a multiple regression analysis but the following points may be helpful.

Number of predictor variables

- If a large number of predictor variables are tested then we expect that some will be significant by chance alone
- When a large number of variables are fitted to a small dataset, it may appear that the fit is very good. Exact prediction can be obtained where the number of factors is one fewer than the total sample size but clearly this would be nonsensical
- For an existing dataset with n observations, Altman, Chapter 12,[1] suggests as a guide that no more than $n/10$ predictor variables should be included at a time

Number of observations

- If the number of observations is large then some very small effects that may not be of practical importance will be statistically significant
- If sample size calculations are based on unifactorial analyses, then a useful rule of thumb is to increase the sample size by 10% for each predictor variable that is to be analysed

Further reading on multiple regression

- Bland, Chapter 17,[2] Altman, Chapter 12,[1] and Kirkwood and Sterne, Chapters 11 and 12[3] give more examples and discussion of multiple regression
- Peacock and Kerry, Chapter 10,[4] show how to carry out multiple regression in SPSS and Stata and also gives examples of how to present the findings in a report or paper

References

1 Altman DG. *Practical statistics for medical research*. London: Chapman & Hall, 1991.
2 Bland M. *An introduction to medical statistics*. 3rd ed. Oxford: Oxford University Press, 2000.
3 Kirkwood BR, Sterne JAC. *Essential medical statistics*. 2nd ed. Malden, MA: Blackwell Science, 2003.
4 Peacock J, Kerry SM. *Presenting medical statistics from proposal to publication*. Oxford: Oxford University Press, 2006.

Logistic regression

Details of logistic regression

- It is used for a binary outcome variable, such as survive yes/no, diseased yes/no, symptom yes/no, satisfied yes/no
- It enables us to disentangle the effects of several predictor variables on a binary outcome, either to test hypotheses about predictive factors or to produce a predictive model
- Predictor variables can be any mixture of continuous, binary, or categorical data
- It uses a logarithmic transformation to allow a linear relationship to be modelled
- It gives a set of regression coefficients that represent the relationship between each predictor variable and the binary outcome, after adjusting for all the other variables in the model
- It fits a model of the form:

  $\log_e[p/(1-p)] = b_0 + b_1x_1 + b_2x_2 + b_3x_3 + b_4x_4 + ...$

where:
- p is the proportion with the outcome
- $x_1, x_2 ...$ are the predictor variables
- b_0 is the intercept and b_1, b_2, b_3, etc. are the regression coefficients (estimates) for the variables x_1, x_2, x_3, etc., which when back-transformed from the log scale to the natural scale are **odds ratios**
- $\log_e[p/(1-p)]$ is known as the **logit transformation**

Approach to the analysis

1. Consider which predictor variables may be important in advance
2. Investigate the relationship between each of these and the binary outcome separately before doing the logistic regression to guide both the analysis and the interpretation:
   - *Binary predictor variables:* calculate the proportions of the outcome in each group, e.g. if the outcome is die/survive and the predictor variable is sex, calculate the proportion surviving in males and females and compare.
   - *Categorical predictor variables:* calculate the proportions of the outcome in each category, e.g. with die/survive and hospital, calculate the proportion surviving in each hospital and compare.
   - *Continuous predictor variables:* divide the variable into categories and calculate the proportion of the outcome in each category, e.g. if the continuous variable is age, divide into age groups and calculate and compare the proportion surviving in each age category. It is not necessary to use the grouped variable in the logistic regression if the relationship with the raw data is approximately linear. In general it is better to analyse the raw data as continuous data rather than grouped data where possible to retain as much information as possible (📖 Outcomes: continuous and categorical, p. 46)
3. Choose the modelling approach to be used (📖 Multifactorial methods: model selection, p. 398)

Tests and estimates

If there is no relationship between y and x_i after adjusting for the other xs, then b_i will be zero on the logarithmic scale. When the b_i are back-transformed to give odds ratios, the null value equivalent to a log of zero is 1, i.e. the null value for the odds ratio is 1. The interpretation of the coefficients depends on whether the predictor variable is continuous, binary, or categorical. The precise meanings are given below.

Interpreting the odds ratios (OR) from logistic regression

- OR measures the strength of relationship and is the ratio of odds in two groups
- OR=1 indicates no relationship
- OR<1 indicates a protective relationship
- OR>1 indicates an adverse relationship
- Note, in general ORs cannot be interpreted as relative risks unless the outcome is rare (📖 Estimates for tests of proportions, p. 268)

- *Binary predictor variable:* OR is the odds of the outcome in one group divided by the odds in the other group
- *Categorical predictor variable with n categories:* gives $n-1$ ORs where each is the odds of the outcome in a particular category versus the odds in the reference category (see Dummy variables for more details on how this works, 📖 Multifactorial methods: overview, p. 396)
- *Continuous predictor variable:* OR is the change in odds of the outcome for a unit change in the continuous predictor variable. A change of two units has an associated OR that is OR $\times$ OR=OR^2 (not $2 \times$ OR), and a change of three units is shown by OR^3 etc.

Assumptions

The principal assumption is that the relationship between the outcome and the predictor variable is linear on the logit scale for continuous predictor variables. This can be tested by categorizing the continuous variable and plotting the logit of the proportion with the outcome in each group to check this is close to a straight line relationship.

Sample size is an important issue for logistic regression. This is discussed in 📖 Extensions to logistic regression, p. 426.

Logistic regression: examples

Using logistic regression to adjust for confounding

A prospective study obtained reports of symptoms and health problems during pregnancy and sought to explore their inter-relationships with social and behavioural factors. Preliminary analyses had shown that both women who smoked and women in manual occupations reported less nausea. Logistic regression was used to disentangle the relationships (Table 12.7)[1]

Table 12.7 The relationships between smoking, occupation and nausea in 1512 pregnant women

Predictor variable	Odds ratio	95% CI	P value
Smoking			<0.001
Non-smoker	1.00		
Light smoker	0.59	0.44 to 0.79	
Heavy smoker	0.51	0.35 to 0.75	
Occupation			0.04
Non-manual work	1.00		
Manual work	0.74	0.55 to 0.99	

Interpretation
- The reference category for smoking was non-smokers and for occupation was non-manual work, and each has OR=1
- ORs for both light smokers and heavy smokers are <1, indicating that smokers have a lower odds of nausea than non-smokers, after adjusting for occupation
- The OR for manual work is also <1, indicating that women in manual occupations have a lower odds of nausea than those in non-manual occupations, after adjusting for smoking
- Both the smoking factor and occupation factor are statistically significant overall
- These data are consistent with there being independent relationships between smoking and nausea, and occupation and nausea

❶ Note
This analysis shows that the risk of nausea was lower in smokers than non-smokers. However, this cannot be interpreted as a causal relationship since the study was observational. It could be that women who felt nauseated in early pregnancy or in previous pregnancies, gave up smoking. Hence the effect might be due to selection and not cause.

Calculating probabilities

The logistic regression equation (not given explicitly opposite) can be used to calculate odds or probabilities for specific combinations of predictor variables, **i.e. for specific individuals**. The following shows the calculations for the nausea data in Table 12.7.

Equation for logit(p) from logistic regression is given by:
$1.6232 - 0.5292 \times smoker1 - 0.6744 \times smoker2 - 0.3013 \times occup$

Where
- *smoker1=1* indicates a light smoker
- *smoker2=1* indicates a heavy smoker
- *smoker1=smoker2=0* indicates a non-smoker
- *occup=0* indicates non-manual occupation
- *occup=1* indicates manual occupation

To calculate the probability of nausea, using the model, for a non-smoker in a non-manual occupation:

- Calculate log odds using the equation by substituting the correct values for smoking and occupation
- Calculate the antilog to get the odds
- Convert the odds to a probability using standard formula:
  probability=odds/(1+odds)

This gives:
- $1.6232 - 0.5292 \times smoker1 - 0.6744 \times smoker2 - 0.3013 \times occup$
  $1.6232 - 0.5292 \times 0 - 0.6744 \times 0 - 0.3013 \times 0 = 1.6232$
- $exp(1.6232) = 5.0693$
- Probability = 5.0693/(1+5.0693) = 0.835 or 84%

Note that the exponential (i.e. antilog) of the coefficients on the log scale gives the odds ratios shown in Table 12.7: i.e. $exp(-0.5292) = 0.59$, $exp(-0.6744) = 0.51$, $exp(-0.3013) = 0.74$

Reference

1 Meyer LC, Peacock JL, Bland JM, Anderson HR. Symptoms and health problems in pregnancy: their association with social factors, smoking, alcohol, caffeine and attitude to pregnancy. *Paediatr Perinat Epidemiol* 1994; **8**(2):145–55.

Logistic regression and ROC curves

ROCs and sensitivity and specificity

These are used to display possible cut-offs for sensitivity and specificity to detect a condition using a diagnostic test, where the test gives a continuous measure (□ Receiver operating characteristic (ROC) curves, p. 348). They can be obtained using logistic regression with the condition as the outcome and the continuous diagnostic measure as the predictor.

ROCs and prediction

ROCs can also be used in a more general way to quantify the extent to which a statistical model predicts a binary outcome. Since the maximum area under the curve is 1, a model with area under the curve close to 1 fits the data better than a model with area under the curve much less than 1. The example in Table 12.8 has used the area under the ROC curve in exploring the effects of baby factors, treatments, and clinical outcomes on bronchopulmonary dysplasia (BPD, yes/no).

Example using ROCs

Table 12.8 Logistic regression models (A,B,C,D) to predict bronchopulmonary dysplasia

Factor	OR	Area under ROC curve
(A) Baby factors		0.94
Birthweight (g)	0.996	
Gestational age (d)	0.924	
(B) Surfactant treatment		0.83
None	1.0	
1 dose	11.9	
2 doses	84.5	
(C) Clinical outcomes		0.94
ETCO 14d (log scale)	570.0	
FRC 14 d (log scale)	0.320	
(D) Combined model (A+B+C)		0.97
Birthweight (g)	0.994	
Gestational age (d)	0.989	
ETCO 14 d	83.2	

Note: 95% CIs and P values have been omitted here to simplify

ETCO, exhaled carbon monoxide; FRC, forced residual capacity; ROC, receiver operating characteristic.

Example using ROCs (continued)

Methods and interpretation
- Four logistic regressions were done, one for each of the three types of variable, and a final model that combined these three
- For each model, several predictive factors were analysed with BPD and used in the model if this gave a significant result
- For each model an area under the ROC curve was reported to indicate the predictive power of the variables included
- The interpretation of the ORs is straightforward for the surfactant doses but is less so for the continuous variables. We illustrate this using birthweight, where the OR is 0.996:
  → The comparative odds of BPD in two infants whose weight differs by 1 g is 0.996
  → The comparative odds of BPD in two infants whose weight differs by 10 g is $0.996^{10} = 0.961$
  → The comparative odds of BPD in two infants whose weight differs by 100 g is $0.996^{100} = 0.670$

Conclusions
These data suggest:
- Birthweight and gestation combined, are powerful predictors of BPD with area under the curve = 0.94
- 14-day measures of ETCO (exhaled carbon monoxide) and FRC (forced residual capacity) combined are also are strong predictors of BPD with area under the curve = 0.94
- When these models are combined a slightly higher area under the curve was given with birthweight, gestation, and ETCO (0.97) suggesting that ETCO improves the prediction slightly

These data come from a clinical study in infants born very prematurely, unpublished at the time of writing (C May, 2010).

Extensions to logistic regression

Interaction terms and non-linear relationships

These can be included, if appropriate, in similar ways to multiple regression (⌑ Linear and non-linear terms, p. 416).

Ordinal logistic regression

Bronchopulmonary dysplasia (BPD) is sometimes analysed as a binary variable but can also be categorized in four groups according to the severity of BPD: no BPD, mild, moderate, and severe BPD. This gives an outcome that consists of four groups with an inherent ordering. These data can be analysed using an extension of logistic regression called ordinal logistic regression. The results of ordinal logistic regression are in the form of odds ratios but the meaning is slightly different due to the ordering and the way the model is fitted. The following example illustrates.

Example

These data come from a study investigating the relationship between bacteria obtained from endotracheal aspirates and the subsequent severity of BPD in infants born preterm.[1] BPD severity was analysed in four groups as: (i) no BPD, (ii) mild BPD, (iii) moderate or severe BPD, and (iv) death. A positive relationship was observed between BPD severity and the presence of *Ureaplasma*, and between the number of days the infant was ventilated and the presence of *Ureaplasma*. An ordinal logistic regression was used to disentangle the relationships to see if the relationship with *Ureaplasma* could be due to infected infants being ventilated for longer. The following results were obtained:

- Before adjustment the odds ratio for BPD or death where *Ureaplasma* was present/absent was 4.80 (95% CI: 1.15 to 20.13)
- After adjusting for number of days ventilated, the odds ratio was reduced to 2.04 (95% CI: 0.41 to 10.25) and was no longer statistically significant
- It was concluded that the relationship between *Ureaplasma* and severity of BPD is partly explained by the length of ventilation either directly or as a proxy for how sick the infant was at the outset

Polytomous logistic regression

The method of ordinal logistic regression can be extended to deal with a multi-category outcome without ordering. For further details see Collett.[2]

Conditional logistic regression

Conditional logistic regression is an extension of the paired test of two proportions, McNemar's test (◻ McNemar's test for paired proportions, p. 276). The analysis gives adjusted odds ratios for paired binary data, such as may be found in a matched case–control study. For further details, see Collett.[2]

❶ Sample size considerations

Logistic regression is a large sample method and so the results will not hold if the sample size is too small. Peduzzi et al.[1] performed simulations which indicated that the **total number of events is the key factor** rather than the total sample size. This means that the number of deaths or survivors, whichever is smaller, must be large enough. The researchers recommend that a sample should contain **at least 10 events (as defined above) per variable** used in a logistic equation. Their study showed that where the number of events was too small, the estimates tended to be biased either upwards or downwards, i.e. they were either too big or too small. This occurs because the estimation methods are unstable when the sample size is too small.

For example, in the study of nausea in pregnancy (◻ Table 12.7, p. 422), the total number of nausea events was 1199 but the number without nausea was 313. It is this number that drives the sample size considerations and so with this number, around 30 variables could be safely modelled at one time.

Further reading on logistic regression

- For more examples, see Bland, Chapter 17,[4] Altman, Chapter 12,[5] and Armitage et al., Chapter 14[6]
- For full details and a more mathematical coverage, see Collett's book, Modeling binary data'[2]

References

1 Payne MS, Goss KC, Connett GJ, Kollamparambil T, Legg JP, Thwaites R et al. Molecular microbiological characterization of pre-term neonates at risk of bronchopulmonary dysplasia. Pediatr Res 22 Dec 2009 [epub ahead of print].

2 Collett D. Modelling binary data. 2nd ed. Boca Raton: Chapman & Hall/CRC, 2003.

3 Peduzzi P, Concato J, Kemper E, Holford TR, Feinstein AR. A simulation study of the number of events per variable in logistic regression analysis. J Clin Epidemiol 1996; **49**(12):1373–9.

4 Bland M. An introduction to medical statistics. 3rd ed. Oxford: Oxford University Press, 2000.

5 Altman DG. Practical statistics for medical research. London: Chapman & Hall, 1991.

6 Armitage P, Berry G, Matthews JNS. Statistical methods in medical research. 4th ed. Oxford: Blackwell Science, 2002.

Cox proportional hazards regression

Details of Cox regression

- This is used for a time-to-event outcome variable, such as the length of survival from diagnosis, the time to recurrence after treatment, time to conception after fertility treatment, and so on
- It enables us to disentangle the effects of several predictor variables on a time-to-event outcome either to test hypotheses about predictive factors or to produce a predictive model
- Predictor variables can be any mixture of continuous, binary, or categorical data
- It uses a logarithmic transformation to allow a linear relationship to be modelled
- It gives a set of regression coefficients that represent the relationship between each predictor variable and the time-to-event outcome, after adjusting for all the other variables in the model
- It fits a model of the form:

$$\log_e [h(t)/h_0(t)] = b_1 x_1 + b_2 x_2 + \ldots + b_p x_p$$

where:
- $h(t)$ is the probability of the outcome at time t – the **'hazard'**
- $h_0(t)$ is the probability of the outcome at time 0, ie the baseline hazard
- $h(t)/h_0(t)$ is the **hazard ratio** which is log-transformed for analysis
- x_1, x_2 … are the predictor variables
- b_1, b_2, b_3, etc. are the regression coefficients (estimates) for the variables x_1, x_2, x_3, etc. which when back-transformed are hazard ratios

Approach to the analysis

1. Consider which predictor variables may be important in advance
2. Investigate the relationship between each of these and the time-to-event outcome separately before doing the Cox regression to guide both the analysis and the interpretation:
   - *Binary predictor variables:* plot the Kaplan–Meier survival curve (📖 Kaplan–Meier curves, p. 320) for each group and calculate hazard ratios, e.g. if the outcome is time to death and the predictor variable is sex, plot survival for males and females, and calculate the hazard ratio for males/females
   - *Categorical predictor variables:* plot the Kaplan–Meier survival curve for each category and calculate hazard ratios relative to the chosen reference category to show the relationships
   - *Continuous predictor variables:* divide the variable into categories and proceed as for categorical variables above
3. Choose the modelling approach to be used (📖 Multifactorial methods: model selection, p. 398)

Tests and estimates

If there is no relationship between y and x_i after adjusting for the other xs, then b_i will be zero on the logarithmic scale. When the b_i are back-transformed to give hazard ratios, the null value equivalent to a log of zero is 1, i.e. the null value for the hazard ratio is 1. The interpretation of the coefficients depends on whether the predictor variable is continuous, binary, or categorical. The precise meanings are given below.

Interpreting the hazard ratios (HR) from Cox regression

- HR measures the strength of relationship and is the ratio of hazards or risks of outcome in two groups
- HR=1 indicates no relationship
- HR<1 indicates a protective relationship
- HR>1 indicates an adverse relationship
- Note that a HR is ratio of risks similar to a **relative risk**

- *Binary predictor variable:* HR is the risk of the outcome in one group divided by the risk in the other group
- *Categorical predictor variable with n categories:* gives $n-1$ HRs, where each is the risk of the outcome in a particular category versus the risk in the reference category (see Dummy variables for more details on how this works, 📖 Multifactorial methods: overview, p. 396)
- *Continuous predictor variable:* HR is the change in risk of the outcome for a unit change in the continuous predictor variable. A change of two units has an associated HR, that is $HR \times HR = HR^2$ (not $2 \times HR$), and a change of three units is shown by HR^3 etc.

Assumptions

The Cox regression method assumes that the hazard ratio is constant across time. This can be checked by calculating the hazard ratio for subjects entering the study at different times, plus there are statistical tests that can be done on the regression residuals (details omitted, see Collett[1]). If this assumption of constancy over time does not hold, the predictor variables are said to be **time-varying** and the Cox model approach needs to be adapted and extended to allow for this.[1]

Footnote

Cox regression was first introduced by Sir David Cox, of Imperial College, London, relatively recently in statistical history in 1972. The paper published in the *Journal of the Royal Statistical Society* has unsurprisingly been cited over 20 000 times![2]

References

1 Collett D. *Modelling survival data in medical research.* 2nd ed. Boca Raton: Chapman & Hall/CRC, 2003.
2 Cox DR. Regression models and life-tables. *J R Statist Soc B* 1972; **34**(2):187–220.

Cox regression: example

Cox regression to disentangle effects of several factors

This study used data from a newly established cancer registry in Southern Iran to investigate survival in women with breast cancer. Table 12.9 shows analyses of effects of distant metastases. Three types of metastasis were statistically significant on their own and so they were modelled together using Cox regression[1], giving the following results.

Table 12.9a Cox regression for factors associated with breast cancer survival: interim model

Factors	Hazard ratio (95% CI)	P value
Bone metastases	2.20 (1.41 to 3.45)	0.001
Liver metastases	1.86 (0.90 to 3.84)	0.093
Lung metastases	2.49 (1.20 to 5.13)	0.014

Interpretation
- Bone and lung metastases were both statistically significant but liver was not (Table 12.9a)
- The model was re-fitted without the factor 'liver' (Table 12.9b)

Table 12.9b Cox regression for factors associated with breast cancer survival: final model

Factors	Hazard ratio (95% CI)	P value
Bone metastases	2.25 (1.43 to 3.52)	<0.001
Lung metastases	3.21 (1.70 to 6.05)	<0.001

Interpretation
- The hazard ratios for bone and lung metastases increased slightly in the second model
- For bone metastases, HR=2.25 indicates that there is a 2.25-fold increase in risk of death for those with bone metastases compared with those without bone metastases
- The 95% confidence interval shows that the true hazard ratio could be as great as 3.52 or as small as 1.43
- The hazard ratio for lung metastases is interpreted in a similar way

Note: the Cox regression method assumes that the hazard ratio is constant across time. Here this means that women who entered the study early had the same hazard ratios as women who entered the study later. The data were checked to confirm this was true.

Sample size considerations

As with logistic regression, Cox regression is a large sample method and the sample size needs to be big enough for the analysis to be valid. Peduzzi et al.[2] performed simulations which indicated that, for Cox regression as for logistic regression, **the total number of events is the key factor** rather than the total sample size. Hence the number of deaths or survivors, whichever is smaller, needs to large enough. The researchers recommended that a sample should contain **at least 10 events (as defined above) per variable** used in a Cox regression equation.

Further reading on Cox regression and its extensions

- Further examples and discussion can be found in Bland, Chapter 17,[3] Altman, Chapter 13,[4] Kirkwood and Sterne, Chapter 27,[5] and Armitage et al., Chapter 17[6]
- For full details and a more mathematical coverage, see Collett's book *Modelling survival data in medical research*[7]

References

1 Rezaianzadeh A, Peacock J, Reidpath D, Talei A, Hoseini SV, Mehrabani D. Survival analysis of 1148 women diagnosed with breast cancer in Southern Iran. *BMC Cancer* 2009; **9**:168.

2 Peduzzi P, Concato J, Feinstein AR, Holford TR. Importance of events per independent variable in proportional hazards regression analysis. II. Accuracy and precision of regression estimates. *J Clin Epidemiol* 1995; **48**(12):1503–10.

3 Bland M. *An introduction to medical statistics.* 3rd ed. Oxford: Oxford University Press, 2000.

4 Altman DG. *Practical statistics for medical research.* London: Chapman & Hall, 1991.

5 Kirkwood BR, Sterne JAC. *Essential medical statistics.* 2nd ed. Malden, MA: Blackwell Science, 2003.

6 Armitage P, Berry G, Matthews JNS. *Statistical methods in medical research.* 4th ed. Oxford: Blackwell Science, 2002.

7 Collett D. *Modelling survival data in medical research.* 2nd ed. Boca Raton: Chapman & Hall/CRC, 2003.

Poisson regression

Details of Poisson regression

Poisson regression is commonly used to analyse data from epidemiological studies such as large occupational cohorts:

- It is used to analyse the number of events as the outcome variable where this can be expressed as a rate. For example, the annual rate of influenza infection in a population, or the rate of myocardial infarction in smokers per 1000 person-years followed up.
- It enables us to disentangle the effects of several predictor variables on a rate, to test hypotheses about predictor factors, or to produce a predictive model
- Predictor variables can be any mixture of continuous, binary, or categorical data
- It uses a logarithmic transformation to allow a linear relationship to be modelled
- It gives a set of regression coefficients that represent the relationship between each predictor variable and the rate outcome, after adjusting for all the other variables in the model
- It fits a model of the form:
  $$log_e (rate) = b_0 + b_1x_1 + b_2x_2 + \ldots + b_px_p$$

where:

- rate is the number of events divided by the population at risk multiplied by the exposure time. For example 'person years at risk'
- b_0 is the baseline rate
- b_1, b_2, b_3, etc. are the regression coefficients that estimate the variables x_1, x_2, x_3, etc. and when back-transformed are **rate ratios**
- x_1, x_2 ... are the predictor variables

Approach to the analysis

This is the same as the general approach for logistic regression (📖 Logistic regression, p. 420) and Cox regression (📖 Cox proportional hazards regression, p. 428).

Tests and estimates

If there is no relationship between the rate and x_i after adjusting for the other xs, then b_i will be zero on the logarithmic scale. When the b_i are back-transformed to give rate ratios, the null value equivalent to a log of zero is 1, i.e. the null value for the hazard ratio is 1. The interpretation of the coefficients depends on whether the predictor variable is continuous, binary, or categorical. The precise meanings are given below.

Interpreting the rate ratios (RR) from Poisson regression
- RR measures the strength of relationship and is the ratio of rates in two groups
- RR=1 indicates no relationship
- RR<1 indicates a protective relationship
- RR>1 indicates an adverse relationship

- **Binary predictor variable:** RR is the rate in one group divided by the rate in the other group
- **Categorical predictor variable with *n* categories:** gives *n*–1 RRs where each is the rate in a particular category versus the rate in the reference category (see Dummy variables for more details on how this works, 📖 Multifactorial methods: overview, p. 396)
- **Continuous predictor variable:** RR is the change in rate for a unit change in the continuous predictor variable. A change of two units has an associated RR that is RR x RR=RR^2 (not 2 x RR), and a change of three units is shown by RR^3 etc.

Assumptions
- The method assumes that the number of events follows a Poisson distribution. A quick check for this is that the mean and variance are similar as would be expected for a Poisson distribution (📖 Poisson distribution, p. 216). If the variance is too big, there is said to be '**over-dispersion**'. This can often be caused by the omission of important predictor variables and so adding more variables may correct the problem. If not, another type of regression may be needed, such as negative Binomial regression (details omitted).
- Rates are often calculated over a time period, and Poisson regression assumes that the rate is constant over time. For example, if age is a predictor variable in a Poisson regression then the assumption would be that the rate is the same for all ages. This may not be appropriate and so it may be necessary in the given example to divide age into categories in which the rate is approximately constant, and calculate the rate ratio for each age category

Link between Poisson and Cox regression
If the rate changes with time, as with age in the example above, and the age categories are made smaller and smaller until each age has its own category, the results of Poisson regression will be the same as using Cox regression.

Poisson regression: example

Using Poisson regression with cohort study data

A national cohort study assessed the risk of venous thromboembolism in women using hormonal contraception (HC) in Danish women aged 15–49 with no history of cardiovascular or malignant disease. Poisson regression was used to estimate rate ratios for venous thrombotic events allowing for the length of time of HC use, age, educational level and, calendar year. Table 12.10 gives an extract of the results.

Table 12.10 Crude incidence rates and adjusted rate ratios of venous thromboembolism in women according to use of the combined pill

Years of combined pill use	<1 year	1–4 years	>4 years
Woman years	684 061	1 449 000	1 031 953
No. with venous thromboembolism	443	787	793
Rate per 10 000 woman years	6.48	5.43	7.68
Adjusted rate ratio	4.17	2.98	2.76
95% CI	3.73 to 4.66	2.73 to 3.26	2.53 to 3.02

Notes: Rates are adjusted for age, calendar year, educational level; Reference category is non-combined pill users.

Interpretation
- Columns 2–4 give results for women who used the combined pill for <1, 1–4, and >4 years
- Row 2, 'woman years', is the sum of the number of years' use for all women and measures the total exposure to the three combined pill categories
- Row 3 is self-explanatory
- Rate per 10 000 years is the number with venous embolisms/woman years
- The adjusted rate ratio comes from Poisson regression. The rate ratios decrease as use increases showing an inverse relationship between length of use and risk
- The rate ratios are interpreted directly, for example the RR of 4.17 indicates an approximately four-fold increased risk of venous embolism in combined pill users for less than1 year, compared with non-users
- The 95% confidence intervals all exclude the null value, 1, indicating that all rate ratios are statistically significant

Conclusions relevant to this extract
- The authors concluded that the risk of venous thrombosis in current users of the combined oral contraceptives decreased with duration of use

Further details of Poisson regression

For more examples see Kirkwood and Sterne, Chapter 24,[1] and Armitage et al., Chapter 14.[2]

References

1 Kirkwood BR, Sterne JAC. *Essential medical statistics.* 2nd ed. Malden, MA: Blackwell Science, 2003.
2 Armitage P, Berry G, Matthews JNS. *Statistical methods in medical research.* 4th ed. Oxford: Blackwell Science, 2002.

Multilevel models

Introduction

Multilevel models are multifactorial regression models in which the data are in different layers or levels. Each level includes a set of units, such as measurements in individuals, or schools within regions, or children within classes. The consequence of this is that the total variability in the outcome is affected by each of the levels separately. In other words, the total variability can be partitioned into a component for each level. There are various types of multilevel model to suit different situations but they all take the layered structure of the data into account. Examples are given below.

Serial lung function measurements on a sample of patients with chronic obstructive pulmonary disease (COPD):
- Level 1: the lung function serial measurements within each patient
- Level 2: the patients

Cluster randomized trial of guidelines for treatment of back pain in primary care, randomized by general practice:
- Level 1: the patients within each practice
- Level 2: the cluster, i.e. the general practice

Dental health of school children in different UK regions:
- Level 1: the children in each school
- Level 2: the schools in different regions
- Level 3: the different UK regions

Fixed and random effects

The predictor variables in a multilevel model can either have fixed or random effects.

- **Fixed effects** are factors where the categories of the factor have specific values which do not vary, such as sex, male/female. With fixed effects, the interest is usually in the factor itself, such as the difference between males and females in some measurements.
- **Random effects** are factors where the categories of the factor are simply a sample of all possible categories that might occur, such as general practices in a cluster trial, where the interest is not in specific practices, but in how the intervention works across different practice settings. Patients are often regarded as random effects if the main interest is in the population from whom they are sampled, i.e. the average effect rather than individual patient effects.

Random effects (mixed) models

A **random effects model** fits a multilevel data structure by explicitly allowing for variability at each level. These types of models are referred to by several different names (see below) but are essentially equivalent.

> **Different names given to the same multilevel models**
> - Random effects model
> - Mixed model
> - Multilevel model
> - Hierarchical model

Choice of outcomes

These models can be used with different types of outcomes, such as continuous, binary or time-to-event data, and since they can fit with standard statistical programs, they are more and more commonly seen in medical research.

Choice of predictor variables

The models can include a mixture of predictor variables that vary at the different levels. For example, if the data are repeated measurements on a sample of individuals in clusters, then the repeated measurements on each individual are level 1, characteristics of the individuals are also level 1, and characteristics of the cluster are level 2. Predictor variables can be continuous, binary, or categorical, as with other multifactorial regression models.

Sources of variability

The degree of variability is determined by the data structure, i.e. the number of levels. For example, if there are two levels: patients (level 1) within clusters (level 2), then the variability at each level will be as follows:
- Level 1, individuals: variability is due to variability between individuals in each cluster and between clusters
- Level 2, cluster: variability is due to variability between the clusters

Random effects models correctly calculate the variability due to the different factors at different levels. If the data were analysed without taking the data structure into account, the calculated estimates of variability would be too small, and so estimates and statistical tests would be incorrect.

Interpretation of estimates

In general, the interpretation of estimates given by these models parallels that of the ordinary single-level models described earlier in this chapter, in that the meaning of the regression coefficients is similar and depends on the nature of the outcome.

Generalized estimating equations (GEEs)

Introduction

Multilevel regression models estimate the model parameters by explicitly estimating the correlations structure from the data itself. While this approach works well in many situations, there can be problems where the data are sparse for some of the levels and this leads to imprecise estimates. An alternative approach was developed by Zeger and Liang,[1] in which the correlation structure of the data is specified by the analyst at the outset, and the model iterates towards a stable set of estimates for the parameters. This approach is known as **generalized estimating equations** or **GEEs** for short.

How GEEs work

When the dataset is reasonably large, the specified correlation structure for the data does not have to be exact because the method gives correct overall estimates. The correlation structure can often be given as one of the following:

- *Independent:* where it is assumed that repeated observations on a subject are unrelated to each other
- *Exchangeable:* where any pair of observations in the same subject have the same correlation as any other pair of observations in the same subject
- *Autoregressive:* where observations that are adjacent in time have the correlation r and observations that are two time units apart have the correlation r^2, etc.

GEEs have been used extensively to model longitudinal data, that is repeated measurements on a sample of individuals.

Choice of outcomes and predictor variables

These can be any data type as with multilevel models but the interpretation of the coefficients is different from that for multilevel models in some situations as described below.

Estimates and their interpretation of coefficients in GEEs

- **Continuous outcome:** gives same estimates and interpretation as multilevel models
- **Binary outcome:** gives different estimates to multilevel models because GEE provides '**population average**' or '**marginal estimates**'. These estimates refer to **average effects for a population** and not the effects for a particular individual and therefore the estimate is different for binary outcomes.
- **Poisson outcomes:** as for binary outcome

---

❶ Missing data
- Multilevel models assume that any missing data is **'missing at random'** (**MAR**) (see 📖 Missing data, p. 402)
- GEEs assume that data are **'missing completely at random'** (**MCAR**) (see 📖 Missing data, p. 402)
- It may not be easy to determine if the MCAR requirement is true and so GEEs may give unreliable estimates when there is a substantial amount of missing data. In such situations, it may be better to use a multilevel model

Reference
1 Zeger SL, Liang KY, Albert PS. Models for longitudinal data: a generalized estimating equation approach. *Biometrics* 1988; **44**(4):1049–60.

GEEs: example

Longitudinal lung function measurements in preterm babies

A clinical study in very preterm babies investigated the relationship between exhaled nitric oxide (eNO) level up to 28 days after birth, and bronchopulmonary dysplasia (BPD) in four groups and as a binary variable.[1] GEEs with exchangeable correlation structure were used to model the relationship. Table 12.11 shows some of the results.

Table 12.11 GEE analysis of the change in exhaled nitric oxide level over time in four bronchopulmonary dysplasia (BPD) groups (model 1) and in two groups (model 2)

	Coefficient	SE	Overall P value
MODEL 1			
No BPD	Reference		0.30
Mild	0.97	0.72	
Moderate	0.61	0.67	
Severe	1.21	0.72	
MODEL 2			
No BPD	Reference		0.08
BPD	0.91	0.52	

Note: the coefficients in models 1 and 2 are the differences in slopes between the reference category and the given category.

Methods
- The model fitted a separate slope to each individual and these have been averaged over all individuals in the given category. For example, for 'mild', the coefficient is the difference between the average slope for all babies with mild BPD, and all babies with no BPD

Interpretation
- For both models 1 and 2 the overall P values are not statistically significant
- There is no evidence that the slopes of the lines are different for babies with differing BPD status
- There is no evidence that the change in eNO to 28 days is related to BPD

Reference

1 May C, Williams O, Milner AD, Peacock J, Rafferty GF, Hannam S *et al.* Relation of exhaled nitric oxide levels to development of bronchopulmonary dysplasia. *Arch Dis Child Fetal Neonatal Ed* 2009; **94**(3):F205–9.

Principal components analysis

Multivariate methods

Multivariate methods are used to analyse multiple outcome variables together, in comparison with all previous methods where there was only one outcome variable. They are used in general to try to reduce a complex dataset to a simpler one which is easier to interpret and understand.

What is principal components analysis?

This method is used to reduce a dataset with many inter-correlated variables to a smaller set of uncorrelated variables which explain the overall variability almost as well. It is sometimes described as '**reducing the dimensionality of a dataset**'. The derived smaller set of variables is then used in later analyses in place of the original larger set.

How principal components analysis works

- The method gives a set of **principal components** (**PCs**), each of which is a linear combination of all the original variables
- If there are n variables in total then a maximum of n PCs can be computed
- Each PC explains a proportion of the total variability
- The first PC is the one that explains the maximum amount of the variance and the second PC explains the next greatest amount and so on

Principal component equations

The following equations show how principal components analysis works mathematically and how the principal components are related to the original set of variables. Assuming that the original variables are:

$x_1, x_2, x_3 \ldots x_p$ the method produces p principal components $y_1, y_2, y_3 \ldots y_p$, which are defined as follows:

$$y_1 = b_{11}x_1 + b_{12}x_2 + \ldots + b_{1p}x_p$$

$$y_2 = b_{21}x_1 + b_{22}x_2 + \ldots + b_{2p}x_p$$

$$y_p = b_{p1}x_1 + b_{p2}x_2 + \ldots + b_{pp}x_p$$

where b_{11}, b_{12} etc. are coefficients.

Practicalities

- It is common practice to include enough PCs to explain at least 80% of the total variability and this often needs only two or three
- Principal components analysis provides a single value for each PC for each subject and therefore each PC is a new variable
- These are then used in further analyses in the same way as other variables are analysed

Interpreting principal components

Specific principal components sometimes usefully represent a particular overarching theme, where several of the original variables contribute to the theme. The example (📖 Principal components analysis: example, p. 442) illustrates this.

Principal components analysis: example

Example

Researchers wished to determine the important features of six lung function tests in 458 coalminers.[1] They used principal components analysis and reduced the six tests to three meaningful respiratory components. The results are summarized in Table 12.12.

Table 12.12 Coefficients for the first four principal components with six lung function variables

Component	1st	2nd	3rd	4th
FEV_1	−0.46	0.18	0.23	−0.26
FVC	−0.38	0.58	0.40	−0.22
FEV_1/FVC	−0.38	−0.57	−0.24	−0.52
$Vmax_{50}$	−0.44	−0.32	0.12	0.05
$Vmax_{25}$	−0.43	−0.21	0.17	0.77
TLCO	−0.35	0.41	−0.83	0.14
% variability	74%	15%	7%	3%

FEV_1, forced expiratory volume in 1 second; FVC, forced vital capacity; TLCO, transfer factor of the lung for carbon monoxide.

- The analysis produces six PCs but the four shown here explain virtually all of the overall variability (99%) in the six lung function measures
- The first principal component is:
  −0.46 × FEV₁ − 0.38 × FVC − 0.38 × FEV₁/FVC − 0.44 × Vmax50 −0.43 × Vmax₂₅ − 0.35 × TLCO
- The largest coefficients for the first PC were for forced expiratory volume in 1 second (FEV_1), $Vmax_{50}$, and $Vmax_{25}$, which measure the capacity of the lungs, and so the authors concluded that the first PC mainly represented **lung size**. It explained 74% of the total variability
- The largest coefficients for the second PC were those for FVC and FEV_1/FVC which relate to airflow through the lungs and so it was concluded that this component mainly represented the **degree of airflow obstruction**. It explained a further 15% of the total variability.
- The third PC was dominated by TLCO (transfer factor of the lung for carbon monoxide) and so this component mainly represented **impairment of gas transfer** and explained a further 7% of the total variability
- The fourth PC explained so little of the variability that it was not considered further

- Hence, principal components analysis was able to reduce six lung function variables to three variables (components), where each represented an important, and different, aspect of respiratory morbidity
- The authors used the components in regression analyses to identify men with different forms of lung function abnormalities (see paper for details[1]). In this way just three variables could be used to encapsulate the key features of lung function just as well as the original six variables
- The authors concluded that the principal components method had provided a '**sensitive method of identifying men with unusual lung function**'

Advantages and disadvantages of PC analysis

- A set of inter-correlated variables can be replaced by a smaller set of independent components which represent all of the key features of the original data
- The problems of colinearity in a complex set of predictor variables may be overcome and the role of possible predictor variables can be more easily examined
- Each component is a new variable that is a linear combination of the original variables, and so the actual values of the components are hard to interpret

Reference

1 Cowie H, Lloyd MH, Soutar CA. Study of lung function data by principal components analysis. *Thorax* 1985; **40**(6):438–43.

Cluster analysis

What is cluster analysis?

Cluster analysis is used to identify groups or clusters of individuals who have common features, in terms of known variables. It is has been used to identify groups at high risk of particular adverse events, as a basis for further analysis of causes and prevention. Clustering may be on a single level or may have a hierarchical structure, where groups are identified within groups.

How does cluster analysis work?

The method is used to identify sets of individuals who are more like each other, than they are like other individuals. Since most datasets include several variables on each subject, it is not straightforward to do this with several variables at a time and so there are several methods that can be used. In general, the approaches are based on the following:

- Determining clusters on the basis of measures of how far apart individuals are for quantitative variables
- Determining clusters on the basis of measures of how similar pairs of individuals are

Further details of cluster analysis are beyond the scope of this book but a simple example is given below and references for further reading are listed.

Example

In a study of factors related to premature delivery, researchers used a simple form of cluster analysis on variables associated with early delivery to try to identify groups of women who delivered too early to inform preventive programmes.[1]

The study reported three clusters of women delivering preterm:

- Younger women, predominantly in manual occupations with low income and minimum years of education and with mean gestational age 34.4 weeks
- Older women who smoked, had manual occupations, mainly had low income and minimum years of education and with mean gestational age 33.9 weeks
- Older women who did not smoke, had higher income, more years of education and were less likely to have manual occupations. These women had mean gestational age 35.0 weeks.

The authors concluded that there were 'three subgroups of women delivering preterm: two clusters were predominantly of low social status and the third cluster comprised older women with higher social status who did not smoke'.[1]

Further reading

The fourth edition of Everitt and Landua's *Cluster analysis*[2] has a comprehensive account of cluster methods.

1 Peacock JL, Bland JM, Anderson HR. Preterm delivery: effects of socioeconomic factors, psychological stress, smoking, alcohol, and caffeine. *BMJ* 1995; **311**(7004):531–5.

2 Everitt B, Landua SLM. *Cluster analysis*. 4th ed. London: Edwin Arnold, 2009.

Factor analysis

What is factor analysis?

Factor analysis is related to principal components analysis in that it attempts to reduce the number of variables in a set of data. It is used commonly in the analysis of psychological tests or the analysis of psychological data where the aim is to identify underlying factors.

How factor analysis works

- The underlying hypothesis is that there are a number of common factors that are hidden among the observed data and the method is used to uncover them
- Each observed variable is assumed to be a linear combination of the (unknown) factors
- There is no unique solution to the factor analysis and so a process called **rotation** is used to rotate to a simple structure that is easy to interpret
- Having discovered factors within a set of data, this may need confirming in a further dataset
- As with principal components analysis, a computer program is used for factor analysis

Example

Establishing new dimensions

An example of the use of factors analysis is the well-known Eysenck personality questionnaire (EPQ), which used factor analysis to demonstrate that personality had three dimensions:[1]

- extroversion/introversion
- neuroticism/stability
- psychoticism/socialization

Further reading on factor analysis

- Article on the use of factor analysis in mental health[2]
- Short textbook account of factor analysis (Everitt[3])
- Longer textbook account of factor analysis (Everitt and Dunn[4])

Further reading on multivariate methods

- *Applied multivariate data analysis*[5] gives a thorough account of all methods outlined in this chapter

References

1 Eysenck HJ, Eysenck SBG. *Manual of the Eysenck Personality Inventory*. London: University of London Press, 1964.
2 Ismail K. Unravelling factor analysis. *Evid Based Ment Health* 2008; **11**(4):99–102.
3 Everitt B. *Statistical methods for medical investigations*. 2nd ed. New York: Oxford University Press, 1994.
4 Everitt B, Dunn G. *Applied multivariate data analysis*. London: Edwin Arnold, 1991.

Meta-analysis

Introduction

In this chapter we describe the statistical issues involved in performing meta-analyses. We discuss the sources and effects of publication bias and consider ways of correcting for it. We also discuss statistical and clinical heterogeneity and consider how these can be addressed in meta-analyses. Finally, we consider individual patient meta-analysis. Throughout, we include both trials and observational studies, discussing the challenges that each study design brings and giving examples.

Meta-analysis: introduction

What is a meta-analysis?
- It is a statistical analysis which combines the results of several independent studies examining the same question
- It is based on a review of all available evidence

Why do meta-analysis?
- To pool all findings on a topic to gain an overall view
- To increase statistical power compared with individual studies
- To improve estimates of effect size
- To resolve controversies when the findings of studies disagree
- To answer new questions not addressed in individual studies

Types of literature reviews
In the past clinicians and scientists have often relied on editorials and narrative reviews to provide a summary of evidence on a topic. However, this is problematic if the reviews do not use scientific methods to assess and present data, since different reviewers may reach different conclusions based on the same data. This is why a formal statistical process of review is needed.

Meta-analysis has been most widely used to pool clinical trial results and this is the most straightforward application. However, meta-analysis is increasingly used to synthesize the findings of epidemiological studies.

Traditional review versus systematic reviews
Traditional or 'informal' reviews are not necessarily systematic. 'Systematic' implies that all available studies are identified so that the evidence base provides an unbiased representation of the totality of evidence. By contrast, informal reviews may be based on literature to hand or on a limited search of studies conducted.

Protocol for meta-analysis
A meta-analysis is a research study in its own right and so needs a protocol. This should include the following:
- Aims of the meta-analysis
- Rules for inclusion and exclusion of studies
- Search strategies
- Statistical methods

What makes a good meta-analysis?
- The meta-analysis has a clear question
- All relevant evidence has been gathered
- The individual study estimates have been evaluated to ensure that studies are sufficiently similar to be pooled
- Publication bias has been considered and addressed as appropriate
- The data have been suitably analysed and presented with a clear description of how the meta-analysis was conducted

Sample size for meta-analysis
- The number of studies in a meta-analysis obviously varies according to what research has been previously conducted in a specific area
- The greater the number of studies, the greater is the precision of the pooled estimate in a meta-analysis
- The most important issue is that the studies represent the **totality of evidence** and so provide an unbiased overall estimate
- It may be perfectly reasonable to pool just three or four studies if they are all that exist

❶ A large meta-analysis that obtains only a subset of all studies because of publication bias may give a very *precise* estimate but it may be **biased**.

Searching for studies

Introduction

A thorough and systematic search includes all relevant publications. Such a search may include the following:

- Computerized databases such as PubMed and MedLine
- Bibliographies of textbooks
- References in published original studies and in review papers
- Archives of studies conducted
- Personal communication with specialists in the field of interest

It is usually necessary to search multiple sources for several reasons:

- Electronic databases are not totally complete due to the accidental omission of a minority of publications
- Studies may only be listed in a specialist database, such as the AMED database for studies in allied and complementary medicine

Search strategy

This needs to be tailored to the purpose of the study. It may be appropriate to include peer-reviewed literature only or to append 'grey' (non-peer-reviewed) literature. It may be necessary to do the search in several stages, for example to:

- Identify abstracts in subject area
- Read and discard those that are inappropriate
- Obtain full versions of all potentially appropriate papers and discard those that are then shown to be inappropriate

Choosing search terms for electronic searching

Search terms need to be inclusive – it may be helpful to get advice from specialists who have done similar work and/or librarians. The **Cochrane Collaboration website** (🖰 www.cochrane.org) has a wealth of information including comprehensive guidelines and databases of reviews. Specific suggestions are:

- **Use a combination of recognized words** – MeSH (medical subject heading) and free text words
- **Watch out for UK versus US spellings** and include both (e.g. paediatric and pediatric, randomised and randomized), and beware of **different versions of the same term** (e.g. randomized trial and RCT)
- **Check that the search strategy has worked** as far as possible. For example, check that studies that are known to be available have in fact been identified by the strategy adopted

Extracting the relevant data

Once the papers have been identified it is important to devise a system for extracting and recording the relevant data. Some of the key points are listed below.

- Consider what information is needed and in what format it should be recorded
- Design paper or electronic forms and test them thoroughly to make sure they work across the a range of papers/studies/estimates and modify them as needed before the 'real' study starts
- It may be helpful to look at forms used in other reviews for tips
- Ensure the data can be easily taken from the form and used in the statistical analysis

Detailed advice is available on the Cochrane Collaboration website: ℘ www.cochrane-net.org/openlearning/HTML/mod7-2.htm

Combining estimates in meta-analyses

Vote counting

The simplest form of meta-analysis is 'vote-counting', in which the numbers of studies showing statistically significant ('positive') results are counted. If the majority of studies are positive then it may be argued that there is 'consensus' in favour of a conclusion that the result is positive overall. This approach is sometimes used as an informal starting point but there are obvious problems with it:

• It treats a non-significant result as indicating that there is 'no effect', which may not necessarily be true
• It fails to take account of the size and direction of individual study effects
• It fails to take account of the precision of the estimated effects
• In its crudest form it takes no account of study design and/or study quality

Borenstein et al., Chapter 28,[1] discusses vote counting in some detail and gives examples to illustrate its problems.

Sign test

This is a better choice than vote counting and is reasonable where no numerical data are provided from studies but the direction of the effect is known, or where studies are so diverse that a pooled estimate makes no sense.

• The test is based simply on the number of studies showing effects in either the positive or negative direction
• It takes no account of sample size, statistical significance, or precision
• It tests the null hypothesis that the mean effect across studies is 0. For more details, see Borenstein et al., Chapter 36[1]

Combining P values

Another way of summarizing several studies is to combine their P values to give a summary P value. It can be useful when combining studies which use different outcomes to assess the same question. For example, when studying lead exposure in children, studies can measure lead in different samples of the body, such as hair, teeth, and nails, and estimates cannot be sensibly combined. It may be informative to combine P values when the P value itself is reported for each study but the sample sizes are not, so that effect sizes cannot be computed.

• There are two relatively easy ways to combine P values, the first based on the chi-squared distribution and the second on the Normal distribution. Both give a summary P value and its statistical significance (see Borenstein et al., Chapter 36,[1] for worked examples)
• Each method takes account of the **direction of effect** in the calculations as well as the actual P value and so this information needs to be available
• Both methods test the null hypothesis that the **effect size is 0 in all studies**

❶ Note that, since the sizes of effects in the studies are not used, it is possible for an overall conclusion to be swayed by a few small and imprecise studies that show a positive finding.

Weighting effect estimates

The simplest way of summarizing a number of study estimates is to calculate the arithmetic mean of all of the individual estimates. The problem with this is that it gives equal weighting or emphasis to all studies, so a small imprecise study with an extreme result can have a large effect on the overall average. (In just the same way as an extreme value can affect a mean calculated from individual subjects.) It is therefore common practice in meta-analyses to weight the individual studies so that bigger and more precise studies have more influence on the final summary value. This can be done by:

• Using the number of subjects in the study to directly weight the results
• Using the inverse of the variance (standard error squared) of the individual study results to directly weight the results

In practice, the second way, weighting by the inverse of the variance, is more often used. Later sections (📖 Fixed effects estimates, p. 458, and Random effects estimates, p. 460) illustrate how this works in practice.

Software

Meta-analysis can be done by hand using standard formulae as referenced above, but it is usually done using specialized statistical software available within standard statistical programs (e.g. Stata) or using a specialized meta-analysis program (e.g. comprehensive meta-analysis: CMA, RevMan. The following references are not exhaustive but may be useful:

• **CMA**: Borenstein et al., Chapter 44[1]
• **RevMan**: Cochrane collaboration, ✍ www.cochrane.org
• **Stata** meta-analysis programs: Sterne[2]
• **SPSS, SAS, R**: meta-analysis programs are referenced in Borenstein et al., page 392[1]

References

1 Borenstein M, Hedges LV, Higgins JP, Rothstein HR. *Introduction to meta-analysis*. Chichester, West Sussex: Wiley, 2009.
2 *Meta-analysis in Stata: an updated collection from the* Stata Journal. Ed: JAC Sterne College Station, TX: Stata Press, 2009.

Heterogeneity

What is heterogeneity?

In the context of a meta-analysis the presence of heterogeneity is usually taken to mean that there is observed variability between study estimates. Consider Figure 13.1 which clearly shows different degrees of variability in the study estimates for different outcomes from the same meta analysis.[1] For example, there appears to be a greater degree of heterogeneity for myocardial infarction and stroke than for major cardiovascular events and all-cause mortality.

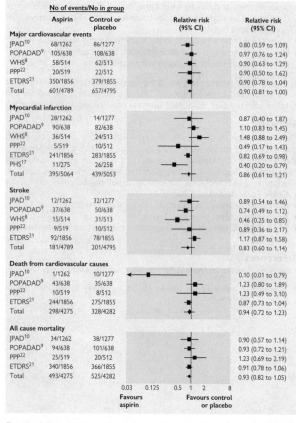

Fig. 13.1 Heterogeneity in effects of aspirin therapy on different outcomes in the same meta-analysis.

Reproduced from *BMJ*, De Berardis *et al*, **339**, b4531 © 2009 with permission from the BMJ Publishing Group Ltd.

Tests for heterogeneity

A statistical test based on the chi-squared distribution can be used to assess the statistical evidence for heterogeneity. The test statistic Q follows a chi-squared distribution (see 📖 Chi-squared test, p. 262) with $n-1$ degrees of freedom where n is the number of study estimates in the meta-analysis.

While the test for heterogeneity can be useful, it should be used with caution because:

- In general the test is conservative and so a non-significant result cannot be interpreted as showing that there is no heterogeneity. For this reason a cut-off of **P<0.10** is commonly used rather than P<0.05 to indicate heterogeneity
- The test itself does not provide an estimate of the degree of heterogeneity (see I^2 statistic below)
- Like all statistical tests, this test is less powerful when the number of studies is small (the sample size), and is very powerful when the number of studies is large
- The test is a statistical tool and does not on its own provide any insight into the reasons for any heterogeneity that exists

The I^2 statistic

This is a descriptive statistic that provides an estimate of the proportion of the total variability between estimates that can be attributed to heterogeneity itself.[2] In other words it indicates what proportion of the observed variability reflects real differences in effect size and so ranges from 0 to 100%. It is based on the test statistic Q, calculated to test for heterogeneity. Hence I^2 is larger when there is more heterogeneity.

Sources of heterogeneity

If there is evidence for statistical heterogeneity, either from a test or from simply observing the individual study estimates, then it is reasonable to consider what the sources of heterogeneity might be. Thompson recommended that meta-analyses should always incorporate a careful investigation of potential sources of heterogeneity.[3] Possible clinical sources of heterogeneity include:

- Treatment differences in randomized controlled trials (e.g. doses, other medications given)
- Variation in patients (e.g. age/sex/diagnosis etc.)
- Variation in study design (e.g. parallel group versus crossover design for trials, cohort versus case–control for observational studies)

References

1 De Berardis G., Sacco M, Strippoli GF, Pellegrini F, Graziano G, Tognoni G et al. Aspirin for primary prevention of cardiovascular events in people with diabetes: meta-analysis of randomised controlled trials. *BMJ* 2009; **339**:b4531.
2 Higgins JP, Thompson SG. Quantifying heterogeneity in a meta-analysis. *Stat Med* 2002; **21**(11):1539–58.
3 Thompson SG. Why sources of heterogeneity in meta-analysis should be investigated. *BMJ* 1994; **309**(6965):1351–5.

Overcoming heterogeneity

Fixed and random effects

When study estimates are pooled in a meta-analysis using the inverse of the variance as the weight, it is implicitly assumed that there is a single underlying true effect that each study is estimating. This type of meta-analysis is known as a **fixed effects** analysis. If, on the other hand, it is more reasonable to assume that the study estimates come from a population of true estimates, then a modified analysis is needed which takes into account this additional variability – a **random effects** analysis (🕮 Multilevel models, p. 436).

Meta-analysis for heterogeneous studies

A pooled estimate may be adjusted for statistical heterogeneity by using a random effects model as described above. When the sources of heterogeneity are known, it may be useful to stratify the meta-analysis by one or more of these sources, if there are enough studies to allow this. See 🕮 Figure 13.3, p. 463 Another way to deal with heterogeneity is to use meta-regression.

Meta-regression

Meta-regression is used to adjust the pooled estimate for known sources of variation in the same way as multiple regression techniques are used to adjust individual data for confounding factors (see 🕮 Multiple regression, p. 406). Meta-regression works in a very similar way to multiple regression in that the study estimates are the outcomes and the sources of variation, such as age of patients and dose of treatment, are the predictor variables.

When considering using meta-regression the following issues arise:

- The number of studies needs to be sufficient in proportion to the number of predictor variables to be included the same way as in a multiple regression analysis
- Information relating to the proposed predictor variables needs to be available for all studies in the same format

For a thorough description of meta-regression and examples see Borenstein *et al.*, Chapter 20.[1]

Reference

1 Borenstein M, Hedges LV, Higgins JP, Rothstein HR. *Introduction to meta-analysis.* Chichester, West Sussex: Wiley, 2009.

Fixed effects estimates

Formulae for meta-analysis

The formulae below can be used to carry out a fixed effects meta-analysis, test for heterogeneity and calculate I^2. These formulae can be used for continuous data, such as mean differences as well as for relative risks and odds ratios (both analysed on the log scale as the example opposite shows).

❶ Note that the formula for the weighted pooled estimate cannot be used if there is evidence for heterogeneity. In such cases a random effects meta-analysis must be done.

---

1. Fixed effects pooled estimate

If there are n studies and each study estimate is E_i with variance V_i then the weight is $1/V_i = w_i$

The pooled estimate E^* is given by:

$$E^* = \frac{\sum w_i E_i}{\sum w_i} \quad \text{with 95\% CI:}$$

$$E^* \pm \frac{1.96}{\sqrt{\sum w_i}}$$

2. Test for heterogeneity

$$Q = \sum w_i (E_i - E^*)^2$$

If there is no heterogeneity, Q follows a chi-squared distribution with $n-1$ degrees of freedom

Note that meta-analysts often use $P < 0.10$ as a cut-off for statistical significance for this test

3. I^2 statistic

$$I^2 = \left(\frac{Q - n - 1}{Q} \right) \times 100\%$$

Calculating a fixed effects pooled odds ratio

The formulae below show how a weighted fixed effects odds ratio is calculated using the raw data from each study. Note that the calculations are done on the log scale and then back-transformed, in common with other calculations that are performed on odds ratios.

Suppose there are n studies to be meta-analysed. Let p_{i1} and pi_2 be the proportions, and ni_1 and ni_2 be the totals in groups 1 and 2 for study i.

The $\log_e OR_i$ in study i is y_i and the standard error is SE_i where:

$$y_i = \log_e\left(\frac{p_{i1}}{(1-p_{i1})} \Big/ \frac{p_{i2}}{(1-p_{i2})}\right)$$

$$SE_i = \sqrt{\frac{1}{n_{i1}p_{i1}(1-p_{i1})} + \frac{1}{n_{i2}p_{i2}(1-p_{i2})}}$$

Each study estimate is weighted by $w_i = 1/SE_i^2$ and so the pooled estimate is:

$$\log_e OR^* = \frac{\sum w_i y_i}{\sum w_i} = y^* \text{ so } OR^* = \exp(y^*)$$

95% confidence limits on the log scale are calculated as:

$$\log_e OR^* \pm \frac{1.96}{\sqrt{\sum w_i}}$$

These are anti-logged to get the 95% confidence interval on natural scale.

Using a statistical program

These calculations can be done using specialized software (see 📖 Combining estimates in meta-analyses, p. 452). This requires the data to be entered in a specified format, which may be:

- Odds ratios: log odds ratio and log standard error for each study or odds ratio and lower 95% confidence limit (from which the standard error can be derived)
- Risk ratios (relative risks): as for odds ratios
- Difference of means: individual group means, n, standard deviation, or difference of means and its standard error or lower confidence limit

Random effects estimates

Within and between study variability

A random effects meta-analysis is used when it cannot be assumed that all studies are estimating the same underlying value. In other words, there are two sources of variability:

- **Within-study variability**: this is the variability between subjects within a study (sampling error)
- **Between-study variability**: this is the variability between study effects in different studies (true variation in study effect sizes)

A random effects meta-analysis takes account of both of these sources of variability and so the overall variability in each study is greater than would be the case for a fixed effects analysis. This leads to different weights and to wider confidence intervals in general. The pooled value is often brought slightly closer to the null value in a random effects meta-analysis than in a fixed effects analysis using the same set of studies.

Random effects weights

Since the total variability has two components, within and between-studies, these must be used to derive the weights for the random effects meta-analysis. The within-studies variability is estimated in the usual way from the variance of the estimated effect in each study. One way to estimate the between-studies variability is to use the DerSimonian and Laird method,[1] which is based on the Q statistic that tests for heterogeneity.

Using a statistical program

Few people with access to a computer would do these calculations by hand, but the steps and the formulae are given so that the interested or more mathematically minded readers can see where the numbers come from. Otherwise the computer program can be a huge black box!

Formulae for meta-analyses

Random effects weights

Assume there are n studies and each study estimate is E_i with variance V_i and weight $1/V_i = w_i$

1. Calculate fixed effects pooled estimate E^*

$$E^* = \frac{\sum w_i E_i}{\sum w_i}$$

2. Calculate Q where

$$Q = \sum w_i (E_i - E^*)^2$$

3. Calculate C where

$$C = \sum w_i - \frac{\sum w_i^2}{\sum w_i}$$

4. Estimate between studies variance by:

$$T^2 = \frac{Q - n - 1}{C}$$

5. The total variance for study i is: $V_i + T^2$

6. Random effects weight w_i^{re} is :

$$\frac{1}{V_i + T^2}$$

7. Random effects weighted pooled estimate E^{*re} is:

$$E^{*re} = \frac{\sum w_i^{re} E_i}{\sum w_i^{re}} \quad \text{with 95\% CI:}$$

$$E^{*re} \pm \frac{1.96}{\sqrt{\sum w_i^{re}}}$$

Reference

1 DerSimonian R, Laird N. Meta-analysis in clinical trials. *Control Clin Trials* 1986; **7**(3):177–88.

Presenting meta-analyses

Forest plots

The results of a meta-analysis are often presented graphically as a **forest plot**. In a forest plot, the individual study results are shown as a circle or square to indicate the study estimate, and a horizontal line to indicate the 95% confidence interval for the estimate. The overall pooled value and 95% confidence interval is shown at the bottom of the graph, usually as a diamond with the width of the diamond indicating the extremes of the pooled 95% confidence interval.

The studies are often displayed in chronological order and, where there are subgroups of patients, a series of plots may be given each with its own pooled value plus an overall pooled estimate. Figures 13.2 and 13.3 show forest plots from a meta-analysis where (i) the outcome was a difference in means from an observational study and (ii) the outcome was a relative risk from a randomized controlled trial.

Example 1

These data are from a meta-analysis of observational studies of passive smoke exposure and baby's birthweight in pregnant women who were not active smokers.[1] The outcome was the difference in mean birthweight (g) between women unexposed and exposed to passive smoke so a positive difference implies an adverse effect of passive smoke.

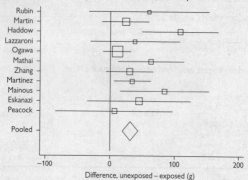

Fig. 13.2 Forest plot from meta-analysis of mean difference on birthweight between women exposed and unexposed to passive smoke in pregnancy.

Q test for heterogeneity gave P=0.23 (I^2=22%) and so the fixed effects estimate was presented
• The pooled estimate was 31 g (95% CI: 19 to 44)
• Note this example is used later in this chapter (□ Detecting publication bias, p. 466)

Example 2

These data come from a meta-analysis of trials of vitamin D and fall prevention in older people.[2] Eight randomized controlled trials were included, some of which tested several doses of vitamin D, giving 11 estimates overall. The pooled relative risk (RR) was 0.87 (95% CI: 0.77 to 0.99) but with significant heterogeneity (Q test P=0.05). The dose of vitamin D was a strong source of variability and so estimates were grouped by dose.

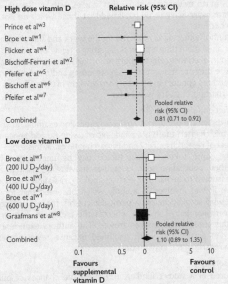

Fig. 13.3 Forest plot from a meta analysis of vitamin D and fall prevention in older people.

Reproduced from *BMJ*, Bischoff-Ferrari et al, **339**, b3692 © 2009 with permission from the BMJ Publishing Group Ltd.

- The white squares indicated randomized controlled trials with vitamin D_2 and the shaded boxes indicated those with vitamin D_3
- The solid line indicates the null value for the RR, 1.0
- The dotted line indicates the pooled estimate
- For high dose: Q test for heterogeneity gave P=0.12 (I^2=41%)
- For low dose: Q test gave P=0.42 (I^2=0%)
- For high dose: pooled RR estimate was 0.81 (95%CI: 0.71 to 0.92)
- For low dose: pooled RR estimate was 1.10 (95%CI: 0.89 to 1.35)
- Note that the authors chose to use random effects estimates regardless of the P value of the Q test for heterogeneity

References

1 Peacock JL, Cook DG, Carey IM, Jarvis MJ, Bryant AE, Anderson HR *et al.* Maternal cotinine level during pregnancy and birthweight for gestational age. *Int J Epidemiol* 1998; **27**(4):647–56.

2 Bischoff-Ferrari HA, Dawson-Hughes B, Staehelin HB, Orav JE, Stuck AE, Theiler R *et al.* Fall prevention with supplemental and active forms of vitamin D: a meta-analysis of randomised controlled trials. *BMJ* 2009; **339**:b3692.

Publication bias

What is publication bias?

Publication bias occurs when the papers that are published on a topic are an incomplete subset of all the studies that have been conducted on that topic. There are several reasons why publication bias happens.

1. Statistical significance

There is much evidence to show that studies with statistically significant results are more likely to be published that those which do not. This can happen because:

- The author either does not write up the work and submit a paper at all, or after submitting a paper and getting a rejection, gives up
- The journal editors reject papers reporting non-significant findings because they are thought to be uninteresting and/or non-informative
- Researchers conduct exploratory analyses on many outcomes and only the significant ones are written up

2. Fashion and popularity

Certain topics are popular at any given time. For example, at the time of writing this chapter, there is a pandemic of swine flu and hence there is a great deal of research activity and research interest in this topic.

By the same token, certain topics may be unpopular which may hinder their publication such as studies showing no harmful effects of agents assumed to be harmful, such as smoking, radiation. As an anecdotal example, JP was involved in a study which observed that for pregnant women who smoked below a particular cut-off, there were no adverse effects on their baby's growth whereas the babies of women smoking above this amount had poorer growth. The authors experienced some difficulty in getting this work published because reviewers expressed concern regarding the implications.

3. Sponsorship

The source of a study's funding may affect the chances of publication. Studies sponsored by some agencies, such as tobacco companies, may be unwelcome. Funded studies, particularly those with commercial sponsors, may be more actively pursued to publication than non-funded studies.

4. Language

The English language dominates the research literature. Hence, papers written in other languages may not be published in prominent journals and so may be missed or omitted from a meta-analysis, particularly where a research team is unable to translate foreign work.

Consequences of publication bias

1. Where there is publication bias, published papers are not a representative sample of all evidence and so the pooled evidence from published papers is biased. This often leads to **inflated estimates** whereby the overall size of effect is exaggerated.
2. The other consequence is **delayed publication** because first choice journals fail to publish the work. This means that, at the point at which a search for studies is made, those that are published quickly will be obtained but studies whose findings are available but not yet published will not be so easily found.

Note: it is possible to include unpublished work in a meta-analysis although this may be questioned because the work has not yet been subject to formal peer-review.

Reducing publication bias

- **Registration of study protocols**: researchers are encouraged to register the protocol for their studies, and specifically the International Committee of Medical Journal Editors (ICMJE; ✍ www.icmje.org) now requires pre-registration of trials as a condition for publication
- **Publication of negative studies**: ICMJE has issued a statement to encourage publication of all sound studies regardless of statistical significance:

'Editors should consider seriously for publication any carefully done study of an important question, relevant to their readers, whether the results for the primary or any additional outcome are statistically significant. Failure to submit or publish findings because of lack of statistical significance is an important cause of publication bias.'

Detecting publication bias

Funnel plots

A funnel plot is a simple graphical method for exploring the results from studies to see if publication bias might be present. It works as follows:

- The magnitude of study effect is plotted against a measure of study precision, such as the inverse of the variance or standard error, or the sample size
- As the precision (sample size) increases, the range of estimates becomes narrower showing a funnel shape
- If there is no publication bias the plot will be symmetrical about the pooled value for all the studies, because small imprecise studies with negative results are as likely to be published as small studies with positive results
- If, however, more small studies with positive findings reach publication than small studies with negative findings, the wide section of the funnel will not be symmetrical – there will be 'holes' in the plot

Is there publication bias or not?

- It will be obvious if there is substantial asymmetry but it may be harder to differentiate between slight asymmetry and random variation
- There are statistical tests, such as **Begg's rank correlation test** and the **linear regression test by Egger**, which are described in Sutton, Chapter 7,[1] and a simulated example is shown in here (Fig. 13.4). These tests can be applied to aid decision making but have limitations in how they perform in different situations and should at best be regarded as a guide[2].

❶ Limitations of funnel plots and tests for publication bias

- A funnel plot is unlikely to be useful unless there are a range of studies of different sizes
- Asymmetry in a funnel plot may be caused by factors other than publication bias, such as study quality or the form of an intervention either of which may differ according to the size of the study (**small study effects**[3]). A new graphical technique to look at this is the **contour-enhanced funnel plot** (details omitted but see Peters et al.[4])

Example

These data are from a meta-analysis of observational studies exploring the effect of passive smoke exposure on baby outcome in pregnant women who were not active smokers.[5] The graph in Figure 13.4a shows a simulated funnel plot where there is no publication bias and the graph in Figure 13.4b is the actual funnel plot drawn from the data.

The outcome was the difference in mean birthweight in grams between women unexposed and exposed to passive smoke. A positive difference implies an adverse effect of passive smoke exposure.

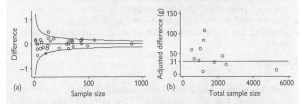

- The simulated funnel plot is symmetrical but the real funnel plot from the data was not – there are too few studies with either very small positive effects or with large negative effects
- This is an example of a typical funnel plot where there is publication bias

Note that these studies were all secondary analyses of larger studies which had investigated factors related to the outcome of pregnancy. It seems very plausible that authors would not bother to publish secondary analyses that did not show a significant adverse effect of passive smoking. See 📖 Presenting meta-analyses, p. 462, for the pooled estimate and forest plot for these data.

Fig. 13.4 Meta-analysis of passive smoke and birthweight: simulated funnel plot (a) where there is no publication bias and (b) actual funnel plot drawn from the data.

References

1 Sutton AJ. *Methods for meta-analysis in medical research*. Chichester, West Sussex: John Wiley, 2000.
2 Sutton AJ, Higgins JP. Recent developments in meta-analysis. *Stat Med* 2008; **27**(5):625–50.
3 Sterne JA, Egger M, Smith GD. Systematic reviews in health care: Investigating and dealing with publication and other biases in meta-analysis. *BMJ* 2001; **323**(7304):101–5.
4 Peters JL, Sutton AJ, Jones DR, Abrams KR, Rushton L. Contour-enhanced meta-analysis funnel plots help distinguish publication bias from other causes of asymmetry. *J Clin Epidemiol* 2008; **61**(10):991–6.
5 Peacock JL, Cook DG, Carey IM, Jarvis MJ, Bryant AE, Anderson HR *et al.* Maternal cotinine level during pregnancy and birthweight for gestational age. *Int J Epidemiol* 1998; **27**(4):647–56.

Adjusting for publication bias

Introduction

Publication bias leads to biased estimates in a meta-analysis and there are several methods that attempt to adjust the pooled estimate for the 'missing' studies.

Trim and fill

This method works in the following way:
- A funnel plot is drawn
- Small studies are removed until the plot is symmetrical
- The true centre of the plot is estimated
- The 'trimmed' studies are replaced with their reflections
- The effect size is re-estimated and the number of 'missing' studies is noted

Example

Figure 13.5 shows data from a meta-analysis of effects of exposure to outdoor air pollution and health. These particular data are from 74 international studies of effects of particulate matter (PM_{10}) on all-cause mortality. Funnel plots and trim and fill were used to investigate publication bias and to attempt to estimate how sensitive the findings were to any such bias.[1]

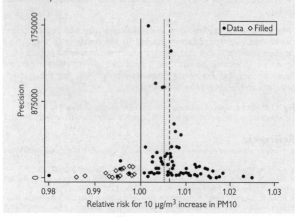

Fig. 13.5 Trim and fill for the meta-analysis of effects of PM_{10} on mortality.

Reproduced from *Epidemiology*, Anderson et al., **16**(2), 155 © 2005 with permission from Wolters Kluwer Health.

Example (continued)

- The solid dots are the study estimates; the open diamonds are the imputed values using trim and fill
- The lack of symmetry suggests the presence of publication bias
- The solid line is the null value (RR=1.0); the dashed line is the pooled value from the reported study data; the dotted line is the pooled value adjusted using trim and fill
- The pooled RR was reduced from 1.006 to 1.005 for a 10 µg increase in PM_{10} level and remained statistically significant
- It was concluded that, although there was strong evidence for publication bias, the pooled estimates remained consistent with a substantial impact of outdoor pollution on mortality when scaled up to population level

Reference

1 Anderson HR, Atkinson RW, Peacock JL, Sweeting MJ, Marston L. Ambient particulate matter and health effects: publication bias in studies of short-term associations. *Epidemiology* 2005; **16**(2):155–63.

Adjusting for publication bias (continued)

Regression method

Regression methods have been proposed to test for publication bias and their use has been extended recently by Moreno and others to obtain an adjusted estimate.[1] The method is based on Egger's test whereby a regression line is drawn through the study estimates in the funnel plot.

Example

See Figure 13.6. These data represent a simulated asymmetrical funnel plot. Egger's regression line is drawn through the points and a negative intercept indicates publication bias. The point at which the precision is infinitely large corresponds to the point 0 on the y-axis and this is proposed as the adjusted pooled estimate – here a log odds ratio (lnOR) = 0.38.

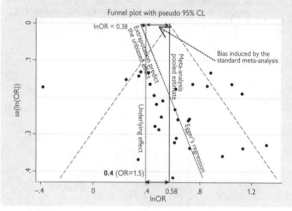

Fig. 13.6 Adjusting for publication bias: Simulated asymmetrical funnel plot and Egger's regression line.
From Moreno *et al.*[1]

Which method to use?

- At the time of writing this chapter, regression methods are preferred to trim and fill
- Moreno and colleagues' paper[1] compared the performance of trim and fill and several versions of the regression method and concluded that regression-based adjustments for publication bias were more reliable than trim and fill methods
- This is a very active and fast-moving area of statistical research and so interested readers are advised to check current research findings

Reference

1 Moreno SG, Sutton AJ, Ades AE, Stanley TD, Abrams KR, Peters JL *et al.* Assessment of regression-based methods to adjust for publication bias through a comprehensive simulation study. *BMC Med Res Methodol* 2009; **9**:2.

Independent patient data meta-analysis

Introduction

Traditional meta-analysis combines summary data from each study to give an overall estimate. This type of meta-analysis therefore uses summary statistics, such as study-level means or relative risks, to put into the analysis. These study-level estimates are reasonably easy to obtain as long as the data are in the public domain, such as in the peer-reviewed literature.

Limitations of study-level meta-analyses

- Individual patient data characteristics that may affect their outcome and contribute to both within and between-study variability, are not available
- Reported analyses are often limited by space and may therefore exclude an outcome of interest

Independent patient data (IPD) meta-analysis

IPD meta-analysis uses the raw patient data from each study that is to be included. It therefore overcomes the limitations of study-level meta-analyses and allows adjusted analyses, subgroup analyses, and new outcomes to be explored.

In order to perform an IPD meta-analysis, it is necessary to contact and obtain all relevant data from the original researchers. This is not a trivial task for the following reasons:

- Data from older studies may have been destroyed
- Authors of original study papers may have moved institutions and/or may not be contactable
- Authors from different countries may store data in different formats and/or languages, which may make it to difficult to share the data
- Some authors may not wish to share their data or may be unable to do so due to contractual or data protection restrictions

For these reasons IPD meta-analyses are relatively uncommon at present.

Example

The PreVILIG Collaboration is a group of neonatologists and trialists who have collated individual patient data from all randomized controlled trials of elective high-frequency oscillatory ventilation in preterm infants with respiratory distress syndrome. The aim was to supplement the findings of systematic reviews of aggregate data concerning trials conducted between 1989 and 2008 by exploring subgroups of infants in whom treatment benefits may vary.

At the time of writing this chapter, detailed data have been obtained from over 80% of all patients entered into trials during the period. A published protocol sets out the aims of the study[1] and analyses are ongoing.

Further reading on IPD meta-analysis

- Sutton, Chapter 12[2]
- Borenstein et al., Chapter 34[3]

References

1 Cools F, Askie LM, Offringa M. Elective high-frequency oscillatory ventilation in preterm infants with respiratory distress syndrome: an individual patient data meta-analysis. *BMC Pediatr* 2009; **9**:33.

2 Sutton AJ. *Methods for meta-analysis in medical research.* Chichester, West Sussex: John Wiley, 2000.

3 Borenstein M, Hedges LV, Higgins JP, Rothstein HR. *Introduction to meta-analysis.* Chichester, West Sussex: Wiley, 2009.

Challenges in meta-analysis

Introduction
Meta-analyses involve many challenges which have not been covered in this chapter so far. A few of these are outlined below.

Trial designs
- Trials of treatments for chronic conditions may include both **parallel groups designs** and **crossover trials**. Combining data from these is not straightforward. See Elbourne[1] for more details
- Some patients are **withdrawn or lost to follow-up** in many trials but this means that published analyses are not strictly 'intention to treat' (see 📖 Intention to treat, p. 22). It is not always easy to determine from papers why patients are missing from analysis and whether it can be reasonably assumed that the analysis presented was conducted on an 'intention to treat' basis.

Observational study designs
- Data may come from a combination of observational studies such as **cohort**, **case–control**, **cross-sectional** and it may not be reasonable to pool estimates across all studies. Even if studies are all of one type, variability between patient groups may lead to heterogeneity and this may make pooled estimates hard to interpret
- A large observational study is not necessarily of better quality than a small one, unlike with randomized controlled trials, where bigger is usually better. A large observational study may provide **big numbers but lower quality data or less detailed information**
- **Diagnostic studies** usually provide several outcomes, such as the sensitivity and specificity of a test, perhaps a receiver operating characteristic (ROC) curve and/or likelihood ratio statistics. The combination of estimates from these studies is not straightforward – see Deeks[2] and Leeflang et al.[3]

Disparate outcomes
- For example, **pain scores** may be measured using a continuous or categorical scale and may reflect current pain, worst pain, pain relief etc. This may make it impossible to combine study results unless strong assumptions are made about the equivalence of outcomes

Number needed to treat (NNT)
- NNT is useful for an individual randomized controlled trial but is **very reliant on the actual rates in the two treatment groups**. Meta-analysis of NNTs is problematic and there is currently no satisfactory way to pool NNTs
- It may be informative to provide a range of NNTs that apply to different baseline risks (see Smeeth et al.[4])

Summary points

When conducting a meta-analysis:

- At the outset, assemble an appropriate multidisciplinary team
- Write a rigorous protocol with detailed methods and data management sections
- Pilot the literature search and data extraction processes
- Allow adequate time for each part of the meta-analysis
- Take time to gain understanding of context-specific issues
- Think about publication bias: if/why it might be there, how it might affect results and conclusions

When reviewing a meta-analysis:

- Check the search strategy and inclusion/exclusion criteria, choice of data to pool, any evidence of publication bias, any consideration of study quality
- Is the analysis reasonable? Has heterogeneity been explored and accounted for in the analysis if present?

Further reading

Meta-analysis, including detecting and correcting for publication bias, is a very active area of statistical methodology research. Key teams in the UK are in Leicester (Sutton and others), Bristol (Sterne and others), and Cambridge (Thompson, Higgins and others). Readers who are interested in this area or who simply want to see current cutting edge research may wish to keep in touch with these teams and their international partners. Some useful books and articles are:

- Sutton (2000)[5] (overall coverage of subject)
- Altman (2001)[6] (overall coverage of subject)
- Petitti (2000)[7] (overall coverage of subject including cost-effectiveness)
- Borenstein et al. (2009)[8] (overall coverage, updated to include recent developments)
- Sterne (2009)[9] (manual for doing a wide variety of meta-analysis tests and methods using Stata)
- Sutton and Higgins (2008)[10] (journal article giving a concise overview of the current state of practice)

References

1 Elbourne OR, Altman DG, Higgins JPT, Curtin F, Worthington HV, Vail A. Meta-analyses involving cross-over trials: methodological issues. *Epidemiol*, 2002; **31**: 140–9.

2 Deeks JJ. Systematic reviews in health care: Systematic reviews of evaluations of diagnostic and screening tests. *BMJ* 2001; **323**(7305):157–62.

3 Leeflang MM, Deeks JJ, Gatsonis C, Bossuyt PM. Systematic reviews of diagnostic test accuracy. *Ann Intern Med* 2008; **149**(12):889–97.

4 Smeeth L, Haines A, Ebrahim S. Numbers needed to treat derived from meta-analyses – sometimes informative, usually misleading. *BMJ* 1999; **318**(7197):1548–51.

5 Sutton AJ. *Methods for meta-analysis in medical research*. Chichester, West Sussex: John Wiley, 2000.

6 Altman DG, Smith GD, Egger M. *Systematic reviews in health care: meta analysis in context*. 2nd ed. London: BMJ, 2001.

7 Petitti DB. Meta-analysis, decision analysis, and cost-effectiveness analysis methods for quantitative synthesis in medicine. 2nd ed. New York: Oxford University Press; 2000.

8 Borenstein M, Hedges LV, Higgins JP, Rothstein HR. *Introduction to meta-analysis*. Wiley, 2009.

9 *Meta-analysis in Stata: an updated collection from the* Stata Journal. Ed: JAC Sterne College Station, TX: Stata Press, 2009.

10 Sutton AJ, Higgins JP. Recent developments in meta-analysis. *Stat Med* 2008; **27**(5):625–50.

Bayesian statistics

Introduction

In this chapter we describe the Bayesian approach to statistical analysis in contrast to the frequentist approach. We describe how Bayesian methods work including a description of prior and posterior distributions. We outline the role and choice of prior distributions and how they are combined with the data collected to provide an updated estimate of the unknown quantity being studied. We include examples of the use of Bayesian methods in medicine, and discuss the pros and cons of the Bayesian approach compared with the frequentist approach Finally, we give guidance on how to read and interpret Bayesian analyses in the medical literature.

Bayesian statistics

Bayes theorem

Bayes theorem (see box and 📖 Bayes' theorem, p. 234) comes from work by the Reverend Thomas Bayes published posthumously in 1763.[1] It is a simple but ingenious statement about conditional probabilities and is widely used in all areas of statistics.

Bayes' theorem formula
- A and B are two events
- *Pr(A | B)* means 'the probability of A happening given that B has already happened'. This is often shortened to 'the probability of A given B' or 'the probability of A conditional on B'.

$$Pr(A|B) = \frac{Pr(B|A) \times Pr(A)}{Pr(B)}$$

This formula therefore allows the calculation of the **probability of event A occurring conditional on the event B having already occurred**.

Bayesian and frequentist methods: two philosophies in statistics

Bayes' theorem is widely used in statistics and is uncontroversial. However the theorem has been used as the basis of an approach to statistical analysis and inference giving rise to two competing philosophies in statistics – Bayesian and frequentist methods. The two approaches differ in their definition of probability. So far in this book virtually all statistical analyses have been based on the frequentist paradigm. Here we summarize the main differences between the two approaches.

Bayesian and frequentist approaches

Bayesian approach

- Probability is interpreted as a **degree of belief that an event will occur**
- This degree of belief comes from past data or past experience
- Unknown quantities, such as means and proportions, follow a probability distribution that expresses our degree of certainty about the true value at any one time
- This degree of belief can be updated when we have further information

Frequentist approach

- Probability is the **long-run frequency of events, r, that occur in n trials**
- Probabilities are estimated directly from samples
- Unknown quantities, such as means and proportions, are considered to be fixed although unknown, and are estimated from data with confidence intervals

The controversy

The frequentist approach is arguably objective and uses only new data to draw conclusions whereas the Bayesian approach uses both new data and past data and belief to provide a fuller picture. It is the choice and use of past data that causes the greatest disagreement. The frequentist statistician argues that it is subjective and therefore may be biased. The Bayesian statistician argues that in practice we use our degree of belief in interpreting new data all of the time – 'the sky is clear blue so it's unlikely to rain'. More seriously they argue that we should use new data to add to, and thus update, what we currently believe.

Which approach to use?

There are some problems that can reasonably be answered by either approach and some for which one or other is clearly more appropriate. In the past statisticians have labelled themselves as frequentist or Bayesian. Nowadays, while many statisticians have a strong frequentist training, they are also schooled in Bayesian methods and so choose the most appropriate method for the problem at hand. The main limitation of the use of Bayesian methods is the availability and use of statistical software. Bayesian analyses cannot be done in standard statistical programs, such as SPSS, Stata, and SAS. Specialist software is required such as WinBUGS (see 📖 Software for Bayesian statistics, p. 492), and this software is not very easy to use and tends to take a long time to run because the method is based on simulations.

Reference

1 Bayes T. An essay towards solving a problem in the doctrine of chances. *Philos Trans Roy Soc* 1763; **53**:370–418.

How Bayesian methods work

Example 1

Suppose we wish to use new data to estimate the prevalence of a condition in an area. The Bayesian approach works as follows:
- Before the data are obtained, the anticipated value or distribution of values for the prevalence is specified, perhaps using national data: this is called the **prior**
- The regional data are collected and the prevalence calculated
- The observed area prevalence is combined with the prior distribution of anticipated values to 'update' the distribution of the true prevalence in the region

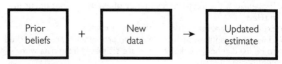

Fig. 14.1 How Bayesian methods work.

Example 2

To illustrate how Bayes' theorem and essentially a Bayesian approach updates an anticipated value according to new data, we return to an example used in ▢ Chapter 7 (p. 203) and present it slightly differently.

A study investigated a new D-dimer test for the diagnosis of venous thromboembolism (VTE)[1] in patients with clinically suspicious symptoms. Here we calculate the updated probability that a patient truly has VTE given that they are positive on the D-dimer test. This is $Pr(VTE+/D+)$ in Bayes' theorem notation.
- $Pr(VTE+)$ is anticipated prevalence of VTE = 14% (0.14)
- $Pr(D+)$ is proportion who test positive on D-dimer = 32% (0.32)
- $Pr(D+/VTE+)$ is probability of positive D-dimer test if the patient truly has VTE = 79% (0.79, the sensitivity)

Example 2 (continued)

Using Bayes' theorem the probability of having VTE is 'updated' using the test result which provides more information about the likelihood that they have the condition than the original prevalence alone:

$$Pr(VTE + |D+) = \frac{Pr(D+|VTE+) \times Pr(VTE+)}{Pr(D+)}$$

$$= \frac{0.79 \times 0.14}{0.32} = 0.346 = 34.6\%$$

So the 'updated' probability that a patient testing positive on D-dimer has VTE is approximately 35%.

Summary

- Before the patient gets tested the best estimate of their likelihood of having a VTE is the population prevalence, 14%. (Note that in this case the 'population' is patients presenting with clinical suspicion of VTE)
- After having the test and testing positive, this information is improved and updated to show their likelihood of having VTE is now higher, 35%
- This is a simple illustration of how the Bayesian approach updates estimates and provides an arguably better estimate
- Note that in this example, the use of Bayes' theorem is not controversial whereas where subjective opinion is combined with new data, there is more debate

Terminology

The following terminology is used in Bayesian statistics and these will be explained in later sections in this chapter.

- Prior beliefs: **Prior distribution**
- New data: **Likelihood**
- Updated estimate: **Posterior distribution**

Reference

1 Kovacs MJ, Mackinnon KM, Anderson D, O'Rourke K, Keeney M, Kearon C et al. A comparison of three rapid D-dimer methods for the diagnosis of venous thromboembolism. *Br J Haematol* 2001; **115**(1):140–4.

Prior distributions

Introduction

The prior distribution is the distribution of the unknown quantity that is combined with new data to provide an updated estimate of the quantity. There are broadly three different categories of prior distribution (taken from Ashby[1]):

- A frequency distribution based on past data
- An objective representation of what it is reasonable to believe about a quantity
- A subjective measure of what a particular individual actually believes

When there is no hard evidence on which to base the prior distribution, subjective judgement has to be used and this is where the approach is most questioned. Opinions can be elicited through informal discussion, expert panels, interviews or questionnaires, or through the pooling of data. For a fuller discussion, see Spiegelhalter et al., Chapter 5.[2]

'Default' prior distributions

The following forms of prior distribution are commonly used. For further discussion, see Spiegelhalter et al., Chapter 5.[2]

- *Non-informative/reference priors:* an example of this is a uniform distribution where all possible values for the quantity over a given range have equal probability. It is used when a range of values can be pre-specified but there is no clear opinion as to which value within that range is most likely.
- *Informative-sceptical prior:* this type of prior distribution is used to express 'scepticism' about the quantity being estimated. For example a sceptical prior distribution may be appropriate if a large effect is considered to be very unlikely. The use of a sceptical prior distribution reduces the chances of a spuriously large effect being found. Its use effectively 'shrinks back' the size of the estimate.
- *Informative-enthusiastic prior:* this type of distribution is the counterbalance of a sceptical prior and is used when a positive effect is expected so that large negative effects are less likely to be found
- *Informative prior based on prior beliefs which are formally elicited:* The actual shape of an informative prior distribution varies according to the context but a Normal distribution is sometimes used

Sensitivity analyses

The choice of the prior distribution can have a marked effect on the final estimate and so it is common and good practice to test the sensitivity of the assumptions for prior distributions by using several different forms. If the choice makes little difference to the updated estimate then all is well. If the choice does matter then a range of results may be presented to demonstrate the sensitivity to the prior.

Key points on prior distributions (Spiegelhalter et al.[2])

- The choice is based on judgement and so a degree of subjectivity is unavoidable
- A range of options should be used as a test of the sensitivity of the choice
- The choice(s) of prior needs to be clearly justified to make the results credible to external consumers

References

1 Ashby D. Bayesian statistics in medicine: a 25 year review. *Stat Med* 2006; **25**(21):3589–631.
2 Spiegelhalter DJ, Abrams KR, Myles JP. *Bayesian approaches to clinical trials and health-care evaluation*. Chichester, West Sussex: Wiley, 2004.

Likelihood; posterior distributions

Likelihood

This is simply a summary of the evidence provided by the new data itself. The likelihood is combined with the prior distribution to give the updated posterior distribution.

Posterior distribution

This is the updated probability distribution for the unknown quantity. It reflects the range of possible values for the quantity and the degree of belief associated with each value.

Since the posterior distribution is found by combining prior evidence with new information, it has less uncertainty than the prior distribution and so the posterior distribution will tend to be narrower than each of the prior distribution and the likelihood (see Fig. 14.2, which illustrates this).

Example

Figure 14.2 shows how the Bayesian analysis has combined the prior distribution (top graph) with the data ('likelihood', middle graph) to give the posterior distribution (bottom graph).

- The prior distribution represents the evidence that was available before the study was conducted
- The 'likelihood' expresses the evidence from the study itself
- The posterior distribution pools the two sources of evidence by effectively multiplying the curves together[1]
- The prior distribution has had the effect of pulling the likelihood towards the null value (0) thus making the final result less extreme. This example is discussed further in 📖 Using Bayesian analyses in medicine, p. 488

Conjugate distributions

Note that it is common for the prior and posterior distributions to be related, i.e. to come from the same distribution or the same family of distributions (e.g. both are Normal distributions but with different means and standard deviations). This makes the calculations more feasible.

Example[1]

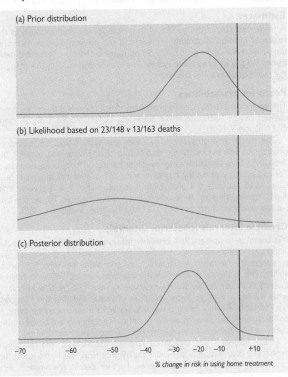

(a) Prior distribution

(b) Likelihood based on 23/148 v 13/163 deaths

(c) Posterior distribution

-70   -60   -50   -40   -30   -20   -10   +10

% change in risk in using home treatment

Fig. 14.2 Illustration of how Bayesian analysis combines a prior distribution (top graph) with the data ('likelihood', middle graph) to give the posterior distribution (bottom graph).

Reproduced from *BMJ*, Spiegelhalter et al, **319, 508** © 1999 with permission from the BMJ Publishing Group Ltd.

Reference

1 Spiegelhalter DJ, Myles JP, Jones DR, Abrams KR. Methods in health service research: An introduction to bayesian methods in health technology assessment. *BMJ* 1999; **319**(7208):508–12.

Summarizing and presenting results

Estimates

A single measure of the middle of the posterior distribution, such as the **mean** or **median**, is commonly presented as a summary. Other estimates are possible for other probability distributions such as the **standard deviation** and the **interquartile range**. The choice depends on the shape of the distribution and the context.

Posterior probabilities

The posterior distribution is a probability distribution and therefore probabilities can be calculated in the same way as for frequency distributions (📖 Chapter 7, p. 203).

One of the strengths of the Bayesian approach is that it is therefore possible to use the posterior distribution to calculate and present the probability for a particular range of values for the quantity being estimated. For example the posterior distribution for the relative risk in a trial could be used to estimate the probability that the relative risk is greater than 1 (i.e. shows efficacy). An example later in this chapter, Paroxetine and suicide attempts, illustrates this (📖 Using Bayesian analyses, p. 488).

Credible intervals (posterior interval)

It is common to present **95% credible intervals** for a posterior estimate. This range is taken directly from the posterior probability distribution and it represents the range within which the true value lies with 95% probability. This is slightly different to the interpretation of a 95% confidence interval as shown below. Bayesians argue that the 95% credible interval is what we really want to know about an estimate, and that the 95% confidence interval while being taken informally to mean the same thing, is not technically the same at all since confidence intervals are based on the sampling distribution of the quantity not the probability distribution.

These intervals are straightforward to calculate if the posterior probability distribution is unimodal and symmetrical, but if this is not the case there is no single unique interval. Further details are omitted here but can be found in Gelman et al., Chapter 2,[1] and Spiegelhalter et al., Chapter 3.[2]

95% credible interval, 95% confidence interval: strict definition

- There is 95% probability that the **true value lies within the 95% credible interval**
- There is a 95% probability that a **95% confidence interval contains the true value**

The difference between these two is that in frequentist analyses it is assumed that the true value is fixed and so either does or does not fall within the 95% confidence interval. In the long run, if it was possible to compute many 95% confidence intervals from a different sample, 95% of them would contain the true value. This is this sense in which a probability of 95% is assigned to the likelihood that the interval contains the true value.

While some statisticians get very irritated when confidence intervals are described as if they were credible intervals, it could be argued that the subtlety of the difference is of no great practical importance in interpreting the data.

Significance tests

Note that these have no formal place in the Bayesian framework since the emphasis is on a distribution of estimates rather than providing a test against a single value. As shown opposite, posterior probability distribution can be used to calculate the probability that the true value takes specific values – such as in the example quoted, the probability that a relative risk is greater than 1.0. Bayesians argue that this form of information is what is needed rather than a yes/no approach that significance testing gives. Frequentists would tend to reply to this that that is why results should be presented as estimates and 95% confidence intervals! So both camps tend to agree that a single value, or a test against a single value by itself, is of limited usefulness.

References

1 Gelman A, Carlin John B, Stern Hal S, Rubin DB. *Bayesian data analysis*. 2nd ed. Boca Raton, FL: Chapman & Hall/CRC, 2004.
2 Spiegelhalter DJ, Abrams KR, Myles JP. *Bayesian approaches to clinical trials and health-care evaluation*. Chichester, West Sussex: Wiley, 2004.

Using Bayesian analyses in medicine

Introduction

Bayesian methods are now used in many areas of research in medicine including:
- Observational studies
- Design, monitoring and analysis of trials
- Meta-analyses
- Missing data imputation
- Decision making
- Health economics

Bayesian methods can be used in many of the same situations as frequentist methods, such as:
- Estimating a single quantity
- Simple regression analysis
- Multifactorial regression with continuous, binary, Poisson, time-to-event outcomes
- Multilevel models

Sometimes a Bayesian analysis is conducted as a secondary analysis after unexpected results have been shown using a frequentist analysis, as shown in GREAT.

Example: GREAT – a Bayesian re-analysis

The original GREAT (Grampian Region Early Anistreplase Trial) examined the effect of thrombolytic therapy, anistreplase given at home in patients with suspected myocardial infarction. The trial included 311 patients and using a frequentist analysis reported a highly significant and large beneficial effect of the therapy on mortality, **13/163 (8%) versus 23/148 (16%), P=0.04**.[1]

This effect size was equivalent to an approximately 50% reduction in mortality. This finding was challenged for several reasons including:
- It was unexpectedly large
- The trial was quite small
- An unpublished bigger European trial found a more modest beneficial effect

- Pocock and Spiegelhalter conducted a Bayesian re-analysis of the trial.[2] At that time it was believed that thrombolytic therapy was unlikely to provide a benefit greater than 40% and that a reduction of about 15–20% was very plausible
- They therefore constructed a prior distribution to express this opinion and combined the prior with the likelihood based on the observed data
- The prior, likelihood, and posterior distributions are shown in Figure 14.2
- The Bayesian analysis showed that the best estimate of the reduction in mortality was **25% compared with the 49% reported** in the frequentist analysis. This reinforced the conclusion that the trial results were over-optimistic, a view that was confirmed in later studies
- This example shows how in the presence of an unexpected result, a Bayesian analysis can be successfully used to pool prior evidence with the new evidence to provide an arguably more reasonable final estimate

References

1 GREAT group. Feasibility, safety, and efficacy of domiciliary thrombolysis by general practitioners: Grampian region early anistreplase trial. GREAT Group. *BMJ* 1992; **305**(6853):548–53.
2 Pocock SJ, Spiegelhalter DJ. Domiciliary thrombolysis by general practitioners. *BMJ* 1992; **305**(6860):1015.

Using Bayesian analyses (continued)

Paroxetine and suicide attempts: a Bayesian analysis

This meta-analysis addressed the issue of whether antidepressant drugs led to increased suicides in adults.[1] The authors included unpublished data that had not been previously included in meta-analyses. They corrected for duration of medication and placebo treatment and performed a Bayesian analysis. There were 7 suicide attempts in patients taking the drug and 1 in a patient taking placebo.

- The prior distribution was assumed to be gamma (a type of distribution which for large numbers is similar to Normal)
- Three different prior distributions were used to test the sensitivity of the results to the prior assumptions, a pessimistic prior, a slightly pessimistic prior, and a slightly optimistic prior (Fig. 14.3)

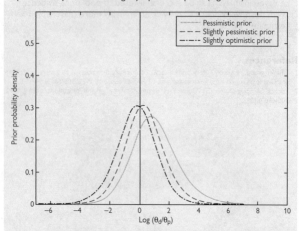

- The outcome was a ratio of the rate of suicide attempts in each treatment group. These are shown on a log scale and values greater than 0 indicate higher probability of suicide attempts for paroxetine
- The pessimistic prior (solid line) was based on prior evidence and referenced in the paper
- The slightly pessimistic prior (dashed line) and the slightly optimistic prior (dashes and dots) were also based on previous studies

Fig. 14.3 Three different prior distributions used in a meta-analysis of antidepressant drugs and suicide in adults.

From Aursnes *et al.*[1]

Posterior distributions

- The three posterior distributions shown below (Aursnes et al.[1]) relate to the three prior distributions shown opposite

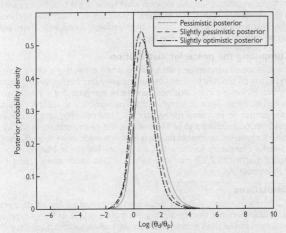

- The bulk of each distribution is greater than 0, the null value, showing that the evidence is weighted in favour of an adverse effect of paroxetine on suicide risk in this group
- The authors reported that these distributions corresponded to the following: paroxetine is associated with an increased rate of suicide attempts (relative risk=2.46, pessimistic prior; relative risk=2.20, slightly pessimistic prior; relative risk=2.34, optimistic prior, after anti-logging the values in the graphs)
- The authors concluded that the Bayesian approach supported the results of recent meta-analyses and that they suggested an increased risk of suicidal activity in adults taking certain antidepressant drugs

Fig. 14.4 Three posterior distributions corresponding to the three priors used in a meta-analysis of antidepressant drugs and suicide in adults.
From Aursnes et al.[1]

Reference

1 Aursnes I, Tvete IF, Gaasemyr J, Natvig B. Suicide attempts in clinical trials with paroxetine randomised against placebo. *BMC Med* 2005; 3:14.

Software for Bayesian statistics

Introduction

This section describes in high-level terms the software that can be used to do Bayesian analysis and also explains what some of the terminology used in the computing means. The technical details are less important to those who only need to interpret (rather than perform) Bayesian analyses but can be helpful to be aware of the terms.

Computing the posterior distribution

In the more straightforward situations as when estimating a single quantity, it may be possible to compute the posterior distribution directly using algebra. However, many situations are more complex and solutions are harder to obtain because integrals that are necessary to do the calculations cannot be evaluated mathematically. Until recently, such situations could not be resolved and so the practical use of Bayesian methods was limited. However, enormous progress has been made more recently using powerful computers to carry out simulations known as Markov Chain Monte Carlo (MCMC) methods, which makes much more complex analyses possible.

Simulations

MCMC methods are a set of techniques to evaluate integrals or sums by simulation rather than by algebra. A simple example of how a type of simulation can be used instead of a formula is when we toss a coin, say 10 times and want to know how likely we are to get 8 or more heads. We could use the binomial formula (📖 Binomial distribution: formula, p. 212) or we could actually toss a coin 10 times, many times over as a simulation to see how often the 10 tosses gives 8 or more heads We could use a computer to do this too quite easily with a random number generator (see Spiegelhalter, Chapter 3,[1] for a worked example). Simulations work in this way, such that many repeats are done to get to the long term and stable solution.

WinBUGS

(📖 http://www.mrc-bsu.cam.ac.uk/bugs/welcome.shtml)
The BUGS (Bayesian inference Using Gibbs Sampling) is a statistical program developed at the MRC Biostatistics Unit in Cambridge and more recently with Imperial College, and with other partners joining to provide extra functions. WinBUGS is available free of charge but as the website says, it comes with a health warning that its use is relatively easy but like many statistical programs needs a high degree of understanding of Bayesian methods to do the right thing and interpret the results correctly.

Gibbs sampling

This is a particular Markov chain algorithm that has been found useful in multidimensional problems and is built into WinBUGS.

New developments

Software to carry out Bayesian analysis is developing all the time, often tailored for a particular situation. Researchers often make their programming code available freely to others and in this way the set of programs grows. For example Keming Yu and Craig Reed are currently writing code to do Bayesian quantile regression and will make this available to the whole research community (Brunel University, personal communication, 2009).

Reference

1 Spiegelhalter DJ, Abrams KR, Myles JP. *Bayesian approaches to clinical trials and health-care evaluation*. Chichester, West Sussex: Wiley, 2004.

Reading Bayesian analyses in papers

Bayesian checklist

Sung and colleagues have generated a checklist of seven items (ROBUST) that should be included when a Bayesian analysis is reported.[1] These are helpful in interpreting a Bayesian analysis.

ROBUST (Reporting Of Bayes Used in clinical STudies)

The box below lists the items included in ROBUST. The checklist can be scored to provide a measure of the quality of reporting, but here it is given as a guide to what points to check when reading an article where Bayesian methods have been used.

> 1. Prior distribution: specified
> 2. Prior distribution: justified
> 3. Prior distribution: sensitivity analysis
> 4. Analysis: statistical model
> 5. Analysis: analytical technique
> 6. Results: central tendency
> 7. Results: standard deviation or credible interval

Each point is now expanded, and the issues that are important to check and understand highlighted.

Prior distribution: specified

It is important to know what form the prior distribution took and its parameters (e.g. Normal distribution with mean 0 and standard deviation 5).

Prior distribution: justified

Here it is important to know where the data for the prior distribution came from (e.g. a previous review, cited papers, cited experts).

Prior distribution: sensitivity analysis

It is good practice to repeat the analyses with different prior distributions unless the form of the prior is certain. We therefore need to know how the results varied with the different choices of prior distribution to gauge the range of true values that might be implied by the analysis.

Analysis: statistical model

As with frequentist analyses, it is important to know what model was fitted, such as what the outcome and predictor variables were, how they were treated (e.g. continuous or categorized), and the type of model (e.g. random effects).

Analysis: analytical technique

What software was used and how it was implemented (e.g. the choice of starting values for the simulations and the number of runs).

Results: central tendency

The main results presented as a mean, median, etc., as appropriate and if sensitivity analyses were performed how these varied according to the assumed prior distribution.

Results: standard deviation or credible interval

Some measure of spread for the main results is needed and again it is helpful to know how this varied with choice of prior.

Key factors still apply

Frequentist analyses will be familiar to many readers but Bayesian analyses may be less so. In many situations a Bayesian analysis is interpreted in a very similar way to a frequentist analysis. Hence, in addition to the specifics listed in the ROBUST guidelines, the same general principles apply for all analyses:

- What is the main question?
- What is the study design and is it reasonable?
- What data were collected?
- What analyses were done?
- What results were found?
- What do the results mean?

Reference

1 Sung L, Hayden J, Greenberg ML, Koren G, Feldman BM, Tomlinson GA. Seven items were identified for inclusion when reporting a Bayesian analysis of a clinical study. *J Clin Epidemiol* 2005; **58**(3):261–8.

Bayesian methods: a summary

Comparison of Bayesian and frequentist methods

Table 14.1 is adapted from Spiegelhalter et al.[1] and gives a helpful summary of the two approaches.

Table 14.1 Brief comparison of Bayesian and frequentist methods in randomized trials

Issue	Frequentist methods	Bayesian methods
Prior information other than that in the study being analysed	Informally used when choosing a model/form of analysis	Used formally by specifying a prior probability distribution
Interpretation of the parameter of interest	A fixed unknown value	An unknown quantity which can have a probability distribution
Basic statistical question	'How likely are the data, given a particular value of the parameter?'	'How likely is the particular value of the parameter given the data?'
Presentation of results	P values, estimates, confidence intervals	Plots of posterior distribution of the parameter, calculation of specific posterior probabilities of interest, and use of the posterior distribution in formal decision analysis. Expected value and credible intervals
Dealing with subsets in trials	Adjusted P values (e.g. Bonferroni)	Subset effects shrunk towards zero by a 'sceptical' prior

Adapted from Spiegelhalter et al. © 1999. Used with permission from the BMJ Publishing Group Ltd.

Strengths of Bayesian methods
- They incorporate prior information – this is something we commonly do in everyday life but is hidden in frequentist analyses
- They allow healthy scepticism to be incorporated to guard against unlikely results, and to avoid false positive findings
- They provide a probability distribution for parameters of interest which is what researchers often want
- They provide a distribution of possible values for all parameters to build in uncertainty in a way that frequentist methods do not
- The interpretation is more intuitive than frequentist methods
- They place less reliance on parameters following a Normal distribution as the sample size increases, as many frequentist methods do, and so can be safely used in wider range of situations

Weaknesses
- The choice of prior distributions affects the results but may be subjective or controversial
- They are computationally complex and require special software and specific expertise to conduct the analyses

Notes
- For large datasets, a frequentist analysis may give similar results to a Bayesian analysis since the prior distribution is less influential
- In small datasets, extreme findings can be tempered by a Bayesian analysis

Further reading
- Introductory articles[1–3]
- In-depth books and monographs[4–6]
- Review of Bayesian statistics in medicine[7]

References

1 Spiegelhalter DJ, Myles JP, Jones DR, Abrams KR. Methods in health service research: An introduction to bayesian methods in health technology assessment. *BMJ* 1999; **319**(7208):508–12.
2 Bland JM, Altman DG. Statistics notes: Bayesians and frequentists. *BMJ* 1998; **317**(7166): 1151–60.
3 Lilford RJ, Braunholtz D. The statistical basis of public policy: a paradigm shift is overdue. *BMJ* 1996; **313**(7057):603–7.
4 Spiegelhalter DJ, Abrams KR, Myles JP. *Bayesian approaches to clinical trials and health-care evaluation.* Chichester, West Sussex: Wiley, 2004.
5 Gelman A, Carlin John B, Stern Hal S, Rubin DB. *Bayesian data analysis.* 2nd ed. Boca Raton, FL: Chapman & Hall/CRC, 2004.
6 Spiegelhalter DJ, Myles JP, Jones DR, Abrams KR. Bayesian methods in health technology assessment a review. *Health Technol Assess* 2000; **4**(38).
7 Ashby D. Bayesian statistics in medicine: a 25 year review. *Stat Med* 2006; **25**(21):3589–631.

Glossary of terms

Analysis of variance See One-way analysis of variance (p. 280) and Two-way analysis of variance (p. 412)

Bayes' theorem A formula that allows the reversal of conditional probabilities (see 📖 Bayes' theorem, p. 234)

Bayesian statistics A statistical approach based on Bayes' theorem, where prior information or beliefs are combined with new data to provide estimates of unknown parameters (see 📖 Chapter 14, Bayesian statistics, p. 477)

Bias Any factor that moves the findings of a study away from the truth

Binary data Data where there are only two possible values such as survived/died; also known as dichotomous data

Blinding in a randomized controlled trial When the treatment allocation is concealed from either the subject or the assessor or both (see 📖 Blinding in RCTs, p. 14)

Box and whisker plot A graph that depicts the minimum and maximum (whiskers), lower and upper quartiles (box) and the median (horizontal line in the box) for a set of data (see 📖 Graphs: box and whisker plot, dot plot, p. 196)

Case–control study Observational study that starts with cases with a disease and compares them with controls without the disease to investigate possible risk factors (see 📖 Case-control study, p. 24)

Categorical data Data where each individual falls into one of a number of separate categories

Census A study that includes the whole population rather than a sample

Chi-squared goodness of fit test A statistical test used to investigate whether a frequency distribution follows a specific theoretical distribution (see 📖 Chi-squared goodness of fit test, p. 364)

Chi-squared test A statistical test used to investigate the association between two categorical variables (see 📖 Chi-squared test, p. 262)

Cluster analysis A statistical method used to identify groups or clusters of individuals who have common features in terms of known variables (see 📖 Cluster analysis, p. 444)

Cluster randomization When groups of individuals are allocated to treatments so that all subjects in a group receive the same treatment

Cohort study Observational study that starts with a sample of individuals who are disease-free and measures possible causal factors at baseline and over time. The cohort of subjects is followed and their disease status is observed to investigate which factors are linked to the disease (see 📖 Cohort studies, p. 28)

Confidence interval (CI) A range of values that indicates the precision of an estimate; for a 95% CI we can be 95% confident that the interval contains the true value (see 📖 Confidence interval for a mean, p. 242)

Continuous data Data that lie on a continuum and so can take any value between two limits

Cox proportional hazards regression A multifactorial regression model used with a time-to-event outcome (see 📖 Cox proportional hazards regression, p. 428)

Cronbach's alpha A statistic used to measure the degree of internal consistency between items in a questionnaire (see 📖 Internal consistency: Cronbach's alpha, p. 93)

Crossover trial A single group study where each patient receives each of two or more treatments in turn so that they act as their own control (see 📖 RCTs: parallel groups and crossover designs, p. 16)

Degrees of freedom (DF or df) A quantity used in statistical testing and modelling that is related to the size of the sample and the number of parameters that have been estimated

Dichotomous data See binary data

Direct standardization Gives a standardized mortality rate in the comparison population that can then be directly compared with the rate in the observed population (see 📖 Direct standardization, p. 372)

Discrete data Data that do not lie on a continuum and can only take certain values, usually counts (integers)

Dummy variables Used in regression modelling to enable a categorical predictor variable to be included, by converting a variable with n categories into $n-1$ binary variables, where one category is the reference category (see 📖 Dummy variables, p. 397)

Equivalence trial A trial that aims to see if a new treatment is no better or worse than an existing one (see 📖 Superiority and equivalence trials, p. 20)

Factor analysis A statistical method used to identify unknown underlying factors within a set of data (see 📖 Factor analysis, p. 445)

Fisher's exact test A statistical test that can be used to investigate the association between two categorical variables when the sample is small (see 📖 Fisher's exact test, p. 266)

Forest plot A graph used to display individual study estimates and confidence intervals, and the pooled estimate and confidence interval in a meta-analysis (see 📖 Presenting meta-analyses, p. 462)

Frequentist statistics A statistical approach where the data alone are used to provide estimates of unknown parameters

Funnel plot A simple graphical method for exploring the results from studies to see if publication bias might be present (see 📖 Detecting publication bias, p. 466)

Generalized estimating equations (GEEs) An alternative approach to multilevel modelling for data with a hierarchical structure or clusters, or serial measurements, that gives population average estimates (see 📖 Generalized estimating equations (GEEs), p. 438)

Gold standard test A diagnostic test that is regarded as definitive, i.e. it gives the correct answer (see 📖 Sensitivity and specificity, p. 340)

Hazard ratio In survival analysis, the ratio of hazards or risks of outcome in two groups (see 📖 Chapter 12, p. 428)

Heterogeneity Where there is statistical variability between estimates such as may be found in a meta-analysis (see 📖 Kappa for inter-rate agreement, p. 454)

Histogram A graph depicting the frequency distribution of a variable, with the area of each rectangle representing the proportion of subjects lying in the category (see 📖 Graphs: histogram, stem and leaf plot, p. 194)

Incidence The number of new cases of a given condition occurring within a specific time period

Independent data A set of separate data values that are not related to each other such as the height of each man in a random sample of men (see 📖 Independence: data and variables, p. 204)

Indirect standardization Gives the standardized mortality ratio (SMR), which is the ratio of the observed number of deaths in the comparison population and the number expected if that population had the same age-specific death rates as the standard population (see 📖 Indirect standardization, p. 374)

Intention to treat analysis Statistical analysis where patients are analysed in the treatment group to which they were originally randomly allocated even if they did not actually receive that treatment (see 📖 Intention to treat analysis, p. 22)

Interquartile range The range of values that includes the middle 50% of values when they are arranged in ascending order (see 📖 Summarizing quantative data, p. 183)

Interventional study A study investigating the effect of a treatment by deliberately exposing individuals to the treatment and observing its effects (see 📖 Interventional studies, p. 6)

Kaplan–Meier curve A graph demonstrating survival probabilities over time (see 📖 Kaplan-Meier curves, p. 320)

Kappa A statistic that measures the agreement between two raters where responses can fall into any of a number of categories (see 📖 p. 354)

Life table A table displaying the mortality experience of a population (see 📖 Life tables, p. 370)

Likelihood ratio A measure of the performance of a diagnostic test; equal to sensitivity/(1 − specificity) (see 📖 Chapter 9, p. 346)

Logistic regression A multifactorial regression model used with a binary outcome (see 📖 Logistic regression, p. 420)

Logrank test A statistical test used to compare time-to-event data in two or more groups (see 📖 Logrank test, p. 322)

Mann Whitney U test See Wilcoxon signed rank test

McNemar's test A statistical test used to investigate the association between two paired proportions (see 📖 McNemar's test for paired proportions, p. 276)

Meta-analysis A statistical analysis which combines the results of several independent studies examining the same question (see 📖 Chapter 13, Meta-analysis, p. 447)

Multifactorial methods Statistical models fitted to datasets with one outcome variable and several predictor variables; used to disentangle effects

Multilevel models Statistical modelling approach for data with an hierarchical structure or clusters, or serial measurements; sometimes referred to as random effects or mixed models (see 📖 Multilevel models, p. 436)

Multiple regression A multifactorial regression model used with a continuous outcome (see 📖 Multiple regression, p. 406)

Mutually exclusive events Two or more events that cannot occur together, such as death and survival

Negative predictive value The proportion of those found negative on a diagnostic test who are truly negative (see 📖 Calculations for sensitivity and specificity, p. 342)

Non-parametric tests Statistical tests which do not require the data to follow a given probability distribution; include tests based on ranks

Normal distribution A continuous probability distribution with a symmetrical bell shape, which is followed by many naturally occurring variables (see 📖 Normal distribution, p. 222)

Null hypothesis The baseline hypothesis that is tested in a statistical significance test and which is usually of the form 'there is no difference' or 'there is no association'

Number needed to harm The number of patients who need to be treated in order that one additional patient has a negative outcome (see 📖 p. 368)

Number needed to treat The number of patients who need to be treated in order that one additional patient has a positive outcome (see 📖 Number needed to treat, p. 366)

Observational study A study in which subjects are observed, with exposures and outcomes measured, without any intervention by the researcher

Odds The probability of an event occurring divided by the probability of it not occurring

Odds ratio (OR) A measure of the difference in odds between two groups, calculated by dividing the odds in one group by the odds in another group

One-way analysis of variance A statistical test used to compare the means from three or more independent samples (see 📖 One-way analysis of variance, p. 280)

P value The probability, given that the null hypothesis is true, of obtaining data as extreme or more extreme than that observed (see 📖 P values, p. 248)

Parallel group trial A trial in which subjects are allocated to receive one of two or more possible treatments and the comparison of different treatments is made between treatment groups (see 📖 RCTs: parallel groups and crossover designs, p. 16)

Pearson's correlation A measure of the strength of linear relationship between two continuous variables (see 📖 Pearson's correlation, p. 290)

Pilot(ing) A small-scale study conducted prior to the main study to check feasibility and/or make estimates of key parameters that are needed to design the main study

Placebo An inert treatment which is indistinguishable from the active treatment

Poisson regression A multifactorial regression model used to model rates (see 📖 Poisson regression, p. 432)

Positive predictive value The proportion of those found positive on a diagnostic test who are truly positive (see 📖 Calculations for sensitivity and specificity, p. 342)

Posterior distribution A probability distribution obtained by combining prior evidence with new information (see 📖 Likelihood; posterior distributions, p. 484)

Power The probability that a statistical test will find a significant difference if a real difference of a given size exists, i.e. the null hypothesis is not true

Predictor variable In regression analysis, a variable which is used to predict the value of an outcome variable

Prevalence The proportion of individuals with a condition within a specific population at a given time (point prevalence) or over a given time period (period prevalence)

Principal components analysis A statistical method used to reduce a dataset with many inter-correlated variables to a smaller set of uncorrelated variables that explain the overall variability almost as well (see 📖 Principle components analysis, p. 441)

Prior distribution The distribution of prior beliefs or existing information that are combined with new data to provide the posterior distribution in Bayesian statistics (see 📖 Prior distributions, p. 482)

Probability The proportion of times an event happens in the long run, which can be estimated from a proportion calculated in a sample

Publication bias A bias that occurs when the papers which are published on a topic are an incomplete subset of all the studies which have been conducted on that topic (see 📖 Publication bias, p. 464)

Qualitative research Research that generates non-numerical data which are not analysed using statistical methods, for example recorded in-depth interviews may be examined to identify common themes

Quantitative data Data which can be expressed numerically and are usually either measured or counted

Quantitative research Research that generates numerical data which can be analysed using statistical methods

Range The interval between the minimum and maximum value

Rank correlation A non-parametric measure of the relationship between two variables, using the ranks of the data rather than the data values themselves (see 📖 Rank correlation, p. 312)

Receiver operating characteristic (ROC) curve A graph plotting the sensitivity against 1–specificity for a diagnostic test at different cut-off points (see 📖 Receiver operating characteristic (ROC) curves, p. 348)

Relative risk (RR) A measure of the difference in risk between two groups, calculated by dividing the risk in the exposed group by the risk in the unexposed group (also known as risk ratio)

Risk difference A measure of the absolute difference in risk between two groups

Risk ratio A measure of the difference in risk between two groups, calculated by dividing the risk in the exposed group by the risk in the unexposed group (also known as relative risk)

Sample A sub-group of subjects selected from a population

Selection bias A statistical bias introduced by the way in which subjects are selected for a research study

Sensitivity The proportion of those who have the disease who are correctly identified by the diagnostic test as positive (see 📖 Sensitivity and specificity, p. 340)

Sensitivity analysis A way of testing assumptions made in statistical analyses by doing several analyses based on different assumptions, and comparing the results

Serial data Repeated measurements taken on an individual or individuals over time (see 📖 Serial (longitudinal) data, p. 378)

Significance level The probability that a statistical test rejects the null hypothesis when no real difference exists, i.e. the null hypothesis is true (type 1 error)

Simple linear regression A statistical method to estimate the nature of the linear relationship between two continuous variables (see 📖 Simple linear regression, p. 296)

Skewed data Data that do not follow a symmetrical distribution (see 📖 Graphs: shapes of distributions, p. 198)

Specificity The proportion of those who do not have the disease who are correctly identified by the diagnostic test as negative (see 📖 Sensitivity and specificity, p. 340)

Standard deviation (SD) A measure of dispersion used for continuous data; is equal to the square root of the variance (see 📖 Summarizing quantitative data, p. 182)

Standard error (SE) A measure of precision of an estimated quantity that is equal to the standard deviation of the sampling distribution of the quantity

Standardization A method of adjusting data to enable mortality rates to be compared between populations with different age structures (see 📖 Other statistical methods, p. 353)

Statistically significant This is when the P value from a significance test is less than the agreed significance level, usually $P<0.05$

Stem and leaf plot A graph which uses the data values themselves to depict the shape of a frequency distribution (see 📖 Graphs: histogram, stem and leaf plot, p. 195)

Subject An individual from whom data are obtained; in medical research this individual is usually a patient

Superiority trial A trial which aims to see if one treatment is better than another (see 📖 Superiority and eqivalence trials, p. 20)

Systematic review A literature review which aims to identify and appraise all published research answering a given question

t test A statistical test used to compare the means from two independent samples (see 📖 t test for two independent means, p. 252)

Transformation A function applied to a dataset to better fit a specific probability distribution, for example applying a logarithmic transformation to skewed data to make it fit a Normal distribution (see 📖 Transforming data, p. 330)

Two-way analysis of variance A statistical method used to investigate the effects of two factors on a continuous outcome (see 📖 Transforming data, p. 412)

Type 1 error Getting a significant result in a sample when the null hypothesis is in fact true in the underlying population ('false significant' result)

Type 2 error Getting a non-significant result in a sample when the null hypothesis is in fact false in the underlying population ('false non-significant' result)

Variable A quantity that is measured or observed in an individual and which varies from person to person

Variance See standard deviation

Washout period The time interval between the administration of different treatments in subjects in a crossover trial that prevents there being any carry-over effects of the current treatment when the next treatment starts

Wilcoxon matched pairs test A statistical test comparing ordinal data from paired samples (see 📖 Wilcoxon matched pairs test, p. 308)

Wilcoxon signed rank test A statistical test comparing ordinal data from two independent groups; equivalent to the Mann Whitney U test (see 📖 Wilcoxon two-sample signed rank test (man whitney U test), p. 303)

z test for proportions A statistical test used to compare proportions from two independent samples (see 📖 z test for two independent proportions, p. 260)

Index